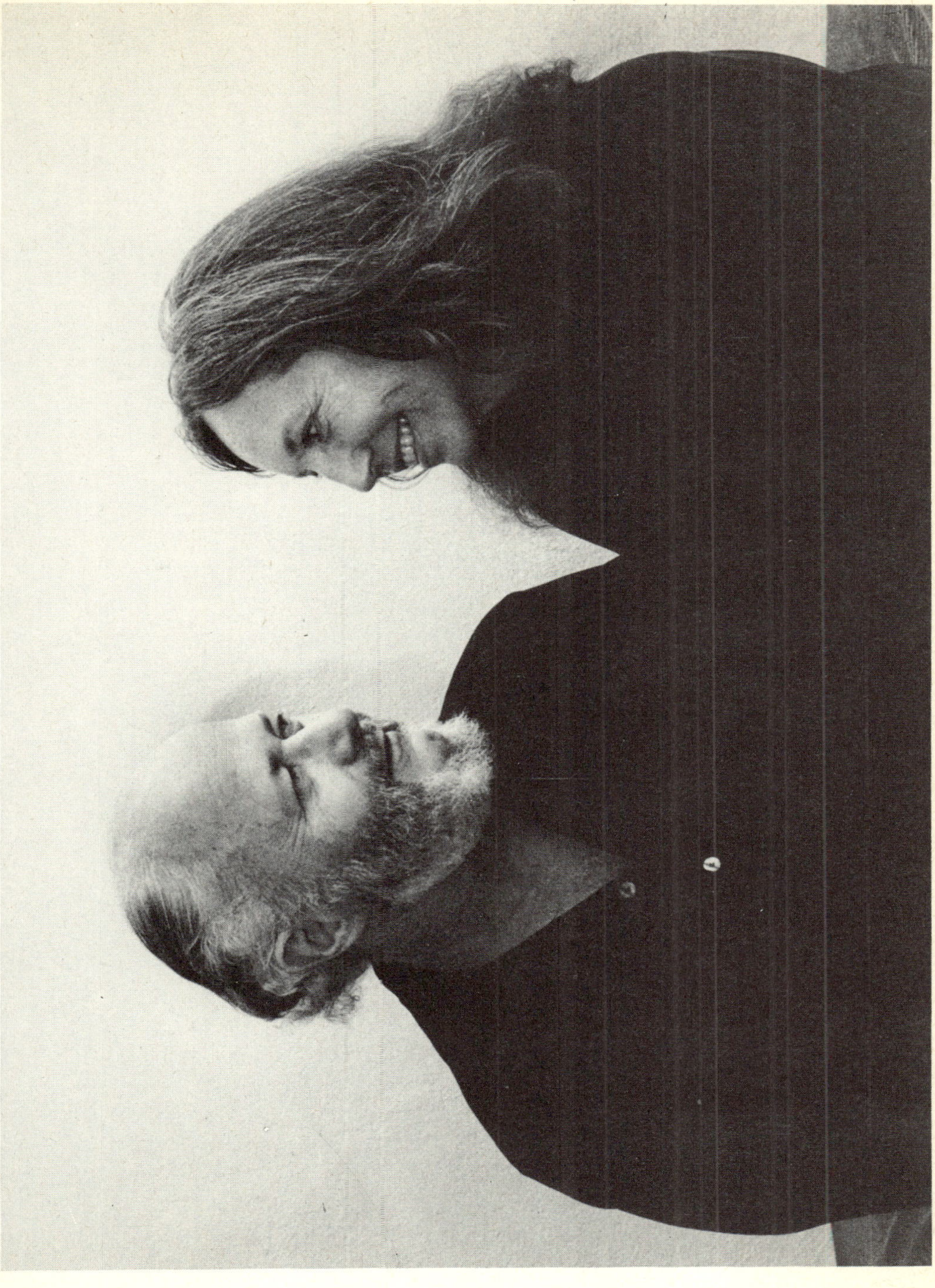

DEDICATION

This book is dedicated to the seven men who have taught me the most about the art and science of body psychotherapy: D. H. Lawrence, Abraham Maslow, Wilhelm Reich, Kurt Goldstein, Carl Rogers, Carl Jung, and Erich Neumann, and to those patients and pupils who have compelled me to put this knowledge into practice.

ACKNOWLEDGEMENTS

To Dr. Susan Persson of Sante Fe, New Mexico, I owe the greatest thanks for helping me to simplify and lighten my heavy writing style. Large parts of this book were edited by her gratuitously.

To my colleague and wife, Katherine Ennis Brown, I am indebted for her encouragement and indispensable criticism throughout the seven years during which this book was being formed. She too has helped me to simplify and condense my writing style.

Thanks are due to: Ursula Keller of Lugano, Switzerland, my private secretary, for her excellent work in preparing a camera-ready copy of this English version, even though her mother language is German; to Dr. Alan Richardson of Chicago, Illinois, for his extremely frank, forthright, and not always compliant observations about some of my basic concepts and clinical perceptions; and finally to Wilhelm Schittek of Essen, Germany, for his disciplined and patient dedication to preparing the illustrations for this book.

Janie Westmoreland

TABLE OF CONTENTS

INTRODUCTION TO BOOK

I was trained in and practiced a humanistic-Rogerian style of verbal psychotherapy for six years before I became clearly dissatisfied with the progress and results of the treatment, particularly with the more severely crippled neurotics. It seemed to me that a more direct and essentially non-verbal interaction with the patient's organism was necessary before any substantial positive changes in the personality structure could unfold. I could dimly sense that the rigidities in the psyche were embedded in and sustained by rigidities in the body, and that the stasis in both must be loosened before a healthy energy flow could be established. However, at that time I did not know how to facilitate such a development and of necessity I resorted to a method of trial and error. So it was that in the middle of the nineteen sixties, while practicing privately in London, I began to experiment with using direct touch and various other energy-mobilization techniques at infrequent intervals during the course of each session. Then, realizing how little I knew, I re-acquainted myself with the thinking of Wilhelm Reich in depth, and studied personally, both as patient and pupil, under Alexander Lowen, Simeon Tropp, Ola Raknes, and Gerde Boyesen.

For the next eight years I developed my sensibilities as a body psychotherapist always aware that I had no substantial scientific knowledge or informed accuracy of intuition about what I was doing. I knew I had to get the energy currents in the patient's body flowing in any way I could find, but I was never sure to what end. Much of the time it seemed like working in the dark. I was never certain what would happen next to the patient or what my own reactions would be after using the body methods. I knew there was indisputable value to using the softer, less threatening styles of direct touch as practiced by Ola Raknes and Gerde Boyesen. I knew there was an equally unique value in using the harder, more threatening techniques of gross energy-mobilization of the total organism as practiced by Alexander Lowen and Simeon Tropp. I also knew there was a unique value to using the confrontive, sometimes attacking verbal techniques of character-analysis as practiced by Wilhelm Reich.

Still I did not know enough to be able to integrate these three different styles of working in terms of the right sequence and amounts of usage. I had to face again and again that what worked for one type of character-muscular pattern of armoring was ineffective for another type. For many years I distrusted my deepest intuitive faculties and overly relied upon the Reichian-Lowenian typologies for providing all the answers. As a consequence, both the soul of the patient and my own suffered unnecessarily. The more my own character-muscular armoring dissolved, the more it became clear to me that no-one can conceptually pigeon-hole another without ignoring altogether the sacred depths of the body and the individual soul. The further my own armoring dissolved, the more compelled I became to resonate to the organism of each patient as an absolutely distinct and uniquely organized being, both when perceived in terms of patternings of tension and energy flow and when perceived as the actual locus of the person's creative soul powers.

Yet I did not understand the interconnections between the two levels of psycho-organismic beingness: the patternings of tension and energy flow and the various dimensions and state of evolution of the person's creative soul powers. Herein is revealed the primary motivation for writing this book: by having to put it down in precise words and concepts I am forcing myself to crystallize my own intuitively filtered clinical experience and to bring to greater rational lucidity the many subtle and unclassifiable inter-relationships that exist between the patterning of energy flow and the waxing and waning of the creative soul powers.

In 1974 Katherine Ennis, now my wife, began to work with me with a few selected patients. We quickly discovered the mysterious, often awesome healing power of the Yin-Yang circuit, especially when we applied our four hands at the same time directly to the body of the patient. With us both working together as energy catalysts the defenses of the patient, both psychic and organismic, seemed to melt and crumble much faster than when either she or I worked separately. We now work regularly as a man-woman treatment couple, and find that this is an optimal arrangement for evoking the emergence of a creative disintegration process in which id-like regressive states of being assume greater and greater prominence during the sessions. The presence of both a man and a woman psychotherapist bestows upon the treatment a special sense of security and containment which the defended patient needs in order to regressively reexperience the emotionally uncompleted past with minimal anxiety and pain.

It is this latter feature which gives our style of body psychotherapy its unique stamp and healing potential: namely, the facilitating of regression to primary-process feeling-centered states without intolerable amounts of anxiety and physical pain. We have discovered how fragile the entire ego-defense network becomes as we gradually cultivate an energetic and emotional field of security around the client which is as organismic in nature as it is psychological. Once this field emerges as a living reality, usually during the long second stage of treatment, whatever id-like states of rational disorientation and feeling insecurity the client happens to fall into can be tolerated, sustained, and creatively confronted for what they are with the supportive direct touch of the psychotherapists.

One of our main therapeutic goals is to guide our clients into their unconscious feeling depths with sufficient fullness of self-absorption that even in our presence they increasingly permit their usual controls to dissolve. This means a progressive loss of their hitherto tight egoic boundaries of self-identity, and with this loss some amount of fear and anxiety, or psychic and physical pain, is usually inevitable. However, we have found that the right kinds of nurturing and catalytic touch, and often the right alternation between the two categories of touch, facilitate the client's falling into feeling depths whose primordiality and boundarylessness is both endurable and liberating even though also somewhat frightening.

It is more important to us that our clients become capable of confronting in the here-and-now in their embodied souls the psychic and physical pain that attends the dearmoring process, or the process of destroying and reconstructing their boundaries of self-identity, than it is that they become immersed and swallowed up in the archaic emotional pain of their earlier years. Regression to the unfinished feeling past can only be healing when there is simultaneously awakened in the client hitherto dormant inner resources by which he or she can consciously face the repressed feeling past. The client's own creative unconscious faculties must be given time and space to emerge within each treatment session before the archaic past can be fully assimilated into a here-and-now opening of the client's healthy feeling capacities to present relationships. For these reasons more than sixty percent of our time during sessions is devoted to spontaneous verbal exploration at the initiative of the client, with or without accompanying direct touch of a supportive nature. Our body-centered energy-mobilization techniques are for us exclusively intermediary in function, and never ends in themselves. They mediate the opening of the client's awareness to his own neglected soul-powers and intuitive capacities for self-evolution and self-fulfillment.

By placing our four hands on those parts of the patient's body that are most likely to produce a widespread simultaneous dispersion of energy flow into distant parts of the metabolism, we stand a good chance of softly challenging the ego-defense network without over-threatening and provoking it to assume a position of defended vigilance. Sometimes this is best accomplished by touching the most tense muscles or regions of the body in a soft, immobile nurturing mode for as long as fifteen minutes. At other times it is best accomplished by touching the least tense parts in a three-phase mobile style, which begins with a purely nurturing mode of touch and gradually converts over to a low-grade catalytic mode invoking movement and pressure and then returns to an immobile, purely nurturing mode. In either event we are concerned to bring about a subtle divergency of energy flow which radiates in several directions at once away from our hands. From experience we have learned that the more the blocked pockets of energy can swim freely in the broad massive streams of the body's main energy currents, those towards the innermost regions of the organism, the more probable it is that the psyche and soul of the receiver can swim freely in the repressed, collective, and personal unconscious networks with a minimum of organismic or psychic pain.

We have increasingly come to reject the goal-directed charging up and discharging of large quantities of stasis energy at the body's surface that so many body psychotherapists aim for in their treatment. Such energetic carthersis must happen spontaneously from within to be of healing value, and even then the most which is accomplished adds up to nothing more than a very brief jolting and shaking up of the intact muscular armoring. Such charge-discharge-driven behavior and feeling has merit only if it develops into far more qualitatively refined and deeper psychoorganismic happenings; more specifically, the quiet awakening of the core longitudinal energy currents and the spontaneous unfolding of the repressed, and later the collective and personal unconscious networks and their accompanying repressed core soul powers of intuition. It follows at the clinical level that a delicate balance must be observed by the practicing therapist between time spent on body centered methods and time spent exploring the patient's psyche and soul. Perhaps the greatest hazard involved in the use of energy-mobilization techniques - and particularly the harder, do-it-yourself ones - is the tendency of the psychotherapist to use them excessively, and thereby neglect the client's psyche and soul and the allowing of time and space during each session for the latter to emerge.

The positive change and growth process for us hinges upon the degree to which the old rigidities, both energetic and characterological, are dissolved and replaced by new forms of beingness-for-self and beingness-for-others that attest to a more integrated differentiation of the person's embodied soul. The latter is a multi-dimensional meeting place of intrinsic opposites which have temporarily found an inner balance and unity of expression. This inner balance and unity is always short-lived and is followed by imbalance and a divergent scattering of the psyche and energy currents into states of non-differentiation. We repudiate any rendering of a solid and permanent consistency of form in the structure of the embodied soul when it is fully alive. We believe, to the contrary, that a process of being and becoming, of integration and differentiation, of autocentric divergency and allocentric convergency, is always in the midst of perpetual alternating change. At best, the most self-actualizing person can know only occasional peak moments of inner-outer unity and a perfected balance of spiritual-instinctual wholeness. Given this continual change and alternation in the soul's structuring of its own boundaries, the wise body psychotherapist will listen increasingly to his clients and allow the latter to initiate and decide what happens in the course of each treatment session.

For these same reasons we tend to avoid teaching our professional students precise rules or sets of sequences in the use of specific techniques. We teach them to risk affirming the repressed unconscious of the client by working directly with the deadest, tightest, or flabbiest parts of the patient's body while simultaneously, or alternatingly, evoking the emergence of the most underdeveloped parts of the patient's psyche and soul. In order to encourage the latter development we believe the creative imagination and its symbol-forming faculties become indispensable to the more advanced phases of the dearmoring process. It is a coming together into a single temporary unity of just such intrinsic opposites as an instinctual impulse and an imaginal symbol that constitutes for us the essence of the higher individuation process after the dearmoring process is mostly completed. The more such temporary meetings of the instinctual-spiritual opposites within occur, the more likely the patient will find the intuitive understanding to appreciate how to love him or herself and others more deeply, and how to creatively act and assert him or herself with a warrior-like self-reliance that trusts the deeper instinctual-spiritual guides within.

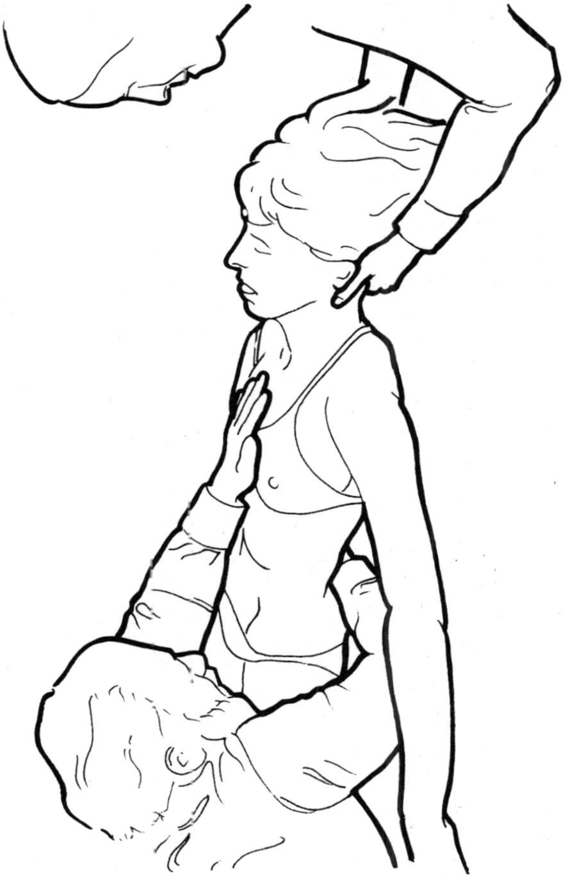

Chapter I

HUMANISTIC BODY PSYCHOTHERAPY : A SCIENCE AND AN ART

I. Introduction

The conventional distinction between consciousness and the unconscious dimensions of the human psyche has been classically rendered as two basic categories of mind. Modern psychiatry and psychotherapy will continue to flounder in misplaced practices and irrelevant theories until they recognize the simple truth that the core of man's psyche is located not in his head, but in his total organism. The unconscious dimensions of the human psyche actually belong more to the kingdom of the body than of the mind. Furthermore, the depths and breadths of the human soul, as distinct from the mind and psyche, find their primary locus in the total organism, in its many and opposing complex fields of immediate responsiveness.

We will present a cognitive map of this marvellously complex territory of the individual human organism, in all its changeability and intuitive subtlety of form. But first, we must stake out the territory. We will look in detail at actual therapy sessions to gain empirical knowledge of the client's experience. Only through experience can we begin to map the differences between the neurotically crippled and fully self-actualizing individual and begin to formulate the theoretical contructs.

Whenever we directly stimulate a client's body, the response is wonderfully spontaneous and unpredictable. This enormously varying response complicates the entire healing and growth process. It becomes so complicated that wisdom prompts the wise body psychotherapist to acknowledge that much of what happens during a treatment session comes as much as a surprise to him as it does to the client, and consequently, it is almost impossible to categorize the subtle differences of feeling expression and outer behavior beyond simply describing them experientially. Only the relatively inexperienced body therapist needs precise procedural rules, tightly conceptualized labels and character typologies in order to assume a directive stance toward the client.

The following accounts of individual sessions demonstrate how a humanistically oriented body psychotherapist will adopt a variety of roles depending upon the client's existential state of being and emotional neediness. Artistic sensibilities are required to assess the client's existential state and to select appropriate body and psychic techniques. But artistic sensibility must balance with the therapist's empirical knowledge -- a legacy from many different sources: a refined knowledge of certain physiological systems; a clinical understanding of how different concrete body expressions reveal certain general psychological as well as organismic patterns of rigidity; and a largely pragmatic clinical knowledge that if one initiates a particular body technique or sequence of techniques, interpenetrated or followed by certain psychological suggestions, then certain processes of progressive breaking down of the client's ego defense structure may possibly ensue. This legacy is scientific in origin and content. But the choice of method with respect to a particular client arises as much from the therapist's intuitively alive creative unconscious as from his clinical knowledge.

In the accounts which follow, it will be almost impossible to determine which methods were dictated by my artistic sensibilities and which by my objective knowledge of the client's mind and body. Nevertheless, I shall attempt to point out the distinctions. In the last analysis, the humanistic body psychotherapist acts according to the subtlest energetic and feeling vibrations emanating directly from the body of the client and the capacity to tune into these messages cannot be quantified.

II. Case of Ronald

Ronald would never have risked entrusting himself to me unless his girlfriend of three and a half years had not finally left him for good. Her departure created so much irrational anxiety that he could not cope alone. A school psychologist, Ronald was not unacquainted with pertinent psychological issues, but he could not manage his gnawing sense of desperation.

Arriving for his sixth two hour session, Ronald slid into a comfortable armchair. I in another, we talked face to face for twenty minutes. Ronald spoke of his most recent attempts to persuade his girlfriend, whom he thought he loved very much, to reconsider her decision to leave him. The fact that his anxiety was notably reduced when he talked about her, compared with the previous sessions, told me he was beginning to adjust to the prospect of living alone without her, but was still hoping intensely that she would change her mind. Ronald said that he realized the situation had reached a stalemate, that he saw little merit in discussing it further, and was ready to begin bodywork. I responded instantaneously to this new and significant declaration thusly:

> So take off your clothes. I want to see you do something on your feet for a change. Take a broad split -- not excessive. Now, watch what I do. As I come down, I bring my elbows in so that my shoulders are pushed up from below and I open my knees... Close your eyes and listen to your breathing... Focus your conscious awareness on sensing your belly region. As you get pain, allow sound, but wait until the pain comes. (see page 4)

Ronald reports feeling stress in his stomach, asking if it should be there. I tell him to wait and see, that the stress could be in any part of the body. After a silence of a minute and a half, I ask him to let his breathing deepen, to stay aware of the front half of his body. Ronald's breathing does indeed begin to deepen, becoming transparently audible. It also begins to manifest a slow, rhythmic alternation, attesting to a noteworthy amount of intact energy flow beginning to circulate freely between the upper and lower halves of his torso.

Seeing this slow rhythm emerging, but also perceiving that he is still unable to allow the slightest vocal sound despite experiencing much physical pain in his lower half, I ask him to make the sound, 'Ah.' Ronald begins to make a barely discernible 'Ah' with each exhalation. Its muted quality tells me that he is unawarefully controlling all of his organism's outlets of primitive self - expression.

I wait another minute before asking Ronald to allow self-images from his earlier years, while

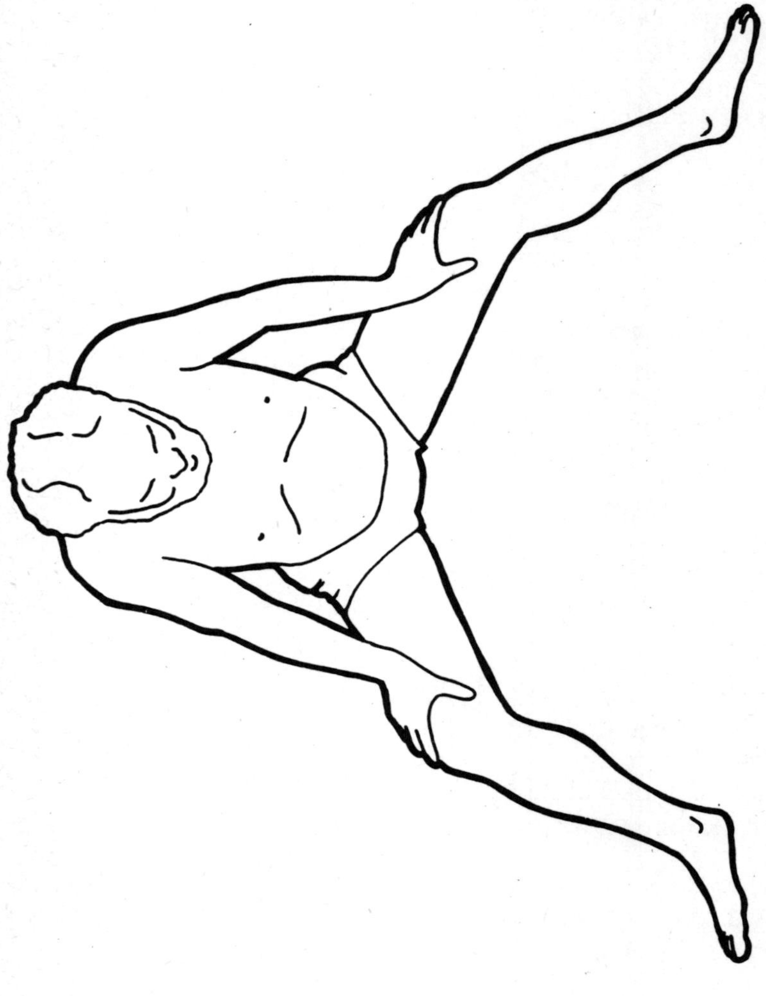

staying in the position. About twenty seconds following this psychological stimulus, Ronald's 'Ahs' begin to assume a definite vocal audibility and dynamism. Initially coming from his throat region, they sound like effort-filled spurts of will struggling to release something buried in his chest. There is a slightly childlike churlish quality to them, half-beseeching and half-defiant. They begin to show much movement in timbre, racing upwards to high scratchy, reedy tones and then abruptly downwards into lower tones, but remaining forced and willful. The length of each sound increases, causing Ronald to increasingly prolong each exhalation.

After the fourth minute, Ronald's sounds begin to intensify into real feeling -- rage and sorrow weave a pattern. After the eighth minute, he stammers thickly, almost inaudibly: "Leave me alone. Leave me alone." Following a brief torrential outpouring of rage and anger, Ronald actually weeps. By now the sounds have deepened, stemming as much from his belly as from his chest. As they deepen into his belly, they become increasingly lionesque, mirroring Ronald's physique: a broad-shouldered torso thickly muscled up and down the back with a massive head and limbs to match. Several times, he repeats: "Leave me alone.".

Tiring slightly, Ronald's breathing cycle quickens a little, but not too much. He mutters: "Oh God, there's no way out of this pain." Intermittently, he bellows rage and weeps helplessly in a high-pitched voice. Suddenly, Ronald yells:

> You bitches. You always hurt me. (He roars, then weeps.) ..... You bitch. (A roar) You asshole. You God-damned bitch. (More roars) Get me out of here. Oh shit..... You bitch.

The accompanying powerful forward and backward thrust of his pelvis and legs crescendoes into explosive spit: "Get away from me. Fuck you. God-damned you." Ronald spits again, a nasty sound issuing from between his lips. There is now a steady humming-like tremoring pervading his entire lower half. He shrieks, "Fuck you... Fuck you," with a screaming intensity, but focused like outer-directed, object-centered rage.

Now, twenty-six minutes since the body work began, I ask Ronald sympathetically to lie out on the mattress. Thanking me, he slowly comes forward and down onto his knees, his leg muscles so stretched he cannot possibly stand fully upright. After lying out on his back, he weeps quietly for several minutes and then, gradually, becomes quiet. "What was it all about ? " I ask.

> My mom. Oh man ! I just got in touch with how much I needed her and loved her and how angry I was at her too. I felt in my legs like a small child who was really helpless and really needed to be dependent upon my mom. Yet I hated her for it too. She's a fucking manipulator. She used me. What flashed in my head was Golden Boy. A fucking perfect kid I was. (He weeps) I could never get angry with her. Oh, God, how she would worship the ground I walked on. She manipulated and controlled me totally with that Golden Boy shit. I hate her for that. (He bellows) I hate her for that !
>
> So I grew up with all my relationships with women the same stuck way : I love and I hate them at the same time. Damn it. God, how it pisses me off.... I do have a fucking lot of anger in me, you were sure right. All the pain was in my thighs, and a little bit in my knees. But mostly right here, right in the center of my crotch.

I asked Ronald what I was right about.

> About a fucking lot of anger in me. With women, I love 'em and I need 'em. I'm dependent on 'em and I'm also pissed at 'em. That's been my stuck place with women for a long time... God! I had a flash while standing there -- Hey, I'm gonna grow up some day. I'm gonna get you back for this because I'm not going to need you at some point and then I'm gonna really fuck you over.

Twenty-six minutes is an uncommonly long time for anyone to maintain this particular position of stress, a position especially difficult for anyone with chronic tension, or what we shall be calling muscular armoring, in their pelvic, lower back and belly regions. People severely armored in any of these three regions usually find this position so painful that they can maintain it for no more than three to four minutes : they either stop, or more likely, they lift their bottom gradually higher and higher so that their pelvis is above rather than on the same horizontal plane with their knees.

The fact that Ronald maintained the position for a very long time without lifting his pelvis even slightly indicated to me that he was not severely armored in his lower half. Another objective indication was the fact that his breathing cycle progressively lengthened and deepened the longer he remained in the position. If he had been severely armored in his lower half, his breathing would have become increasingly rapid, superficial and survival-oriented.

Another indication that Ronald carried only moderate chronic tension throughout his body was the manner in which his vocal sound production slowly shifted its center of gravity from his throat to his belly. As it moved into the lower regions of his torso, it moved inwards as well as outwards : it became progressively more substantial the longer he remained in the position, almost as if more and more parts of his total organism were participating in the production of sound. The resonance grew and grew, swelling outwards to his peripheral metabolic layers and at the same time inwards to his deepest regions. What is more, the flow became increasingly longitudinal. As he began to vibrate with tremendous purring dynamism throughout his lower half, his vocal tones became richer and more gargantuan, filling the room with their power.

I asked Ronald to assume this particular position because I believed from previous sessions that whatever armoring he had was located in his pelvis and belly. My deductive elimination was coupled with my clinical knowledge that Ronald could be classified as partially crippled by a chronic psychic conflict, often labelled 'phallic-narcissistic'. This syndrome is characterized by a striking compartmentalization and dynamic opposition between tender feelings and sexual desire. It is difficult for the 'phallic-narcissist male' to extend both tender loving and sexually erotic feelings towards the same woman.

Split between his tender and sexual dimensions, his genitals compel him to aggressively overwhelm the female even when he is spiritually invested.

Integral to this chronic internal conflict between different parts of his soul's feeling capacity with respect to women is a chronic blockage of energy flow between Ronald's genitals and his heart. As with any neurotic syndrome if the 'phallic-narcissist's' energy block is severe, it will extend deep into the muscular wall which divides the chest from the abdominal cavity, the diaphragm. Ronald's diaphragmatic armoring was minimal; his armoring lay hidden deep inside the pelvis itself, in the iliopsoas muscle complex. This muscle always armors whenever there is some form of chronic blockage of energy flow between the genitals and the other feeling centers of the torso, even when no other part of the body is significantly armored, as was true of Ronald.

Such clinical knowledge prompted me to place Ronald in one of the most demanding do-it-yourself stress positions I know. Intuitively, I realized that his total energy economy might awaken and mobilize enough for him to experience the archaic withheld emotions intimately intertwined with his chronic pelvic and abdominal muscular tensions. Loosening the somatic counterpart to an underlying chronic impasse between opposite emotional inclinations might be sufficient to release the psychological repression of these emotions and to resurrect in consciousness the actual source of chronic inhibition.

The combination of objective and intuitive evaluation of Ronald's armoring enabled me to select the right body technique, a technique powerful enough to catalyze the most loaded repressed psychological material. If I had chosen a less demanding energy mobilization technique, Ronald might have retained his customary ego control from his head. The right method enabled him to become progressively identified with a kind of feeling consciousness largely centered in the release of energies in the pelvic and genital regions. This physical loosening and partial release of energy flow triggered a release of rigid feelings in consciousness.

Consequently, for the first time in his adult

life, Ronald was able to experience in full consciousness how his mother's manner of relating to him as a young boy double-binded his own soul's feeling needs. For the first time in his thirty-four years, he could feel the anger and rage toward his mother which he had been harboring unconsciously since early childhood. Simultaneously, he began to sense how his enormous need for her love caused him to restrict himself from seeing how she played upon his need in order to control him to execute her will. Now, Ronald could actually feel in his pelvis and upper legs how she had somehow seduced him into submissively obeying her every request without a murmur. Now, he could sense how she used him like an object, rather than unconditionally affirming his deepest feeling needs. And finally, he could perceive without the slightest ambiguity how his boyhood relationship to his mother was directly connected with his adult love-hate response to women.

This is a rather impressive set of new discoveries during twenty-six minutes while standing in a physically painful position. If Ronald had been severely armored, he could not have moved so completely into an altered state of consciousness in which the chronic emotional conflicts locked into his pelvic muscles assumed such dominance. Unless the dynamic feeling centers in his body were alive and in internal communication with his rational self-awareness, he could not have experienced in this brief period the powerful repressed feelings of rage, hatred, enormous dependency, and determination for revenge. To be sure, he could not directly experience the great sexual frustration sustained by his chronic genital-pelvic tension, but the fact that he could experience the other repressed feelings so fully was indispensable to subsequent discoveries of how his mother had cultivated in him a love so intense for her that it resembled that of a little male adult rather than that of a needy child.

I had but a glimmer of what was happening to Ronald psychologically and emotionally as he stood before me in the broad split position. Although I suspected and hoped that he was raging against his mother, I could not be sure it wasn't against his girlfriend. I was not sure what his conscious feelings were when his vocal expression became weepy and especially when it became regressed and helpless.

I could only perceive beyond doubt his increasingly lionesque mobilization of anger and rage. I had to wait until he spoke after lying out on the mattress to learn his psychological space. Such sizeable lapses of immediate intuitive contact with the psychic space of the client frequently occur when using body techniques and represent one of many adventuresome risks of body psychotherapy. The humanistic practitioner must be prepared to give his clients a very loose rein: to allow them to enter spaces not clearly known by the therapist, and to let them stay there freely and responsibly until ready to share subjective experience.

III. Case of Gayle

Gayle is a female rigid compulsive type already on the road to loosening her armoring. We need to take a closer, more individualized look at Gayle to transcend the stereotyped conceptual models such labels inspire.

The body psychotherapist could hardly regard himself as existentialist or humanist in his clinical orientation if he used a medical model of labelling to understand human uniqueness. To be sure, initial labels do help the clinician engage in a more discriminate and actively catalytic stance towards the client's body, thanks to the characterological typologies worked out by Wilhelm Reich and Alexander Lowen. But once treatment has begun to affect the core, the value of such typologies rapidly diminishes. In fact, they become a positive liability if the clinician continues to rely upon them, simply because they can never fathom the unconscious depths of the human organism and soul. At best, they enable the clinician to superimpose stereotyped intellectual categories upon the visible frozen outer forms and movements of the client's mesodermal voluntary musculature.

With Gayle, for instance, it was obvious that her manic restlessness, combined with a certain chronic intensity and lability of affect, went hand in hand with a body structure defined as rigid in the Reichian-Lowenian framework. Her tight, flat-chested upper half and narrow tube-like torso conveyed a well-coordinated volitional aliveness up and down her back from her feet to her head. Her entire upper half was girlish, from her large but harrassed eyes and baby-face volatility to her underdeveloped front half and doll-like rigidity. Except for a steely, overdeveloped back, she looked like a lost street urchin who never wanted to grow up.

A closer, more subtle look at Gayle's manner of being and potential for wholeness reveals, however, that her psychological maturity far surpassed her bodily maturity. Gayle displayed a degree of psychological sophistication and richness of feeling capacities that far exceeded Ronald's, a professional psychologist. Gayle's body did show signs of a severe neurotic splitting of her soul and a severe amount of chronic muscular armoring which would take several years to eliminate. Nevertheless, she intuitively knew what she needed to do psychologically and emotionally to facilitate her own healing.

Gayle mailed us a description of her emotional space during the three days immediately following her tenth hourly session. She described with gripping incisiveness the maelstrom of contradictory feeling states. With unrelenting honesty and objective awareness, she shared her terror-filled swift changes in feeling regarding her boyfriend and two children by an estranged husband. Gayle was able to feel fully and to describe with intuitive accuracy her irrational, murderous impulses toward her two children -- feelings she was just beginning to allow herself to experience consciously. She catapulted from the wildest, craziest impulses to kill them on the spot to feelings of acute shame and remorse as she cried profusely until completely emptied of any feeling. For limited periods of a few hours, she described feeling good about herself as a mother. She expressed amazement at the good feelings, since only three months previously, she had come to us in a state of almost total despair and paralysis, arising from her sense of imprisonment by the responsibility of raising two children alone without a husband's supportive presence.

Gayle had come a long way out of her compulsive-hysteric paralysis to allow conscious murderous impulses. Her psychological maturity and resiliency of feeling flow enabled her to rise to any occasion requiring a reality-centered approach and allowed her to risk such a letting go. I reassured her that she needed to disintegrate creatively in tolerable doses before she could reconstitute her false role of the perfect mother.

In her next session with us, Gayle described her crazy, mixed up constellation of emotions which she experienced as both frightening and exciting. While Gayle was speaking, Katherine and I have been holding one of her hands from behind, with her arms extended over her head and backwards along the mattress as she lies in the spread-eagle position. We have been alternately pulling one arm at a time, causing her severely armored arm-shoulder joints to loosen to the point where she will be compelled to kick and to scream frantically in order to discharge the energy being polarized in her upper half through her lower half.
(see page 13)

I am so impressed with Gayle's acceptance of my clinical advice to allow herself to creatively disintegrate that I suddenly propose: "Let's hear what happens to you when you go crazy. Tell us about this past week. You say you were sitting alone in the living room with your children."

> They were like birds. Everytime I wanted to be still and just be with me, they wanted to peck at me. I wanted them to leave me alone, and then when I tell them, they escalate a whole bunch of shit around that naturally. I become more angry and I get all kinds of phantasies of wiping them out by throwing them against the wall. I just hate them.

Me: All right - talk to them.

> I hate you when you do that. I hate you when you are constantly needling me. You can figure it out yourselves.

Gayle speaks in a voice that perpetually wails, soars and dives rapidly to many different pitches within the duration of a single sentence. This vocal hyper-resiliency indicates considerable dearmoring in her throat and chest. Gayle manifests anger, self-doubt, fear and a forced aggressive hostility as she speaks to her children:

> I want to take you by your feet and just throw you against the wall. I want to hurt you..... I just want to hurt you.

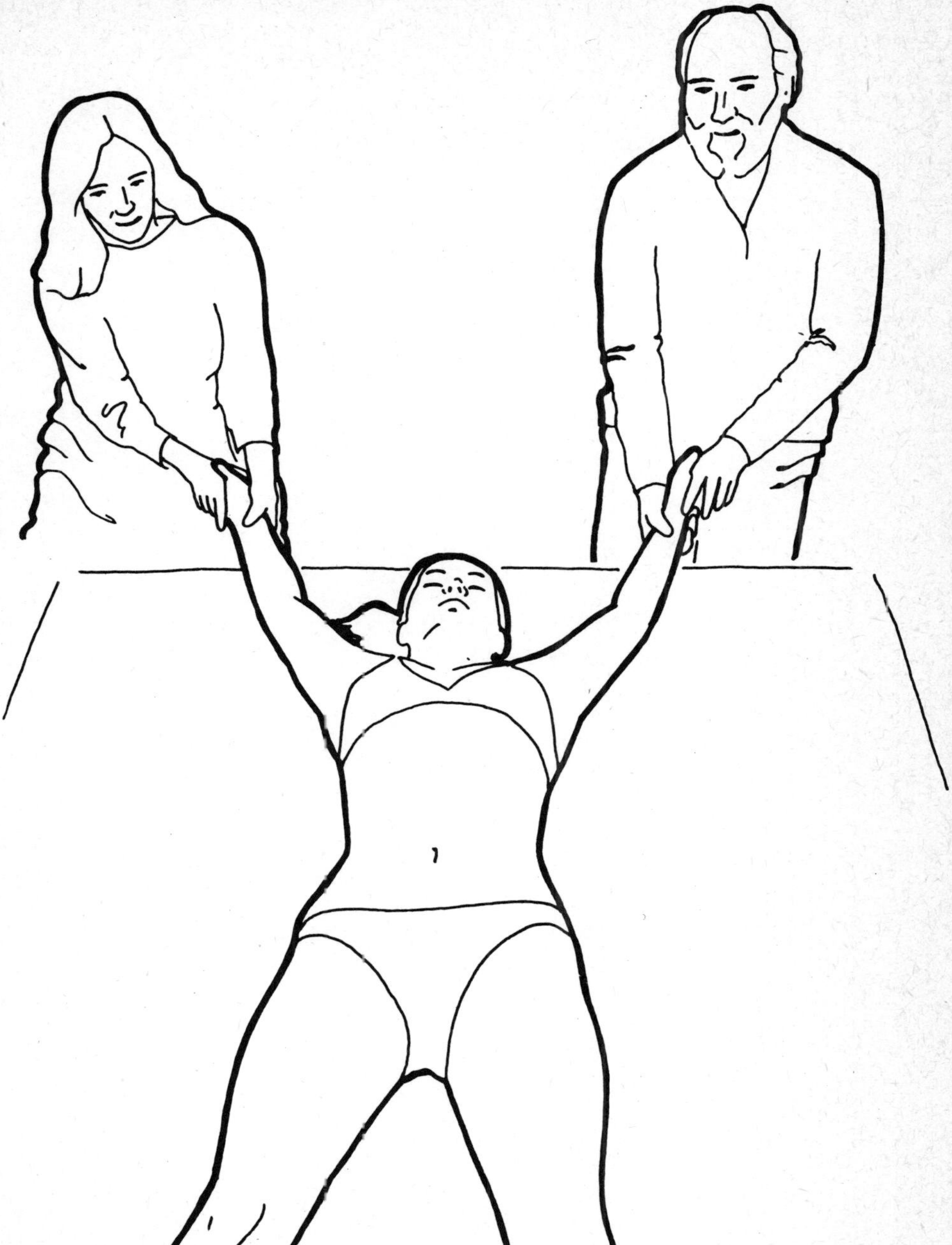

I ask Gayle to squeeze our hands as she tells her children she wants to hurt them, so that we can catalyze an energy buildup which can only find release in some form of immediate primitive discharge.

> I want to hurt you, because I do not know the answers. (Her voice begins to rise in pitch, energy-release, and intensity.) I do-o-o-n't know ho-o-o-w to be a m-o-o-o-o-o-ther.

From the moment Gayle begins to say "mother", she dramatically shifts from yelling to frenzied shrieks--her voice literally skyrockets into extremely high registers. And then, she lets out a few deep breaths, sobbing quickly in between. Catching her wind, she bellows: "I don't want to be your m-o-o-o-o-o-ther".

I ask Gayle to bounce her pelvis. This exercise, designed to catalyze the energy metabolism in the lower half of the torso, is intended to affirm Gayle's further skyrocketing of her cathartic discharge of repressed feeling bound by chronic tension.

> I don't know how to be your mother. I don't know. I don't want to be your mother anymore. I don't want to be your m-o-o-o-o-o-ther anymore.

Gayle stops screaming hysterically and simply breathes deeply. After thirty seconds, I inquire: "How do you feel?"

> Good... Feels good. I mean I know a lot of stuff they don't know, but I don't know a lot of other stuff too. I don't have to be perfect. I don't even know what perfect is. Somehow, I thought I had to do all the things my mother didn't do. I've given up all that power. I can't do what she did.

Directing Gayle to become her mother, I ask her what she sees.

> She worries a lot that she's not doing it right. She knows she's not. She's alone. She's sitting in her house, watching me all the time. She's hoping that she will see signs that I am really O.K., but everytime she does, she rips it off. She doesn't really know what O.K. is. It's somehow being happy. I've got to be happy. Not like poor little sister Jessica and brother Erwin who

> didn't have half of what I have, and deserve a lot more.

I tell Gayle that her blood has been retreating from her hands since she's been speaking about her mother. I urge her to speak to her in the way she spoke to her children to get the blood flowing back into the periphery.

> I don't want to be your daughter, and I don't want to be your mother. I don't even want to know her. I don't want to know you. God, I wish you would die! There's just nothing you can do for me... Nothing... Absolutely nothing! God, I've learned all I need to learn from you.

I take both of Gayle's hands now and ask her to put her hands on my wrist. I must have anticipated some impending expression of aggression which would be more effectively contained if she had a firm grip around both my wrists, while my hands simultaneously gripped her wrists.

> God, I was supposed to have learned a lot from you, tons of things, but name just one I really should feel grateful for. Just one. (A toughly defiant tone) I don't want to go through anymore with you in me. I really hate you. I hate having to be your mother. I hate having to be your daughter. I hate having to kno-o-o-o-o-o-o-ow yo-o-o-o-o-o-o-o-u.

Gayle's voice catapults rapidly upwards into the higher registers; she begins to kick extremely rapidly with both legs while screaming hysterically. I was right that she needed containment rather than further catalytic stimulation : gently, but firmly holding her wrists gave her total organism enough security to let go of all controls completely, and to move with total abandonment.

Shortly after Gayle stops kicking and screaming, she says in a surprisingly cool voice, almost as if she were watching herself from outside of herself:

> It feels really less real. It doesn't feel real. I don't know if it is real or not. She doesn't feel real... Wow, that feels yucky. I can talk like that to my kids because I really love them, but it's hard to say that to my mother because I

hate her.... I don't know if I do or not. I guess I do, and I sure don't want to see her... I want to hate her. But I don't want to hate her either.

The capacity to scream primitively is of little consequence for Gayle. The currently fashionable belief in the capacity to scream as a cure for neurosis is a lamentably exaggerated half-truth, if not outright falsification. Gayle did a lot of screaming, and much of it did help to reduce her transient tension level, but it is difficult to know to what extent it lowered her chronic tension level.

Much more to the point is the partial emergence of hidden unconscious psychological material which immediately evoked a skyrocketing polarization of Gayle's whole energy economy with an intensity great enough to momentarily obliterate her psyche and soul. The most significant healing process occurred when Gayle's profound ambivalence about the mothering role (whether in her real mother or in herself) emerged on a half-conscious feeling-centered level. The ambivalence is so powerful it reeks of great self-hatred. It is so great that it is still too painful and catastrophically disintegrating for Gayle to experience it except tangentially and in the form of brief surries into her chaotic emotional depths. It is not accidental that she plunges into uncontrollable shrieking the moment she utters the word 'mother'. The whole mothering process is really anathema to her at an unconscious feeling level. Therefore, she has had to compensate psychologically by willing herself to become an idealized mother, who behaves according to a cerebrally controlled image of perfection.

The outstanding clinical technique used with Gayle is the interpenetration of psychological and bioenergetic methods with identical intent: to catalyze a primitive emotional release which serves to loosen her repressive ego defense network. Sensing her ripeness to let go, I deliberately polarized in particular her cathartic release of what I intuitively sensed was a chronic unconscious hostility toward her feminine sex. I knew that her rage towards her two children was largely a projective displacement of rage with herself and her mother. By endorsing her expression of irrationally intense negative feelings towards her two children, I realized she might come in touch with her destructive unconscious attitude towards herself as woman.

Before this could happen, her congealed energy circuits needed enormous shaking. If I had not asked Gayle to squeeze our hands each time she expressed a sadistic sentiment towards her children, she might not have moved right out of her head into her sick hatred of herself as a woman. The transition from the reality centered perspective of the rational ego into a feeling centered realm dominated by the irrational id, I call a movement out of a convergent into a creatively divergent mode of being. When there is a lot of armoring, such a movement is always extremely anxiety arousing, if not catastrophically overwhelming. Gayle experiences acute anxiety from the moment she starts to say 'mother', and slides into her chaotic feeling depths below her head.

I had no clear idea what would happen when I asked Gayle to squeeze our hands -- certainly no idea what would happen psychologically. What did happen was more than I could have even hoped for because she herself was able to fall into her hitherto denied hatred of her own perfect mother self-image and begin to explore its connection to her multifaceted relationship with her mother. Both the hand-squeezing and pelvis-bouncing techniques were necessary to mobilize enough freely fluid metabolic energy flow to upset her tight ego defense network from underneath her head. The flow mobilized had to be more powerful than the fear of catastrophic anxiety belonging to her defense network. The fact that this very fear of experiencing anxiety in the here-and-now is one of the key devices by which the intact psyche maintains a state of chronic emotional repression and conflict provides one justification for using directive catalytic bioenergetic and psychological methods.

Asking Gayle to identify herself with her mother revealed how extraordinarily well and easily she could do it mentally. This attests to the unconscious primary-process feeling fixation which she still had towards her mother, a fixation and identification process which was powerfully intact because of the determination of Gayle's rational consciousness to deny its existence. This represents perhaps her primary neurotic conflict, which is frequently the case in the compulsive hysteric syndrome. It is not difficult to understand, therefore, why Gayle could not believe in the authenticity of her expression of hostility towards her mother: a large part of her soul was still closed to anything but total feeling paralysis. Consequently, she could not marshall all of her dynamic feeling centers when she addressed her mother directly. She would only be able to do so after most of her chronic armoring had dissolved. Until then, it would be premature, indeed reckless, to bulldoze her into fully facing her murderous feelings towards her mother and herself which sprang from the poisonous impact of mother upon child.

These observations are directly supported by two incidents which occurred at the bioenergetic level. When Gayle projected herself into her mother's image and verbalized what her mother thought and felt, her peripheral blood flow noticeably diminished. As Katherine and I held Gayle's hands, they dramatically changed their temperature and texture, moving from warm and charged to cold and somewhat dead. The most probable explanation is that talking as if she were mother generated a great deal of unfelt anxiety and fear. It is a well known physiological mechanism that the presence of anxiety tends to constrict the peripheral blood vessels while accelerating the heart, resulting in a massive withdrawal of blood flow from the periphery to the center of the cardiovascular system. The generation of anxiety clearly indicates the existence of some kind of chronic psychic impasse between opposite feeling tendencies, the precise nature of which is discussed above.

Once Gayle addressed her mother directly and began to experience her intense hostility, her peripheral blood vessels flowed vitally again. But it took violent primal screaming and kicking before she managed to break out of her ego defenses. The reversal of energy flow from periphery to center to a centrifugal flow from center to periphery was probably the basic bioenergetic reason why Gayle needed to experience her encounter with her mother as unreal. And indeed it was, but for self-protective reasons: complete dissolution of Gayle's severe intact armoring would either kill her biologically or plunge her into a psychotic episode. Mother nature always moves at a slow, conservative pace of change, and by the same token, an intact ego defense system serves the invaluable function of preserving a certain necessary degree of psychological equilibrium and continuity of identity.

The other bioenergetic support for my observations occurred later in the session. Gayle discussed the tragic experiences of her mother's life which her mother had often talked about with Gayle. But Gayle also knew that her mother would suck off of others until she drove them away, so desperate were her needs for love. These remarks confirmed my earlier impression that Gayle had a powerful unconscious feeling identification with her mother.

On a rational level, Gayle had always and was still actively affirming a heart-felt sympathy and understanding of her mother's fate. But this very sympathy and understanding required her to maintain rigorous repressive defenses against her murderous impulses toward her mother. Gayle needed to externalize and fully express these hostile feelings before she could free her deepest self-assertive and self-reliant feeling centers from the insidious chronic psychological impasse at whose nucleus seethed a generalized hatred of woman. To enable Gayle to focus on the hostile side of her fluctuating feelings, I used her own lability as follows.

Gayle is talking about how her mother cannot stand Gayle to be angry with her :

> And of course I can't stand being around her without getting angry at her, so it's an impossible situation... She wants to want to see me. She feels guilty. She feels lonely. She wants so much. She has a sense of how things could be, and she reaches for them. I am how they should be. I'm the last one, and so all her other children are more casual in meaning for her.
>
> It's like she could watch her daughter die -- my daughter, whoops, I mean my sister who is almost twenty-five years older than I am -- watch her die of alcoholism and could cry and feel bad for a while. But wow! There's still me around. I'm like she put all her last-ditch efforts into me. Oh God, I hate it. She can't just let me be! But neither can she like what I'm doing. I want to give her up... I want to either...

Interrupting her, I say, "Tell her".

Sighing deeply, Gayle speaks :

I either want you to die and forget it and realize that this life is over for you, that you can't get any more out of it, you've milked the last bit of growth you can possibly get out of it.

Go away and die and leave me alone! (Her voice begins to soar and dive with intensity.) Or either I have to do something. I have to give you up in some way I don't understand. If I get angry, it doesn't work. I can't love you because I can't stand being around you. How can I love you if there's nothing to love? I can just watch you and not feel anything, but I tried that and I don't want it. So my problem now is how to get to be a whole person -- ahow.

The sound of 'ahow' expresses the real physical pain that I am deliberately giving Gayle by placing my index and middle finger of one hand into the center of the back of her neck just at the edge of the base of her skull. While my other hand firmly holds her head still, I palpate my two fingers and move slowly into the tight knot of muscle at this particular neck juncture.
(see page 21)

This is one of the severest direct touch methods we use, and because it can be so painful, we administer only one such touch per session. The point in her neck described is what I have come to call 'the paranoid button': clients who exhibit a character-muscular rigidity of an extremely rigid type, have an especially hardened neck at this point. I have discovered that if I slowly screwdriver my two fingers into this particular spot on the neck to the edge of intolerable pain, this often loosens the deeper layers of repressed hostility and frustration which cripple most kinds of rigid types.

Gayle continues her verbal confrontation :

and have you still hovering on the edge and hanging onto me like a fossil... I don't want to feel my feelings. (She cries openly.) I

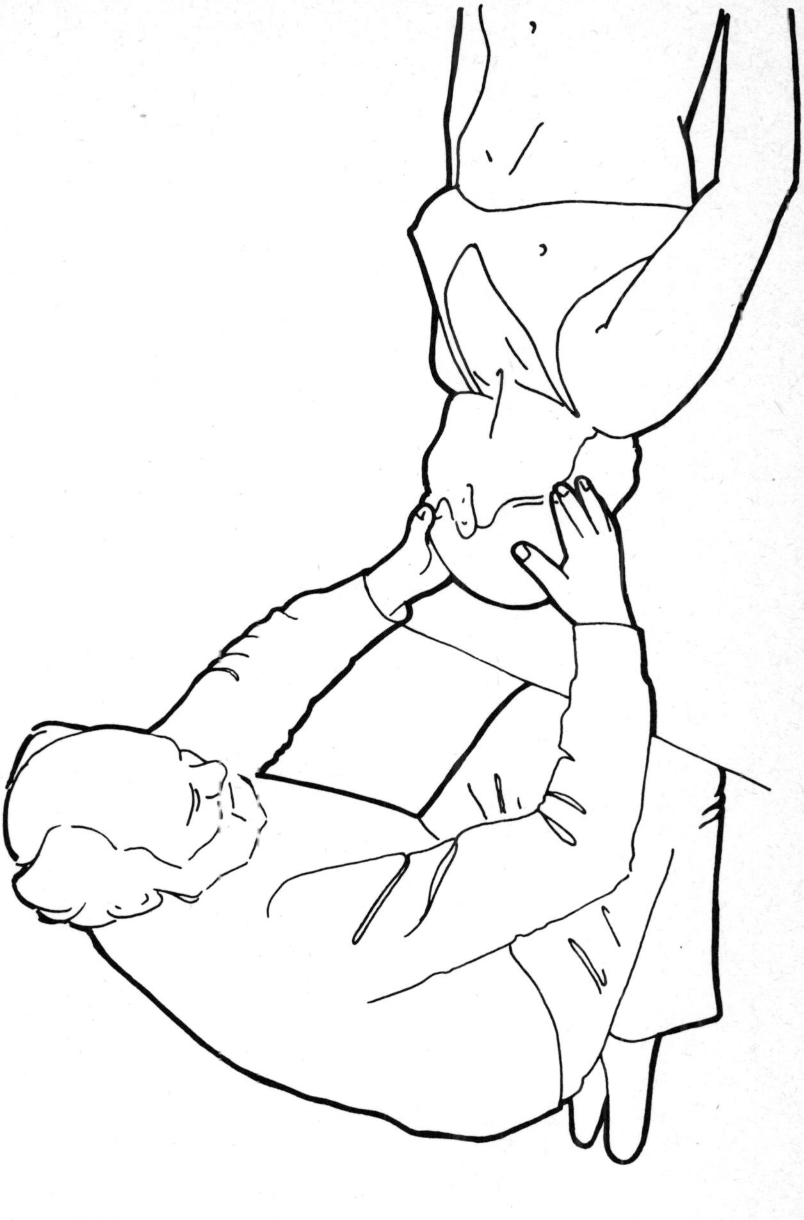

don't want to feel my feelings.

Gayle's voice begins to deteriorate, losing its normally vibrant youthful resonance. There are not exact words for the sound. Uttering only 'ah', Gayle's voice slowly metamorphoses into the half-animal cackling of a witch. The sounds resemble a drowning animal in the last throes of anguish. Rasping, clawing, hoarse and abnormally deep, her voice sounds more like that of a man as her face simultaneously twists into an ugly, horrifying grimace. Gayle has become totally possessed by this eerie voice and grotesque facial contortions. Extremely desperate, she manages to force through her lips once more, "I don't want to feel it", before disintegrating again into complete incoherency. This involuntary process continues for a minute and a half before she suddenly becomes still and quiet.

After a few seconds, Gayle murmurs: "That sounds just like my mother when she cries. I hate that sound". She then becomes quiet except for a deep breathing whose mechanical rhythm tells me there is something abnormal about it. I am holding her head gently but firmly in my two hands; her scalp sends messages into my hands communicating half-crazy alertness. I sense that she is watching herself like an object, the wonder of what is happening to her has paralyzed her with fear. She does not move a muscle in her whole body for several minutes.

I remove my hands. Several more minutes pass in silence. And then Gayle begins to whimper -- the sounds are of a severely panic-stricken two-year-old child. As her cries diminish, I ask, "What"? She sobs uncontrollably: miserable, alone, helpless. Later, she replies: "I don't know what's happening to me". She resumes her regressive weeping, involuntarily drawing her two legs up into her belly and turning on her side in the foetal position. She remains, crying for a long time. When I ask her some five minutes later what's happening, she says she can't stand women like herself with bloated bellies and then rambles on half-mindlessly about how she wants to kick every woman she sees who has a flat belly. In other words, she completely avoids the reality of what she has just been living through on a feeling level, spending the remainder of the session talking about women's bellies.

Again, both psychological and bioenergetic techniques spearhead the excruciatingly painful breakthrough into repressed feeling. The psychological technique consists of asking Gayle to address her mother in the first person singular rather than from the more detached perspective of a third person. This shift in perspective is often sufficient to alter the subject-world interaction from a rational to an emotional level of encounter, by virtue of the greater subject-centeredness of perception generated by a first person singular stance. As a result of this shift in perceptual perspective, we see how Gayle's sympathetic identification with her mother's pain-filled life gradually recedes into the background as her own sense of having been used to satisfy her mother's insatiable neurotic needs emerges in the foreground.

But it is the intertwining of this psychological technique with the direct catalytic touch applied to the back of her neck that sends Gayle into a process of disintegrative divergent functioning which is almost more than her psychic balance can tolerate. Her first wail, "I don't want to feel my feelings", initiates a dangerous stretching of the emotinal polarities within her to the edge of an emotional breakdown. There are many signs that she experiences almost more than she can bear : a total loss of control over her body's behavior which resembles a complete disorganization and loss of identity, followed by a total petrification of her feelings in a state of suspended shock, and terminated by a complete splitting off in consciousness from facing her own disintegrative experience and its emotional significance. Because I clearly sensed the brinkmanship assault to her integrated psyche, I deliberately did not ask about her experience for the remainder of the session.

The body psychotherapist who could not intuitively sense Gayle's need to escape at this time from facing her own internal world would be guilty of the most monstrous insensitivity to the client's core state of being. But if the therapist had already been in touch with the highly developed capacity for living both sides of the core soul's feeling polarities which Gayle is capable of, and recognized how resiliently she can move from one end of the continuum to the other, there would be no question but to appreciate Gayle's need to flee from the horrifying aspects of her still encapsulated inner world. The delicacy and brittleness of her metabolic condition is sufficient reason to let her alone to work out the psychological implications of the session's experience by herself in subsequent days and months. I knew Gayle could do this when she was ready, without needing my actual presence.

IV. Case of Eldridge

The bioenergetic and psycho-dynamic processes that occurred within Ronald and Gayle are relatively straightforward. Such is not always the case. Some clients have become so fragmented in their psyches and twisted in their normal energy currents that their responses to concrete body methods are as bizarrely incomprehensible and distorted as their labyrinthine interiors. Working with such a person creates its own special difficulties -- the greater the severity of the armoring, the greater the challenge to unravel the complicated psychic and somatic knots within.

Body psychotherapy shares with every other style of depth psychotherapy the preliminary task of putting together the pieces of an elaborate jigsaw puzzle before the singularity of the psychopathological complexes crippling the client can be perceived by either therapist or client.

I stand with those who ultimately must reject all efforts to scientifically categorize the various styles of psychopathology, including the Reichian-Lowenian formulation of the various character-muscular typologies of armoring. They ignore the vast number of different possibilities that each psychopathological syndrome assumes. And it is the gradual unraveling of the individual peculiarities of each syndrome in each human being which constitutes the real beginning to the identification of the pathology. One must adopt a metaphysics of radical empiricism and absolute relativism if one hopes to do justice to the objective complexity of each psychopathological syndrome as it exists within each person.

Let us explore a session with Eldridge as an example of the more convoluted process just described. Eldridge came to California for an intensive with us just after successfully completing his medical training and exams in Europe. Despite such success, he felt like "nothing" : "hopeless, helpless, and damned". Desperately split within, he had never felt satisfaction from any accomplishment.

Part of Eldridge's excessive guilt came from his puritanical Roman Catholic upbringing. Schooled in German and Swiss monasteries, he had been trained to cultivate the "Christian virtues" of self-sacrifice and self-deprecation. Medical training helped Eldridge to overcome his early indoctrination into the wickedness of the human flesh, but he was still too incapacitated emotionally to even recognize his inadequate sexual satisfaction.

Responding to Eldridge's masochistic character-muscular armoring, Katherine and I began applying tremendous amounts of physical pressure to his body. For three weeks, both of us would regularly lie on top of him with our whole bodies. But even our combined weight of nearly 325 pounds, applied for half an hour, had scarcely any apparent loosening effect. At best, he would collapse into pathos-dominant feelings of longing and mourning for his dead mother, experiencing some comfort as he remembered how he had loved his mother and suffered with her in common allegiance against an unpredictable, brutally insensitive, hardworking and authoritarian father. Only twice had Eldridge spontaneously experienced any mobilization of negative feelings against his father, but these were quickly aborted by feelings of guilt and anxiety.

During his fourteenth three - hour session, Eldridge addressed his father and mother :

> Yes, I see the split because I love you both, but I cannot be so angry as you have been with me. You have been so terribly angry.

At this moment my two hands, which have been pressing firmly downwards on either side of his spinal column between the shoulder blades about two to three inches below the cervical vertebrae, begin to exert greater pressure in an on-off rhythm. Each time I press squarely downwards, Eldridge groans. (I have already given Eldridge all the catalytic direct touch he can comfortably tolerate by sitting for ten minutes on the lower end of his spinal column where the pelvic bone protrudes.) I continue the rhythmic pressure until I decide to come away from his body completely. Eldridge stops groaning almost instantly: I realize that the pain has not been great, nor the methods very fruitful. But I know that for an organism as tightly armored and densely hardened as Eldridge's to elicit the slightest spontaneous expression of pain is noteworthy.

After a few seconds of silence, Eldridge says:

> Malcolm, I am afraid to tell you -- terribly afraid to say that you must now hurt me. You must pull me down and suffocate me. You must strangulate me. You should take my throat and stop all of my breathing. I should not be able to move or to defend myself. But a moment before I die, you then have to leave me alone. Then I think I will become healed.
>
> I am waiting to live these terrible things. Somewhere in me I am persuaded I must go through this. I want to be killed before I can become alive. You have to put me on a torture wheel. Not so obsessional, like the one I'm on, but a wheel where my hands are tied and bound and I am laid out. A wheel with metal swords, which will then cut me to pieces. The idea is that I have to be destroyed again before I can be healed. Somebody has to do it to me and with me. I cannot do it alone.

Normally, when I have been sitting on a client's lower back for several minutes before applying strong pressure to their upper back, they reach their threshold of pain and ask me to get off their back. (I weigh over 175 pounds). By contrast, Eldridge seemed to positively invite the pressure and pain, so much so that it seemed to whet his appetite for a greater intensity of pain which he intuitively sensed he needed to experience. Such an abnormal response is typical of a masochistic type of character-muscular armoring. But this statement merely begins to designate the unique formation of Eldridge's psycho-pathological complex. Eldridge's request for torture would have been absurd from an average masochistic client. By contrast, Eldridge was deadly in earnest when he asked me to almost kill him.

Eldridge's request told me how desperate was his

need to be penetrated psychologically and bioenergetically from within. He needed quite literally to be beaten, punished, wounded, lacerated, suffocated, and in essence, tortured physically in any way I was willing in order to feel something coming alive deep within his soul and organism. I was thrilled that Eldridge could make such an explicit request, because it told me that he was at last becoming intuitively aware of his inner psycho-biological condition of unreleased chronic deadness. An unconscious need to burst through and thereby free himself from this tension was finally surfacing in consciousness. But he could not marshal the necessary internal energy flow to liberate himself from within.

I was prompted to rhythmically pressure Eldridge's upper back largely because of his own recognition that his love and his anger towards both of his parents were severely split. I must have already crystallized his primary psychic impasse: he was still actively embedded within a love-hate relationship to both of his parents. Furthermore, he would not become free until he could face his father, the more aggressive and actively tyrannical, with his underlying feelings of anger and rage which he never was able to express directly to anyone throughout his life. Masochists who are not severely armored are hung up on finding ways to let go sexually. More severely armored masochists, like Eldridge, have a basic identity problem, one so desperate that they have little sense of self-worth, no matter how Promethean their daily achievements very often are.

Eldridge's experience of worthlessness follows from the bioenergetic reality of the extremely high level of pressure sustained internally by a tight holding in of his very alive endodermal layer (or core fluid energy currents). His armoring in the mesodermal layer, which forms the peripheral voluntary muscular sheath just below the surface of the skin, was extraordinarily effective at maintaining a massive collision of energy currents between the surface and the central regions of his metabolism. In every masochist, there is a chronic collision of energy currents between the front and back halves of the body. But with Eldridge, there was such an enormous compression of jammed counter - currents throughout his body in every direction, that the only really fluid alive part of his soul was confined to a small area deep inside the very center of his belly. Large quantities of physical pressure superimposed from without loosened the massive walls of jammed energy currents which had established themselves around the alive center nucleus of his belly. They loosened these walls to the extent that they began to decompress from within this immense compression of muscle and nerve located around the alive center of the belly.

Eldridge's wish to be tortured from without, when analyzed phenomenologically, amounts to a request to be pricked, poked, prodded and lacerated at the surface of the skin while not being allowed to move or struggle free. This combination of circumstances will unconsciously produce at the bioenergetic level a forced and explosive awakening of the alive fluid energy currents encapsulated deep within the center of his belly. But such an awakening cannot occur until the panic level of the organism has reached such a survival-motivated extremity that it will mobilize last-ditch reserve forces while attempting to flee overwhelming external stimuli. Fighting to escape a death-threatening situation mobilizes a secretion of adrenalin and other organismic emergency resources greater than those already operating below the threshold of consciousness in the form of a low-grade chronic emergency patterning.

Eldridge unconsciously longs to break out of the massive stalemating of his self-regulatory bioenergetic resources which he had to erect in order to hold in the feelings of humiliation and shame induced by both parents since childhood. He had reached the plateau in his treatment with us of realizing how deadened and locked in he is at his energetic-emotional core, and wants to risk his life to blast open this core.

The humanistic body psychotherapist must be able to understand both the psychodynamic and bioenergetic truth which underlies every request a client makes of him. Some deep unconscious truth underlies even the most bizarre request. I was quite unwilling to risk my life or Eldridge's, and besides, torturing him would only have reinforced his chronic predisposition to passivity and helplessness. What we really needed to find was a compromise structure in which the three of us together could accommodate our mutual energy flow to his chronic condition of depersonalized deadness. The following transactions between Eldridge, Katherine and me reveal how we did succeed in awakening Eldridge's alive visceral belly currents without forcing the fabrication of a death-defying situation.

Eldridge speaks of how he walks the streets, "with my jaws and face held tightly together, I think I am dead. It is dark around me and I feel like someone with rigor mortis." As I direct him to go into rigor mortis, Eldridge instantly contracts every muscle in his body and holds his breath. Beautifully, even brilliantly, he simulates a state of frozen deadness throughout his organism. He maintains this massive clonic contraction of his total musculature for about a minute and then releases his breath convulsively. His breathing is very heavy as he coughs slightly. When I ask what happened, Eldridge says that he had to cough, that his upper chest was itching. We continue in the following interchange:

Me: The body has to go into a rigor-mortis-like state in order to reclaim the psychological parts of you which have become identified with your mother in her coffin -- in order to reclaim those encapsulated parts of your psyche which have been buried alive with your mother.

E : And father ?

Me: Yes, and father.

E : Yes. Yes. Yes. (A minute of silence). How can I do it ? I can only pretend.

Me: I'm trying to suggest that there is a wisdom about going into the feeling as if you were dead, feeling it fully, that the body and the psyche both are asking for. How can we do this, using Katherine and me ?

Asked to make some vital decisions for himself, Eldridge is at a loss for words. His head and neck make spontaneous circular movements which are the body's way of offsetting the exaggerated muscle constriction while stimulating rigor mortis. Grunting, he ponders the matter. And then, speaking in a soft, curiously depersonalized voice :

Katherine is living. She should be dead if she would play my dead mother. If you could both be dead, and hold me down, and keep me imprisoned.

Me: Let's put the mattress in the center of the room. Lie down in the middle on your back. How can we lie on top of you as mother and father ?

E : I thought that I was between and you were on both sides.

Me: Who is in front and who in back ?

Lying on his side, Eldridge beckons me to lie on my side facing him: "I think you are the stronger and so I want you here... and I should be held tightly imprisoned. I want to feel you holding me down very strongly."

I grip Eldridge by holding one wrist of one arm underneath me while my other arm lounges across his chest and pins down his other arm at the wrist. After I have firmly positioned myself across half his body, Katherine lies down on the other side, placed longitudinally alongside of his body and over my extended arm. (see page 31) After several minutes, Eldridge says, "I cannot go into my feelings because of your warm bodies." I direct him to use his warmth to talk to his mother and father.

Pausing briefly, Eldridge addresses both parents, imploring them to free him from their haunting presence. After a few sentences, it is clear that he is talking to his father exclusively. He says that he has always wanted to love him openly and to be held by him as I am holding him. He says he never could understand or even feel what his father was thinking and feeling, that his father never spoke voluntarily about his inner self. Eldridge's voice shows excitement as he recalls how his father's nearly omnipresent anger always filled him with fear of unpredictable beatings. (He often was actually beaten.) Eldridge's excitement peaks: "I should kill you, but I love you and so I think I cannot."

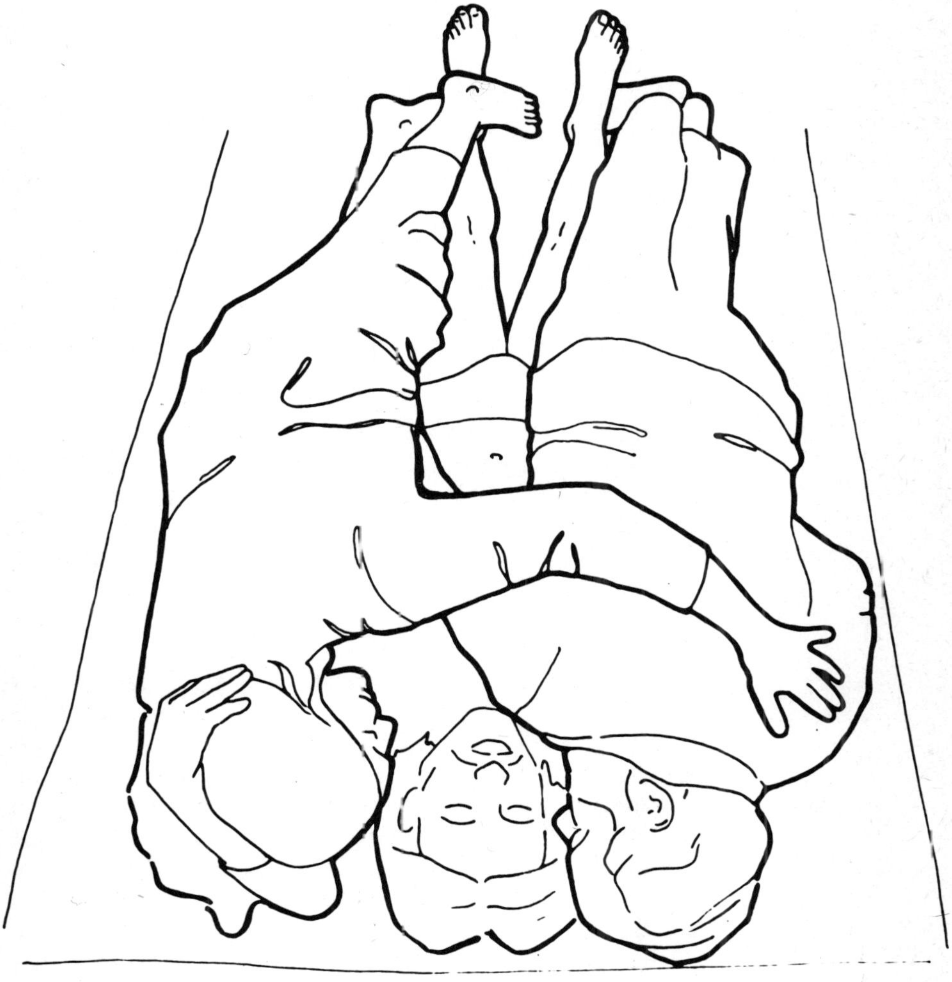

After a brief silence, Eldridge tells his father how preoccupied he was with his father's genitals, their size, and how his father always hid them so carefully. Eldridge sensed his father's antisexual attitude and remembers how he was never able to masturbate without imagining his father discovering and thrashing him. Innumerable times, his father would come in with a terrifying facial expression as the rest of the family waited at the dinner table for him to sit down. His father would look at each one of them with a face filled with hate, as if he wanted to kill each of his children who cowered in terror before him. At this point, Eldridge's voice assumes a more active vitality and raises slightly as he says :

> Oaw! Oaw! Oaw! Yes, you have killed me many, many times, father. Many times you have killed me. You have taken even your shoes and kicked us in the ass with them. Oaw! Oaw! You have never given me self-confidence. Never. You have always showed me how small and impotent I was. You know if my anger could come out I think I would have to kill you. Because you have destroyed me. All in me you have destroyed. (He weeps with anguish.) You have destroyed my soul. (His weeping turns into open vocal sounds of quiet crying -- his voice has a whimpering quality.)
>
> Even in my dreams today you are still so brutal. I see only your brutal hands, and your powerful force. You are for me like a rock, and made of stone, metal and iron. An iron father. Like a brutal machine you were sometimes. The most terrible thing is that sometimes you could show your feelings and you allowed my confidence in myself to come out and then my love came out and I turned and went towards you. Then you suddenly became angry and I didn't know what happened.
>
> Oaw! Oaw! I was growing up like a flower and then you came and smashed me. (He breaks into open weeping.) You have smashed me! You have smashed me! (His voice assumes a growing animation and fervor.) You have annihilated

me hundreds of times. You always told us that if we didn't like it, we could leave because it didn't matter to you if we left. You were so brutal that you didn't know you had children...

You are a devil -- a real devil. A demon black as hell for me. I wanted to love you. I needed love. I showed you that I loved you. I was off my guard and then you nearly killed me for nothing. I could never trust you. You never knew who I am.

From this point, Eldridge's voice loses its flat, monotone quality, taking on greater variability as it increasingly conveys more feeling. For twelve minutes, Eldridge reviews other horror-filled memories of his father and mother, but his attitude has shifted from entreaty to righteous rage. He focuses on his father's sexual adequacy, newly contemptuous as he recognizes with some objectivity that his father could not possibly have been an adequate lover to his mother, that his rage-filled hands could never have been capable of expressing tenderness.

I think that even if your hands were ever extended towards me with good feelings it was the same thing as if you were beating me. You were so full of a terrible force. Your hands have suffocated me at the same time as they have been loving and warm towards me because of their terrible force. They gave me only paralyzing feelings. In all your feelings you were paralyzing me. And so you killed me.

Oaw! Oaw! Oaw! You made me dead -- and mother too. You both made me dead. I have no real feelings. I am functioning like a machine. I am going around and around, doing, doing, doing, and not feeling. I only feel sometimes that I have a stomach, but it's empty. Only my brain is working, but it's like an entangled machine. It's making noise, but metal sound only.

I am a man, but I only let out metal sounds. I am not lubricating. Everything heats up in me as I go around and around. Enjoyment heats me up to a point where I cannot afford the risk of it because it's like the sun were burning on me. I am like a machine going from morning til night heating up, and in the night I am cooling down a little. Then I see you in my dreams again. Then I go on functioning because you told me I had to function. So I am functioning like a machine until I die. If somebody gives me love or enjoyment it's only like a drop of water on a head of hot metal. It evaporates. I have to be immersed in a flood of water before I can cool down. Yes, you killer, you killer, you killer. You killer with your lead hand. Oaw! Oaw!

(These sounds are responses to the painful sensations being generated by my thumb and forefinger pressing against the sternocleidomastoid muscles on both sides of the back of his neck. Katherine and I are both still lying on top of Eldridge, but my hand, now on the back of his neck, has been gradually exerting greater and greater pressure.)

Yes, you have killed me. But I could have given you love. There was love in me. (He cries openly again, but with greater pathos and agony.) I am dead now. There is nothing in me. Oaw! Oaw! (These cries are self-generated -- I have withdrawn my hand from his neck altogether.)

I have always to be your car and you run it, you bloody bastard. Yes, you are still killing me. Oaw! Oaw! Oaw! Oh yes, Malcolm, I always wanted to go into a rage but I could not. I should have killed him. (His voice rises and falls with each statement, giving emotional punch and vivacity to every word.) Now I feel me dead. Dead by my father. I have no feelings at all. (He cries loudly.) I perceive myself to be a metal man. Or almost metal. A machine. No soul. Oaw! Oaw! Oaw! (His words accelerate and become increasingly frenzied.) And I cannot kill him. Why? I should have. He is always haunting me in my dreams. I am so terribly fixed on all this -- on him -- so terribly fix-x-x-x-x-x-x-x-ed .... A-h-h-h-h-h-h-h.....
a-h-h-h-h-h-h-h-h. A-h-h-h-h-h-h-h-h-h........

The moment he began to say the word "fixed", Eldridge lost all his controls. After forty-five minutes of us lying on top of him, he finally let go of his reason, continuing to yell and scream Ah-h-h-h-h-h like a crazy angry animal for the next twelve to fifteen minutes without uttering a single discernible word. With Katherine and me still lying on top of him, holding his arms pinned to the mattrass, he began kicking spasmodically with his legs. Each time he kicked or yelled, we intensified our grip on his arms, trying to prevent him from lifting them off the mattress. He was a very strong man, however, and was able to lift the upper halves of our bodies off the mattress by a few inches whenever he screamed or kicked.

Katherine and I tried to restrict Eldridge's movements because he needed to actively struggle with our physical bodies and yet not be overwhelmed in order to release his pent-up primitive emotions. He needed to feel our resistance to his movements in order to continue to polarize his core energy currents deep inside his abdominal cavity. We could tell this from the manner in which he struggled -- never so desperate as to even approach a survival-driven life-and-death interaction. Whenever he stopped yelling and kicking, we completely released our tight grip. Our continued resistance, only when he was yelling and kicking, successfully awakened more and more of his dormant fluid energy reserves. With his feet on the mattress, the released energy enabled him to lift his entire pelvis upwards to successively bang it hard into the mattress, carrying Katherine and me with him. After this pelvic bouncing, Eldridge's animal cries became ferociously abandoned, sounding like "Wahs" instead of "Ahs." These "Wahs" had the expressive overtones of a two-year-old child, roaring like a chained beast in his crib. After fifteen minutes of this primitively aggressive catharsis, Katherine and I slip off of him, as I say excitedly, "Speak to him."

After a few more "Wahs", Eldridge, as if leading a charging army, says in a demonically inspired and impressive out-of-character manner:

> You are a devil! You're not a man. You are a beast. You have to be killed. You killed me. You killed me. You ha-a-a-a-a-a-a-ave.....

> ..... (His voice wavers up and down, much like a wail. It is eerie and more high-pitched than usual.) to be killed because I love you. And you didn't, didn't, didn't, didn't love me. (He pounds the mattress with both arms with each "didn't")...
>
> I hate you, hate you, hate you, hate you. (He is now up off his back crouched forward on his bended knees pounding the mattress in front of him, lifting up from the middle of the torso both arms and bended back. He interrupts his pounding and yelling to cough up mucous, but then resumes immediately both the mattress pounding and the words.)
>
> Kill you. Kill you. Kill you. Kill you. You have destroyed me. Now I am destroying you. (He collapses forward on his face and chest while still on his knees. Recuperating, he suddenly rises up onto his feet and off the mattress. He begins to pound the mattress with both hands, but from an erect position, pounding faster and more furiously.) Yes -- stay buried... All is dark. I see only you. Wah! Wah! (He jumps onto the mattress and starts jumping up and down with both feet together, yelling, "Wah!" each time he collides with the mattress, finally stopping and standing indecisively.)

I ask for feelings and Eldridge responds between gasps for air :

> It's a feeling that it has to go out -- all. He's dead, but I couldn't get rid of all because I am so filled up... It's coming out but there's so much of it... I saw darkness, my rage, and my dead father... I enjoyed my rage and sank into it, the same rage he put in me.

Eldridge's simulation of rigor mortis when perceived as a psychological stage of being-in-the-world gave me some clear idea of how his vital energy flow had been neutered to the point of deadness at his skin's surface. He was so exclusively identified with his chronically contracted voluntary musculature that his skin had lost the ability to respond to any sensory stimuli. Hence, the world around him seemed dark. He felt locked into the death grip of clenched muscles, unable to yield to aliveness either within or without. I realized that he needed to be warmed at the surface of his skin with a minimum of external threat and a maximum of internal emotional security. He also needed to lie immobile long enough to mobilize some internal energy flow, in positive response to the warming stimulation at the skin's surface.

Encouraging Eldridge to behave as if dead, while requiring him to directly address a symbolic rendering of his dead parents, provided yet another source of emotional-energetic stimulation. We might call this the stimulation of cognitive consciousness, which is merely one additional channel for self-generation of affect which enabled Eldridge to gradually alter his mode of orientation towards his dead parents. The longer he addressed them, the more he discarded a false set of attitudes which he had initially adopted to keep his repressed negative feelings from ever reaching the threshold of conscious awareness. His initial attitude was one of supplication as he begged them to leave him alone. But the longer he talked, and the more he remembered the objective and feeling past, the more actively aggressive he became.

The longer he addressed his father, the more his primary feelings broke through his false self-image of Christian-loving son. In a sense, he talked himself into a frenzied rage against his father's indifference to the inner psychological space of those around him. He progressively managed to project himself inside his father's inner self, thereby arriving at cause-and-effect relationships between his father's habitual attitude and behavior and his own present psychological condition. These cognitive connections were indispensable to his eventual divergent movement out of consciousness into an id-dominant, primitive feeling place.

This stimulation of cognitive consciousness, however, was secondary to the energetic stimulation provided by our direct touch. The fact that Katherine and I both lay on either side of Eldridge's chest and belly in a non-threatening manner gave him a sense of nurturing directly to regions of his torso which rarely received such support. This non-erotic contact slowly seeped into his very bloodstream and spread through his front half, radiating subtly in all directions, until it encountered the walls of armoring deep inside the center of his abdominal cavity and along the back half of his body. In other words, our nurturing direct touch facilitated the more subterranean process of slowly melting his heart, enabling him to reexperience on a feeling level how inhumanly impervious his father's response had been to his own love needs.

From the moment he began to cry with deep anguish, Eldridge was beginning to move out of his head into his body and soul. Simultaneously, he experienced the capacity to empathically feel his father's metallic heart. Eldridge could also reexperience his own enormous pain on those occasions when his father abruptly beat him for approaching him in a loving manner. He could feel how such experiences caused his own heart to close, sealing itself from further hurt and pain.

By allowing himself to contemplate the various parts of his father's body, Eldridge could feel the demonically destructive forces at work within his father. He had remembered how preoccupied he was with the size and adequacy of his father's genitals. But seeing the brute force of his father's hands was the fresh revelation which sent him into a complete emotional tailspin. He contemplated his father's hands several times until he could finally make distinct connections between the way those hands struck his body, the absence of any primal sympathy for his children and Eldridge's own present state of metallic soullessness.

Eldridge was able to face the significance of his father's insensitive, bullying hands because he had the protective affirmation of our two bodies lying against his whole torso. Our nurturing warmth facilitated a mobilization of energy currents within his body whose circulation throughout his metabolism undermined the muscular armoring from within. The disintegration of armoring coupled with the recognition of his father's soul-killing hands generated Eldridge's understanding of his own transformation into a machine so as to tolerate living with his father. Eldridge's subsequent focus on his own metal being, bloodless and devoid of feeling, catapulted him into regressive disintegration.

Eldridge displayed a release of energy almost superhuman in its quantity and intensity. We stayed on him for quite a long time after he went into his infantile state. We deliberately held his arms down, actively resisting his movements, until we sensed that he was becoming so aggressively charged that he would shortly break our bonds. We removed ourselves just in time for him to externalize the aggressive impulses bursting to release themselves in his hands and arms. This was the first time he had ever been able to express his aggression in our presence. We held his arms as long as we could in order to polarize his fluid energy flow into them. We did not attempt to restrict his leg movements because we knew them to be less chronically inhibited than his upper limbs. We knew that the free movement of his legs would loosen and awaken his core longitudinal energy currents at their primary source in the belly region, the seat of the visceral effector organ network. This network consists of an amalgamation of autonomic nerve centers, hormonal glands, blood vessels, and innumerable different organs involved with the generation of fluid metabolic energy designed to cleanse the body of all impurities.

Eldridge soared to new heights of primitive abandonment once we removed ourselves from his body's surface. He gradually rose to an upright position without losing any sense of animal ferocity and forcefulness. He looked possessed while jumping wildly on both feet, smashing his imagined father's body deeper and deeper into his grave. He did not know when to stop, so total was his self-absorption. Eldridge could go creatively beserk because his soul's needs blossomed in consciousness while our alive and compassionately touching bodies polarized his blood-flow.

The healing value of Eldridge's experience is conveyed in his final words: "I enjoyed my rage and sank into it, the same rage he put in me." His experience was much more than simply venting hitherto repressed feelings, or discharging a chronic excess quantity of pent-up metabolic energy. He was actually able to disembowel his very soul of some of the deadened feelings and memories fixating him since childhood. These feelings formed a complex constellation of frozen affects, the nucleus of which consisted of a chronic binding of an instinctive impulse to express himself with an anger and an aggressiveness which matched his father's and a mental inhibition of the instinctual impulse, in the form of the Christian moral principle that one must love one's mother and father at all times, regardless of the terrible abuses they may be imposing upon one's very soul.

V. Case of Ruth

There are many different ways of allowing the ego structure to creatively disintegrate. Eldridge's way of going beserk was somewhat hysterical largely because of his severe armoring. If one is not so bound, it is possible to go completely out of one's ego with a minimum of outer drama and hysterical intensity of affect. For example, Ruth who was far less armored in her body and soul than Eldridge, was able to move out of her ego consciousness into states of being which were singular for their absence of hysteria and manic discharge of primitive affect, and at the same time, authentic relivings of actual events from early childhood. Generally speaking, the more unarmored a person is, the more our methods facilitate a full feeling regression to the earliest years of infantile development.

A professional psychotherapist, Ruth had never been exposed to bodywork, and yet she sensed her need to experience such methods. She also wanted to incorporate bodywork into her own practice. I had planned to do the intensive for the most part without Katherine's presence, a decision I was to radically alter. This was back in 1974 when Katherine and I were still groping with the possibilities of forming a man/woman treatment team. We realized from our exciting experience with Ruth that working together we could facilitate creative encounters of the most growth-enhancing nature.

Severely blocked against expressing anger directly, Ruth felt giddy and nauseous when her energy flow became more mobilized than normal. These traits indicated the need to proceed cautiously for fear of frightening her unnecessarily. I also recognized many bioenergetic and characterological signs of a history of depression. After going on the Lowen stool for the first time, she began to experience acute dizziness and a generalized anxiety attack, characterized by a numbing paralysis of her peripheral metabolic flow, rapid heart palpitations, exceptionally cold hands and feet, and an interval void of consciousness. Such reactions seemed to confirm my diagnosis of a well-compensated oral-depression in view of the extreme flaccidity of her muscular mesodermal sheath.

But I became confused when I touched her belly area in a nurturing mode after she came off the Lowen stool. To my amazement and hers, a four inch column of hard, knotted muscle extended from her pubic bone to her navel. Ruth could feel it as vividly as my hands. Apparently, the catalytic work on her feet and on the Lowen stool had polarized her abdominal area to the point where this hitherto hidden mass of hardened muscle surfaced from deep inside.

Since armored muscle in this part of the body often denotes severe sexual repression, I asked Ruth at once to describe her sex life which she had never mentioned. She blushed, hesitated, and finally blurted out with extreme embarrassment that she was still a virgin. I was quite amazed to hear this from an attractive forty-year-old woman. Quickly offering explanations, she tried to dismiss the subject.

I was rather dogmatic and excessively goal-directed in telling her that her virginity probably represented her primary unresolved psychological and bioenergetic problem. I had been also rather one-dimensional at mobilizing her aggressive self-assertiveness and anger towards both of her parents during the first two sessions, even though her father had been an alcoholic throughout her childhood and her mother largely unavailable for tender caring contact. I sensed an encompassing emotional anesthesia and denial system of ego defenses which went hand in hand with her outer cooperation with everything I asked her to do. I was puzzled by her relative absence of armoring except for a tight neck and the columned formation which had just appeared. I knew that if I willfully bulldozed her into confronting anything psychological, she would outwardly comply, but that her core regions of energy or feeling flow would remain unaffected.

Ruth's imagination and verbal acuity could endlessly weave mental patterns of her own subjective experience without ever touching dynamic emotional material. I would not be able to perceive the state of her body and soul until something happened to her in the sphere of concrete subjective immediacy at a primary organismic level. At the opening of the third session, I asked her to relate what had happened since the previous session which deeply affected her in the immediate moment. Reluctantly, Ruth confessed that she had been preoccupied with being massaged by Katherine the day before:

> I just could not throw that off. I can't get into anything in my past. I can't have any feelings about the past. It's like everything is fine in my past. (She laughs easily.) I've never had an experience like that before. I've been obsessed with it.

Encouraged by me, Ruth assesses her experience:

> There are three things. First, that feeling I had when Katherine was touching me. I felt like a child at times. When she took my hand at one point after finishing my leg, I felt like I was going to cry. I had my eyes closed and she reached up and held my hand, and I felt like I wanted to cry. I felt just like a little girl. It somehow felt familiar to me. I wondered who had once ever held my hand like that. I asked myself when did mom take my hand like that, or when did dad take my hand like that and I couldn't remember that they ever did...
>
> The whole experience was a regressive one for me. At one point Katherine asked me to turn over on my belly. She said, 'Ruth, I want you now to turn over.' And she brushed my forehead lightly with her hand when she did that and it made me feel like a little first-grader. Somehow the way she did that was so wonderful. There's a part of me who wants to be held by her, but another part of me would be very scared. There's a part of me who would like to be her little girl. She'd be a beautiful mother.

For a forty-year-old woman who takes great pride in her independence to experience clearly such regressive feelings in a single massage told me how her psyche and consciousness were open to her soul's deepest needs at the pregenital level. Consequently, she could not be very armored, despite the rock-like formation which had emerged in her abdomen. Ruth and I continued to work upon the mobilization of her capacities for aggressive self-assertiveness with mediocre success for the remainder of the session. She mobilized some anger towards her alcoholic, largely inadequate father but without depth or vitality. Perhaps Ruth's most valuable self-revelation was that she had never felt enough unconditional affirmation and direct loving contact from her mother. This recognition accompanied the realization that she had wanted to kiss Katherine's face on several occasions during the massage, like a daughter seeking tender contact with her mother.

The session convinced me that Ruth did not need an adequate grizzly-bear of a father to polarize her anger and self-assertive instincts. Except in intimate man-woman relationships, she was plenty self-assertive in her daily life: she was a successful psychotherapist and leader of many social groups. Her will-power, responsibility and competency enabled her to handle any outer-world situation with pragmatic effectiveness. Yet at the same time, there was an overtone of forced jolliness whenever she spoke of her personal life.

When Ruth had described her preoccupation with the massage, I sensed an enormous emotional deprivation and largely repressed emotional insecurity beneath her jolly, self-assured facade. More importantly, I realized that no amount of ego-affirmation would be able to satisfy this particular lack in her being. Only a man or woman psychotherapist who could assume the role of a mother could satisfy this particular need. I asked Ruth to allow Katherine to participate in the next session despite her strong ambivalence about working with Katherine in the role of a female psychotherapist. I intuitively knew that Ruth's ambivalence masked an enormous, and largely repressed, longing for mothering which must first be satisfied before she could face the gaping problem of her denied sexuality.

Ruth stayed awake throughout the night following the third session. She had diligently done the energy-mobilization exercises assigned during the previous sessions. The effects were positive: major convulsions throughout her organism of such vividness that she had to restrain herself from screaming for fear of waking neighboring lodgers. Lying down to sleep, she found herself wide awake and strangely excited by the prospect of Katherine's presence the following day. She also was flooded by memories from the first seven years of her life, memories she had blocked from consciousness throughout her adult years. Her body was wracked with acute pain during these memories -- she cried out several times. Nearly all of the memories related to not getting enough tender contact from her mother. The only time her mother was tender was when Ruth was physically sick, so she often got sick as a child. But the greatest pain was attached to the memory of when her mother was sick for several months and she was not permitted even to enter her mother's room.

After Ruth describes these memories during our fourth session, I propose that initially Katherine alone should touch Ruth. Katherine suggests giving contact to the full front of Ruth's torso. They both lie on their sides, facing and embracing each other. Immediately, Ruth lets out a muffled cry: "Oh Mother, how I've always wanted this." Ruth cries silently, embracing Katherine in total silence for the next twenty-two minutes while I look on. Ruth then asks for a tennic racket to hit the mattress with in order to churn up some aggression against her real mother. Her performance is astonishingly alive -- she is able to express twice as much anger than previously, and to express it both primitively and with rational clarity of communication. She is like a being transformed.

But Ruth senses from inside that it is not releasing enough. She asks Katherine to do something quite new for us -- to imprison her arms and hands behind her back. Ruth goes down on her knees so that Katherine can maintain a dominant stance over and behind her. Ruth begins to address her mother in an incriminatory manner, reaching a new plateau of anger. She displays a moderately dynamic feeling of resentment against her mother, while using the struggle with Katherine to catalyze the anger. Discontinuing the exercise at her own initiative, Ruth collapses on the mattress sobbing deeply, an indication of much here-and-now tension reduction

Ruth's tears prompt me to tell her to hold Katherine once again along her torso. But she chooses to position Katherine so that her own front is placed against Katherine's back. Ruth continues to weep audibly and continuously this time. Allowing herself to enjoy the greater softness of Katherine's front would probably be too stimulating to her energy flow, as well as too painful emotionally. Ruth must have sensed that embracing Katherine's front would flood her body with excess sensations. Her choice correlates with body wisdom: a premature expansive movement of the core longitudinal energy currents from within outwards will flood the energy metabolism.

Even with her front half against Katherine's back, Ruth's body begins to recoil from direct touch: periodic contractions of her front half harden it against feeling Katherine's back in a nurturing mode. Katherine encourages her to accentuate the contractions by deliberately squeezing her muscles. After three or four contractions, Ruth experiences a progressive paralysis in her legs which moves upwards to the middle of her back. Her entire lower half grows cold and dissociated, as she feels nausea in her belly and a void in the mind. As the paralysis intensifies, Ruth panics, screaming wildly and then coughs. This forces her to disengage from the direct touch and to stand on her knees. When torrential coughing stops her breath, Ruth's entire body involuntarily jerks wildly in order to break through the paralysis and congestion in her chest and lungs. She collapses on the mattress after she can easily breathe again, now alone because Katherine has risen.

After lying out to recover from the muscular seizures, Ruth feels marvellous, as if she were drugged or drunk -- she has never felt like this before. Beginning to feel a tingling all over, she describes her general state of being: "I feel full, like I'm gaining weight. Does that make any sense?" Ruth is experiencing a massive organismic expansion of her surface skin tissues following their previous massive contraction. The expansion relates to the abnormally enhanced vasodilatation of her peripheral blood vessels with increased quantities of fluid blood flow. Both the massive contraction and subsequent massive expansion represent essentially unrepresentative bioenergetic conditions, and therefore, are transient states of altered consciousness, with no intrinsic value except insofar as they usually are a precondition for the lifting of the repressive agents of the psyche.

In Ruth's case, the lifting of her repressive ego defenses did not occur until many hours after the session ended. They were as much triggered by Katherine's observation, "You have a beautiful body and it's not going to let you push it around," as by the entire sequence of direct touch exercises with Katherine during the fourth session.

At the opening of the fifth session, Ruth looked inspired, almost triumphantly happy, as she described her newly discovered capacity to have waking phantasies. Even her dreams were especially rich in feeling and symbolism. Staying alone throughout the weekend, Ruth had suffered a lot of depressive feelings and physical exhaustion. But she also had a deeply moving encounter with her own body, experiencing both its beautiful fluid and ugly armored parts. After doing her energy-mobilization exercises for over an hour, she enjoyed a long bath and then massaged herself with baby oil. She talked out loud with each part of her body as she massaged it tenderly. The experience left her feeling so positive about her body, which in itself was a totally new experience, that she decided to take a phantasied journey throughout her entire body. Entering her mouth, she went immediately to her favorite place, her heart. She dashed upstairs to her head after it started feeling strange. Then she made the connection between her body's physiognomy and a beautiful home she had purchased in a dream the night before. A low ceiling in the second story correlated with her low forehead and heavy pressure in her head. But the second story was the most beautiful part of the house, containing the best designed and best furnished rooms.

Ruth describes her descent into the lower parts of her body :

> I made my way back into the abdomen area, which seems tight but pleasant and down into the pelvic-genital area. It was warm there and I could feel a gentle pulse beat. It was a pleasureable place to be so I rested there for a while. Then I journeyed over to my right leg and I discovered this huge door blocking

the front entrance. There were padlocks on the door made of wood. I couldn't get through at all -- completely blocked. Then I went over to my left leg and found the same situation: big doors, blocked, I could not get in.

I then remembered that my house had no foundation in the dream, none which I could explore at least. The implication is that my body does not have much of a foundation and thus I am a pushover. This also correlates with the fact that my feet are cold most of the time and the circulation is poor in that area. It also has been my legs that have been the most rebellious to this therapy in terms of prolonged pain after the session. It was in my legs during the last session that I became numb and a great sense of coldness swept upwards into the lower back and spine.....

I then went back up through my stomach. It was full of battle scars and I felt sad. At the entrance of both of my arms were small trap doors. With some difficulty I managed to get through the doors and to slide quickly down the arms and fall into the palm area. My hands seemed pleased to see me and I them. I took a quick peek into each finger and thumb and told them that I would be back for a bigger tour at a later time.

I noticed in the palm room a small heater and a small refrigerator. When I inquired as to their meaning, they responded that they took turns turning on, depending upon outer circumstances involving the battlefields of the abdomen, the diaphragm and the back muscles. I understood fully what they were talking about. I told the refrigerator that I would not regret the day that I put it in storage.

The trip up the arm was slow because the passageways were narrow and dark. When I got to the elbow there was a small wooden landing, where I rested for a few seconds. The trip up the rest of my arm was the same as the lower part and I had to squeeze through the trap door.

It was a journey and a dream I will probably

never forget. My work now seems so clearly cut out for me: making a foundation which I believe will relieve the battlefield blocks and vice-versa.

This richly alive imaginal consciousness was made possible by the considerable loosening of Ruth's ego defense network and its corresponding repressive controls. She had never before been able to find her body beautiful in the way that Katherine had suggested. Both the powerful verbal suggestion and the nurturing, other-affirmative direct touch had an unquestionably transforming effect upon both Ruth's soul and body, enabling her to enter the very depths of her own metabolism and make so many astonishingly accurate discoveries about her organismic patterns of energy flow.

Ruth's journey is rather extraordinary for its interpenetration of vivid imagery, objective understanding and courage to face the painful unknown before the full illumination of consciousness. Two outstanding features deserve comment. The first is the interconnections Ruth made between her dream and her waking phantasy the succeeding evening. To be able to link these two distinct levels of imagery -- those experienced during sleep and those occurring in the here-and-now waking consciousness -- presupposes an especially fluid flow of mental and organismic energy currents along the same pathways of movement. And this flow between the unconscious and conscious levels of psychic phenomena is not possible without a total transcending of repressed unconscious material, plus a certain tendency to transcend all internal barriers of the psyche in a broader movement towards a congruence of functioning at both psychological and organismic levels. We will explore the implications of these generalized statements later in the book. They relate to what I believe to be a deep convergence between different levels of psychic awareness when the individual is for the moment more or less armorfree and self-actualizing.

The other outstanding feature of Ruth's journey is its accurate rendering of the blocked internal energy flow patterns of the oral-depressive personality structure. This syndrome is distinguished bioenergetically by what Lowen calls a chronic 'disjointedness' between the limbs and torso. This 'disjointedness' is represented by the padlocked wooden doors barring access to Ruth's legs and the smaller trapdoors preventing easy access to her arms. Significantly, the lower legs are more severely cut off from any fluid energy flow between themselves and the torso that the two arms. This greater alienation from the legs and feet than from the arms and hands is consistent with another distinguishing characteristic of the oral-depressive position -- an insufficient groundedness of the core longitudinal energy currents in the feet and legs. Lacking such grounding, most oral-depressives find it very difficult to stand firmly and substantially on their own two feet and to take a stand in active interaction with the outer world. Hence, Ruth describes herself as a pushover.

Still more amazing is Ruth's revelation about the connection of her cold hands and feet to "the battlefields of the abdomen, the diaphragm and the back muscles". In the oral-depressive, this proclivity to cold feet and hands relates to a chronic lack of blood circulation from the heart into the peripheral arteries on account of the chronic endodermal-visceral energy blocks which constrict the fluid metabolic flow between the heart and the limbs.

In every oral-depressive, the regions of the belly and diaphragm are a battleground of warring forces. Usually, any sensation in these regions is anesthetized until the armoring begins to thaw when an increased amount of endodermal-visceral energy flows through the joints into the extremities. It takes many months of therapy --certainly many weeks-- before the depressive can sense the deep bioenergetic interconnections between the feet, the hands, the belly and the diaphragm which Ruth dirctly senses after a week of body psychotherapy. Her chest must have little blockage and her arm-shoulder joints cannot be severely blocked to register with such intuitive accuracy the essential outlines of her warped core longitudinal energy currents. The severe holding in her legs is another matter.

Much additional thawing is also required to understand how the conflicting forces in Ruth's belly and diaphragm have their historical roots in her emotionally deprived relationship with her mother -- an anesthetized or tightly armored belly region always connotes inadequate vital interaction with mother. In Ruth's case, as is typical of the oral-depressive, her belly is not constantly armored, but to the contrary, extremely vulnerable to feelings of fear and anxiety, forever vacillating between contracting and loosening. When the level of fear reduces to a certain point, her belly automatically relaxes and loosens, but then, she experiences inexplicable feelings of hunger, overwhelming emotional insecurity and internal emptiness. Quickly, she must engage in some objective world activity which produces enough fear and flow of emergency-oriented adrenalin to re-anesthetize her belly and diaphragm. A pattern of extreme lability between good and bad feelings is thereby set up which connects with the equal lability between warm and cold hands and feet.

Ruth could never have dived into the depths of her central metabolic patterns of energy flow without Katherine's massive holding of her front half to significantly thaw the holding in her chest, belly and diaphragm. This direct touch, combined with the catalytic energy-mobilization work with me and alone in exercises, managed to stimulate her organismic rate of energy circulation.

Both kinds of bodywork continue in the sixth session. Initially, Katherine focuses her touch on Ruth's abdominal area and legs, producing a return of a feeling of paralysis to Ruth's legs, from the soles of her feet to her pelvic-leg joints. This in turn precipitates a feeling of nausea in the belly. Interrupting, I force Ruth to stand on her feet. My intrusiveness is mostly deliberate, but in part an expression of my insensitivity to Ruth's womanly need for extremely soft handling and energy-polarization from the hands of another woman. Since I cannot provide this extreme softness directly with my own hands, I structure energy-mobilization work through do-it-yourself exercises.

I have Ruth assume the starting standing position, placing her feet parallel about two feet apart, closing her eyes and dropping her head comfortably forwards. Asking her to listen to her breathing without interference, I let her stand for a couple of minutes before I ask her to put her head straight back and remain as long as possible. Then, I direct her to bend forward from the waist, dangling her arms and head freely underneath her shoulders. After she adjusts to this position, I ask her to shake her head vigorously with each exhalation. (see page 52) Ruth experiences a second wave of severe nausea, but this time not accompanied by paralysis in the legs. She stands upright when the nausea becomes too threatening. Directed to assume the standing stress position again with her head back, Ruth begins immediately to display considerable tremoring in her lower half. For about a minute, the tremoring intensifies until Ruth, crying out, comes out of the position. Describing the tremors as the first she has known to be more friendly than frightening, Ruth explains that it was not the tremors, but their impact upon the hard ball of muscle in her lower abdomen which made her stop the exercise. Ruth's capacity to sense the tightness in her belly is a promising sign that her energy flow is becoming increasingly vitalized, both in quantity and quickness --a movement away from the chronic anesthesia throughout her lower half.

After the nausea abates, I insist that Ruth take the standing stress position again. The tremors appear still more rapidly and with greater flow throughout her torso, breaking through the middle back and diaphragm. Yelling vitally, Ruth collapses on the mattress and then describes the tight constriction in her chest. We have Ruth lie with her head falling over the end of the mattress but not touching the carpet. Katherine and I both touch her simultaneously for the first time in the session. I am a little behind and above her head with my hands pressing against her outer shoulders, while Katherine holds her feet in both hands. After a minute, I ask Ruth to move her head from side to side with each exhalation. She complies with strong sounds, before stopping in less than a minute because of the pain in her neck. I continue to palpate her chest region between her outer shoulders and center breast-bone, taking care not to press her breasts directly so as not to stimulate them sexually. Spontaneously, Ruth brings her two feet up, sounding wonderfully primitive as she pushes them against my chest. I am surprised, having never seen this response to my direct touch.

After disengaging ourselves, Ruth describes the experience :

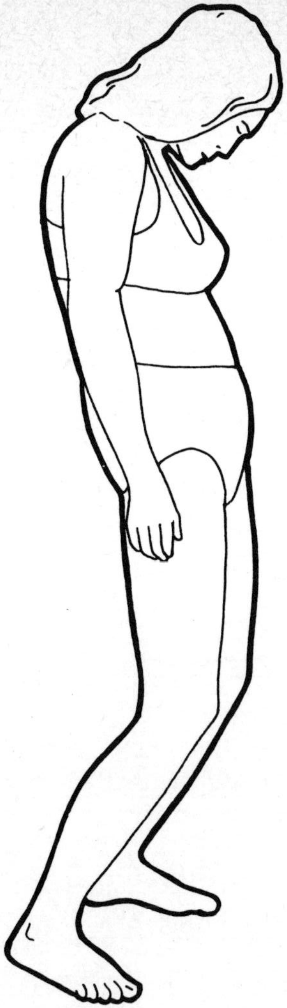

A. Starting Standing Position

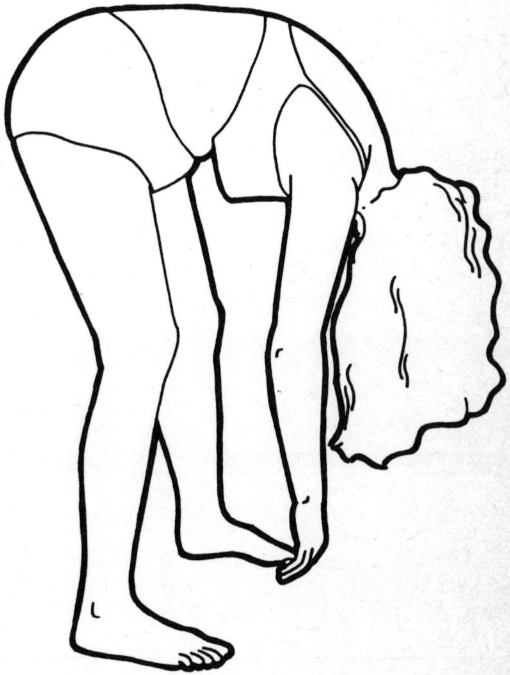

B. Forward Collapsed Position

I had a phantasy of going back and I have my feet in the bars of the crib and I'm on my shoulders and I'm pushing the top of the crib bar as hard as I can. I'm back to the earliest years and it's like they've got to give. Ahhhh. Ahhhh. Ahhhh.

Ruth begins to push again, beckoning me to push my chest downwards into her feet. (I am now standing behind her so that it is less awkward for her to place her feet and legs against my chest). She pushes her legs almost violently against my body, by far the most aggressive action thus far. Her pushing movement becomes increasingly faster in its forward and receding action against my body. Her sounds become increasingly transformed, unmistakably infantile, as high-pitched screeching alternates with lower angry wails. Ruth stops after a minute to breathe deeply. I suggest that she bounce her pelvis while I continue to hold her feet against my chest in order to help stabilize them. She intensifies the pelvic bouncing and then ceases. She says that she is suffering much nausea, but renews the bouncing at a slower, more aggressive rate, managing to thrust her pelvis vigorously downwards into the mattress five times with accompanying sound, before siezed by a massive coughing attack. I release her legs, letting her fall to one side while she coughs, chokes and struggles for breath.

After Ruth regains her breathing cycle, I ask her to call for someone.

Mother...Mother...Mother...Mother...Mother...
Mother...Mother...

The first two 'mothers' come from the voice of a little girl, the next three from the exaggeratedly forced and low-pitched voice of an adult woman. The remainder are spoken with increasing frustration and frantic resignation, diminishing in feeling quality until silence dominates the room.

Ruth begins to mumble inaudibly to herself in a soft, slurred voice. Lying in the foetal position, her body begins to rock very slowly and gently from side to side. Her remarks seem related to her mother in some way, yet essentially directed to herself, as if she is consoling herself that her mother did not come. After three to four minutes, Katherine quietly comes behind Ruth, pressing her front half closely against Ruth's back and placing both hands over the top of Ruth's head, intertwining her fingers to form a solid cup. Katherine accomodates her own movements to the rocking motion of Ruth's body, as the two women flow together as one body.

After about three minutes, Ruth begins to make strangely primitive sighs of exertion. As I look more closely from my chair, I realize that Katherine is now exerting an enormous pressure downwards from the top of Ruth's head with both of her hands, while simultaneously lifting her legs and knees upwards and against Ruth's legs from below -- Katherine is forcing Ruth to increase her efforts to free herself from the pressure being superimposed from both directions at once. Ruth's sighs grow louder as her movements assume greater dynamism. The concentration of her musculature increases as she tries to thrust her head upwards through Katherine's hands. Not for several more minutes do I recognize what is unfolding before me. The two women are engaged in a tremendous struggle the likes of which I had never witnessed. Katherine had only recently begun to work with me and I was not accustomed to seeing client's relive their birth. (see page 55).

After Ruth's head begins to emerge from between Katherine's two hands, separating Katherine's hands further and further apart as she progresses upwards, Katherine begins to make strangely captivating breath sounds unlike any I have ever heard. Slower than Ruth's sighs, Katherine's sounds are so deep and full in their intonation, they must be originating deep within her belly -- they resemble a regulated grunting. Then it dawned within my consciousness that Katherine was emulating the sounds of giving birth, facilitating Ruth's continuing struggle to push her head through Katherine's hands. Katherine's production of the labor sounds caused her to contract and release her own diaphragm, the movement of which must have been directly communicated to Ruth's body.

I felt wonderfully strange to behold these two women wrestling with each other in a primordial harmony of concentrated effort. They were emanating not conflict, but a mindless subterranean self-absorption and mutual investment. They looked like two

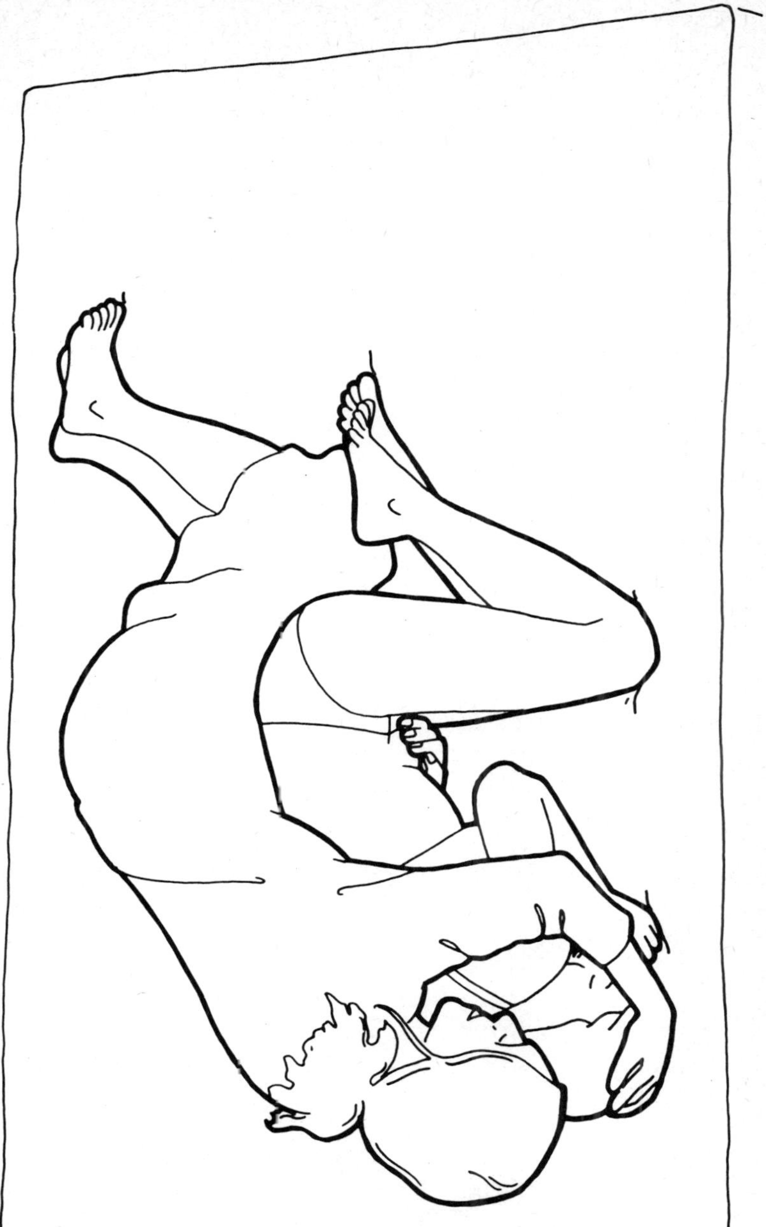

creatures of the oceanic depths, swelling and receding, surging and falling, in a slowness of rhythm that suggested tumescence and softening rather than contraction and tightening. This utterly womanly transmission of energy flow between two separate organisms filled me with wonder, making me appreciate anew how incomparably different the male and the female circuits of organismic contact are from each other. My body could never have breathed and moved, heaved and rolled, as Katherine's was now doing. I felt momentarily so limited, so superfluous and so finite as a male. At the same time, I felt humble in the presence of this beautiful and wholly alien process. Men could never resonate with eath other's bodies with the same subtlety and mutality of containment. The male energy pattern is too abrupt, too actively charged, too thrusting, too muscle-bound and nerve-sensitive to be able to reproduce the voluminous suffusion and diffusion of energy currents operating between two female organisms in synchronous flow. Nothing less than a marvellously resilient and fluidly warm blood flow circuit could permit the birthing process between Katherine and Ruth.

The effect upon Ruth is shattering. She cries like a child afterwards -- cries not of fear or pain, but of gratitude and self-fulfillment. Lying perfectly still for several minutes after separating from Katherine, Ruth speaks with her eyes closed: "My legs and feet feel like a million pins -- almost like they're paralyzed." She continues to lie still, breathing with tranquillity and completeness. To verify my perceptions, I ask her if she has just experienced her own birth. Smiling ecstatically as she confirms it, Ruth relapses into peaceful silence. Several minutes later, after rebuffing my suggestion that she stand up, she says primarily to Katherine :

> I could really feel myself pushing against you. That's why I was caught in the muscles and she was holding against me and I couldn't get through. I tried to get through. I just had to get through. Then when I made it through I was so sick to my stomach. Legs were stiff. Wanted to sleep. It was such a struggle pushing... My legs were pushing hard compared to my head... (There is a long pause between each statement now -- thirty seconds to a minute.)

I'm still feeling sick............. My head hurts.............. Top of head.

Ruth takes forever with every utterance, or so it seems from my detached masculine perspective. I cannot empathize with her total surrender to her feelings of sickness, her need to lie quietly immobile, wanting to languish in a state of choiceless, unmotivated awareness. I continue to prod her with questions, primarily to keep some kind of mental control over the situation and to bury my own previous feelings of superfluity. If I had been more in touch with the desirability and rarity of her now mindless state of undifferentiated being, I would have said nothing and continued to live with my feelings.

It is precisely such states of undifferentiated beingness that presuppose an enormous integration of hitherto divided parts of the psyche and organism. Reliving the struggle of her birth fully entitled Ruth to lapse into a state of relative harmony of being, akin to that of a newborn child. Her lassitude, amounting almost to a stupor, was itself an eloquent indication of her state of creative disintegration as rare for her as it was valuable for her body and soul. For the first time in her adult life, she felt fulfilled and satisfied -- absolutely satiated with tender affirmation from another human being. She was now simply enjoying each moment for what it brought without trying to organize and control what happened with her chronically active mental consciousness. She was steeped in what I have later come to appreciate as a floating state of undifferentiated beingness, which is another form of creative disintegration of the cerebral ego.

I am also unable to fathom the virtual disappearance of the hard columned muscle in the center of Ruth's belly, when I palpate her abdomen with my hands some twenty minutes later. Ruth herself is not surprised as she casually explains that her legs and feet must have been locked in against the rest of her body since birth. She recalls her mother telling her how she was forced to actively inhibit her labor pains. When the pains started, she had to wait for a taxi because her husband was inebriated. And when she arrived at the hospital, the nurses threatened her not to allow the baby to come until after she was taken to the proper delivery room at the other end of the hospital.

Ruth then describes how much relief she felt from being able to push full-strength with both feet against my chest and shoulders. The next moment, she raises her legs in the air, asking me to repeat the exercise with her. As soon as Ruth begins to push against me, we are both astonished that her feet have become so hot. Inviting both of us to feel her feet, Ruth chuckles whimsically as she declares with an air of self-assurance designed to provoke me gently, that the lump in her belly had little to do with sexual abstinence but relates to a deep freezing of her pelvic-leg joints during her prolonged birth struggle. She then reasons more soberly that she must have inhibited her legs from pushing her head against her mother's cervix until they reached the delivery room. Since then, she never had the occasion or the body-awareness to push her legs full-strength against another human body. I can remember standing there as she made these connections, with my mouth open in amazed admiration at the probable intuitive truth of her words.

Ruth learned how to inhibit the freedom of vital movement in her legs before she was born and to anesthetize her consciousness to the primary motoric needs of her legs and feet thereafter. Not until she spontaneously initiated pushing against me, and then later with Katherine, was she able to relearn how to push with her own energy resources upwards against Katherine's grip, to liberate her padlocked legs. My firm male strength actively resisting Ruth pushing against me was a necessary catalyst. But the decisive interaction was between Katherine and Ruth. The initial massage captivated Ruth precisely because it had overtones of what Ruth needed to do more than anything else in order to affirm her body and her fullness of soul: to regress to the earliest years to reclaim her body's integrity in the care of a mother who touched her tenderly and lovingly.

Throughout the remainder of the session, as well as the two final sessions, Katherine continued to give Ruth the kind of tender mothering and soft sustenance of direct touch that was like pouring life-giving oil into Ruth's disjointed limbs and insecure psyche. Later for instance, when Ruth felt extremely thirsty and hungry while longing inordinately for affection, it seemed natural for Katherine to breastfeed Ruth by placing the side of her hand at the base of the thumb in Ruth's mouth. (Ruth's real mother had never produced milk). Shortly after Katherine fed her to satiation, Ruth moved quickly through maturing feeling states until she reassumed her actual age.

Our intensive with Ruth taught me conclusively that the healing forces of direct nurturing touch cannot be replaced by more dynamic energy-mobilizing and muscle-polarizing techniques. No male-dominant circuit of resonance can ever replace a female-dominant circuit of resonance in administering a nurturing touch in the face of a client's yawning psychological need to regress into infancy in order to complete the unfinished processes of early tender maternal caring and sustenance. More indirectly, this intensive taught me that the depths and breadths of the human soul will sometimes be more effectively opened and transformed by the elemental powers of water and earth, of which the feminine circuit is the primary mediator, than by the elemental powers of fire and air, of which the masculine circuit is the primary mediator. The competent body psychotherapist is capable of providing both kinds of circuits of resonance once he or she becomes self-actualizingly grounded in the core self's hierosgamos principle of Yin-Yang complementarity.

Chapter II

AN ONTOLOGICAL THEORY OF CHARACTER-MUSCULAR ARMORING

I. The Four Dynamic Being Centers of the Embodied Soul

Character-muscular armoring develops as the ego defenses begin to extinguish our feeling capacities for interpersonal relatedness. Therefore, we must explore the organismic and psychodynamic foundations of interpersonal well-being which mediate most contactful relationships. The next step is to present an ontological theory of character-muscular armoring.

At the nucleus of our human condition, there are four regions of the body which mediate distinct modes of feeling-cognitive subject-world contact. The four regions are the chest, the belly, the upper back, and the lower back. The chest region includes the face and throat and extends to the diaphragm ; the belly region includes the entire abdominal cavity and genitalia ; the upper back region includes the cerebral cortex (or back half of the head), the two arms and hands ; and the lower back region includes the legs and feet.

Each of these regions mediates entirely unique circuits of subject-world contact. The chest region mediates a positive turning towards the outer world in a primary-process circuit of sympathetic engagement and immediate union. It mediates here-and-now direct contact between self and others. Its most significant feature is a quality of surrender to the momentary being with the other.

The belly region is equally sympathetic in its turning inwards towards the breadths and depths of the inner world of soul and body. Our abdominal viscera provide us with those proprioceptive messages by which we sense the truest state of being of our embodied soul from moment to moment. Such messages are originally conveyed from the bones and muscles and then filtered through the viscera internally. The belly region mediates our participation in and liking of ourselves in the most enlightened ways. It mediates a profound self-love and self-acceptance from moment to moment. Finally, it is the primary-process source of an inner serenity when we reach total centeredness of psyche and soul. (see page 63)

By contrast, the two back regions are both will centers. They are also more secondary-process. This results from their closer connection to the central nervous system and the cerebral cortex. The upper back is the more closely connected with the cerebral cortex for self-evident structural biological reasons. Therefore, it mediates meaning-making, cognition-oriented contact with outer and inner worlds. This region is responsible for higher cognitive differentiations of inner and outer worlds. It superimposes rational structures upon both worlds as part of the wider process of adjusting to the objective realms.

The lower back region mediates more earth-and-body polarized accomplishments of the will. It provides the seat of purposeful action designed to execute practical objectives. This center enables a person to persevere in the pursuit of long or short-range objectives in the face of outer obstacles and inner conflict. It is the primary locus of the enduring, task-oriented integrated ego. When fully alive and functioning, it enables us to complete whatever goals we have committed ourselves to. It mediates those subject-world transactions prompted by a growth-motivated conquest of new worlds as well as a more survival-motivated adaptation to outer world demands.

We are born with these four distinct modes of subject-world, self-other contact. However, initially they are instinctual potentialities which require a favorable environment before they can emerge as achieved capacities. At birth, they are merely inherited primary instinctual potentialities for relatedness which may or may not be actualized. As these instinctual modes awaken and evolve, they become differentiated modes of individuated Being-in-the-World and Being-for-Others and Being-for-Oneself. This process provides the thread of continuity behind the personality development process during the first half of life.

My portrayal of the four dynamic Being centers of the human organism was inspired by D. H. Lawrence. My indebtedness to Lawrence's intuitive thinking accentuates the fact that this model of healthy psychological functioning is anti-academic and re-

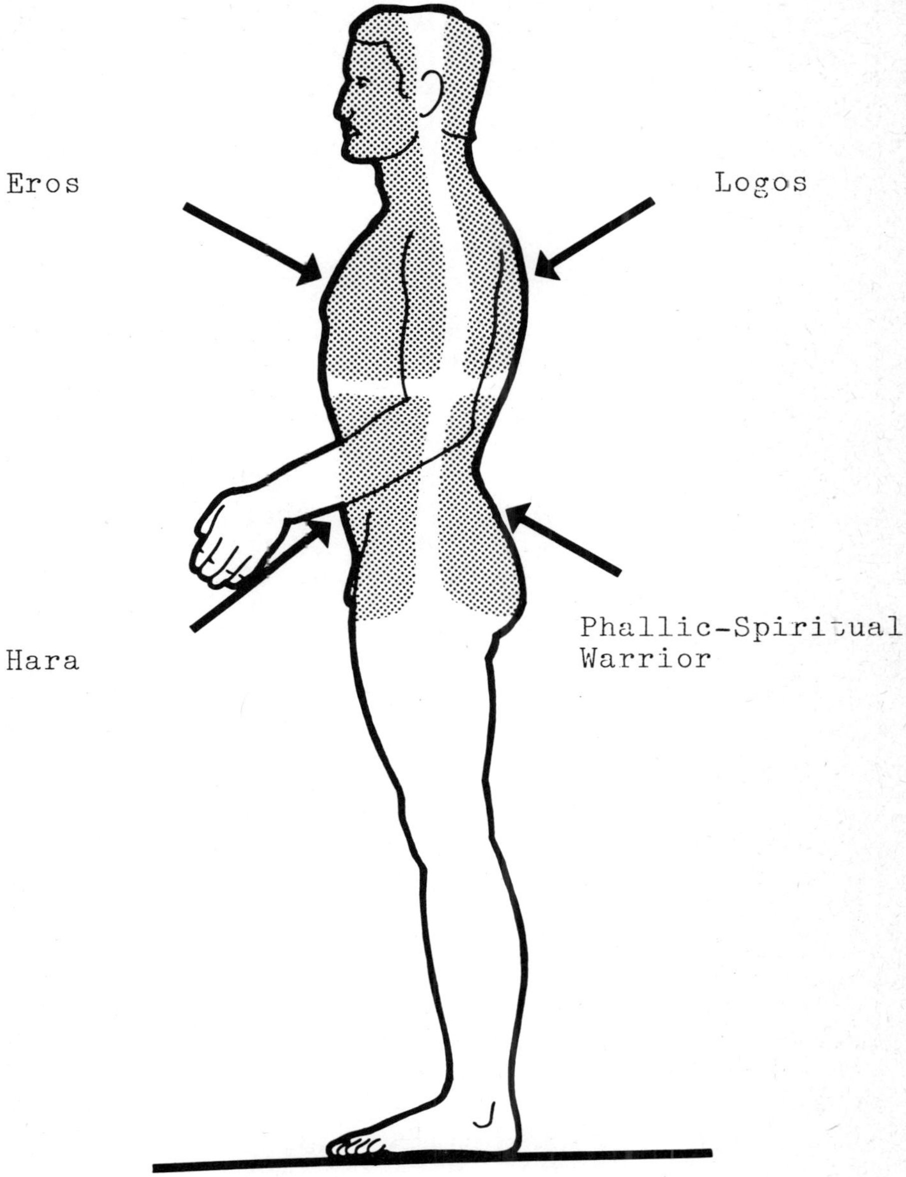

The Four Dynamic Being Centers of the Embodied Soul

volutionary. It is also supremely humanistic. For me, Lawrence's portrayal of the human condition is the most profound intuitive and humanistic rendering of man yet formulated in the West. Lawrence's model of healthy psychological functioning provides a critical antidote to the appalling rigidities inherent in both behaviorist and Freudian portrayals of human potential. Lawrence's sophisticated understanding of the complexity of human relationships sparks his novels. And Lawrence outlines the four primary Being centers which provide the foundation for this sophisticated complexity in his <u>Phantasia of the Unconscious.</u>

This model enables us to fully comprehend the phenomenon known as character-muscular armoring. Reich's tendency to reduce it to an embodied set of psychic defenses against full sexual orgasm is a gross simplification. It gives too much priority to raw sexual orgasm in and for itself. In all their adult complexity, human beings are not reducible to the satisfying or non-satisfying of their sex drive as an explanation for psychopathology.

The emergence of armoring, like healthy psychological functioning, can only be understood after an examination of how the organismic energy fields of the parents directly resonate with the undifferentiated energy fields of the child during the first eight years of life. The most critical period is the first one to two and a half years of life. During this time and also during the intrauterine months (especially the last five), the child's psychological well-being is totally dependent upon the mother's organismic energy fields as mediated by her four dynamic Being centers. There are four kinds of energy fields which radiate outwards from the mother's body from each of these centers. Each energy field has a distinctive rhythm of pulsation. The front half emanations are slower and surer than those emanating from the back half. The emanations from the upper Being centers are lighter and more changeable than those emanating from her two lower Being centers.

From the beginning of life, the child receives such different rhythms of pulsation on both a feeling and an energetic level. At the energetic level, the child is utterly at the mercy of the energy currents radiating from the mother. The result is a psychobiological process of imprinting, or veritable reduplication -- the mother's rhythms of pulsation are reproduced and imitated in the child's unformed organism. At the feeling level, a circuit of vibrations is established between the body of the mother and the body of the child. This circuit resembles the two poles of an electromagnetic field. The magnetic attraction of two separate organisms accounts for the resonating and feeling aspects of the preverbal transactions between mother and child from the beginning, and between father and child after the first year of life.

This organismic resonating process postulates an approach to the parent-child relationship which goes largely against the grain of contemporary orthodox psychiatric thinking. Orthodox thinking tends to be hopelessly entangled in a dualistic set of psychological categories which totally ignores the energetic aspects of the transfer of learning between mother and child which goes on at preverbal, unconscious levels.

By contrast, we postulate that the child lives in a unitary energetic field of continual synbiotic fusion with the mother throughout its first year of postuterine existence. During this year, the mother represents the totality of the child's existence, including its very self and body. The child is so absolutely dependent upon the mother's beingness-for-herself, and so devoid of any sense of separateness as a psyche or a body, that it is projectively identified with the mother's body and Being. The dual union between mother and child creates a circuit of participation mystique which enables the child to feel and be itself exclusively by living in and through the mother.

During this period of absolute dependency, the undifferentiated energy fields in the child's front half become differentiated. They are imprinted by the rhythms of pulsation and patterns of energy currents emanating from the two dynamic energy fields in the front half of the mother's organism. The healthy mother's belly region radiates the preverbal message: "I accept you unconditionally just as you are, regardless of what demands you make upon me." This message is indistinguishable from diffuse feelings within the child of an unconditional self-acceptance and an elemental, mindless sense of ongoing security, unity, and harmony of beingness. The healthy mother's chest and facial region conveys a similar message: "I love you unconditionally just as you are." Combined, these messages fill the child with a sense of being securely protected and actively contained within the mother's energetic-feeling field of Beingness, just as if it were still inside her womb. (see pages 67 and 68).

Erich Neumann's analysis of the mother-child relationship echoes our position and that of D. H. Lawrence :

> When child and mother still form an undifferentiated identity, the primal relationship stands at once for the child's relations to its own body, to its Self, to the thou, and to the world. The primal relationship is the ontogenetic basis for being-in-one's-own-body, being-with-one's-Self, being-together, and being-in-the-world." (*)

In order for a mother to guarantee the child's sense of being fully contained and protected, her own fluid energy flow must emanate from the very depths of her chest and belly regions, and not from her head-and-cortex or peripheral voluntary muscular regions. Her two front half Being centers cannot be fully functioning until an ongoing circulation of energy currents is established between the central and peripheral regions of her body. This circulation is regulated primarily by an unimpeded vegetative nervous system capable of mobilizing an inexhaustible,perpetual fountaining of expansive energy flow which moves from within outwards. This fountaining from the chest and belly regions of the healthy mother is precisely what generates the energetic-feeling field circuits of Beingness which alone can transmit to the child the sense of absolute security.

By contrast, an armored mother's being is partially or totally alienated from fluid energy currents emanating from her front half. In the usual situation, therefore, no form of stable rhythms of pulsation or self-and-other-affirmative energy currents are communicated instinctually from her body.

(*) Erich Neumann, <u>The Child</u> (Harper-Colophon), p. 26.

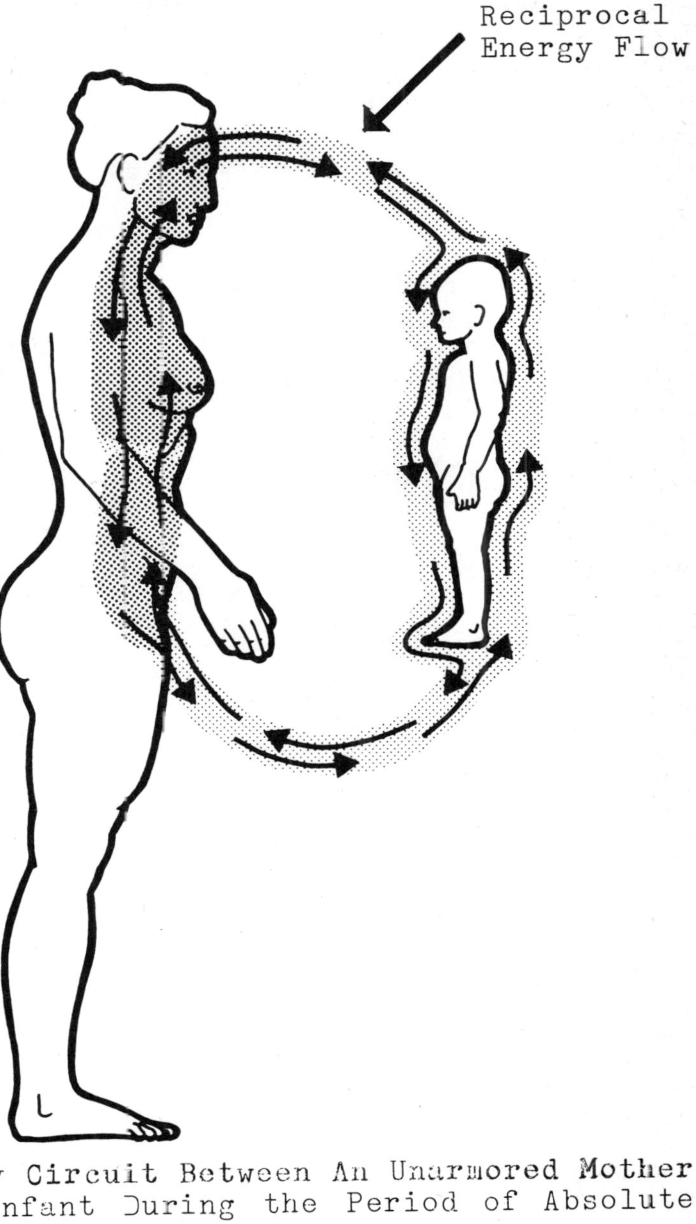

The Energy Circuit Between An Unarmored Mother and Her Infant During the Period of Absolute Dependency

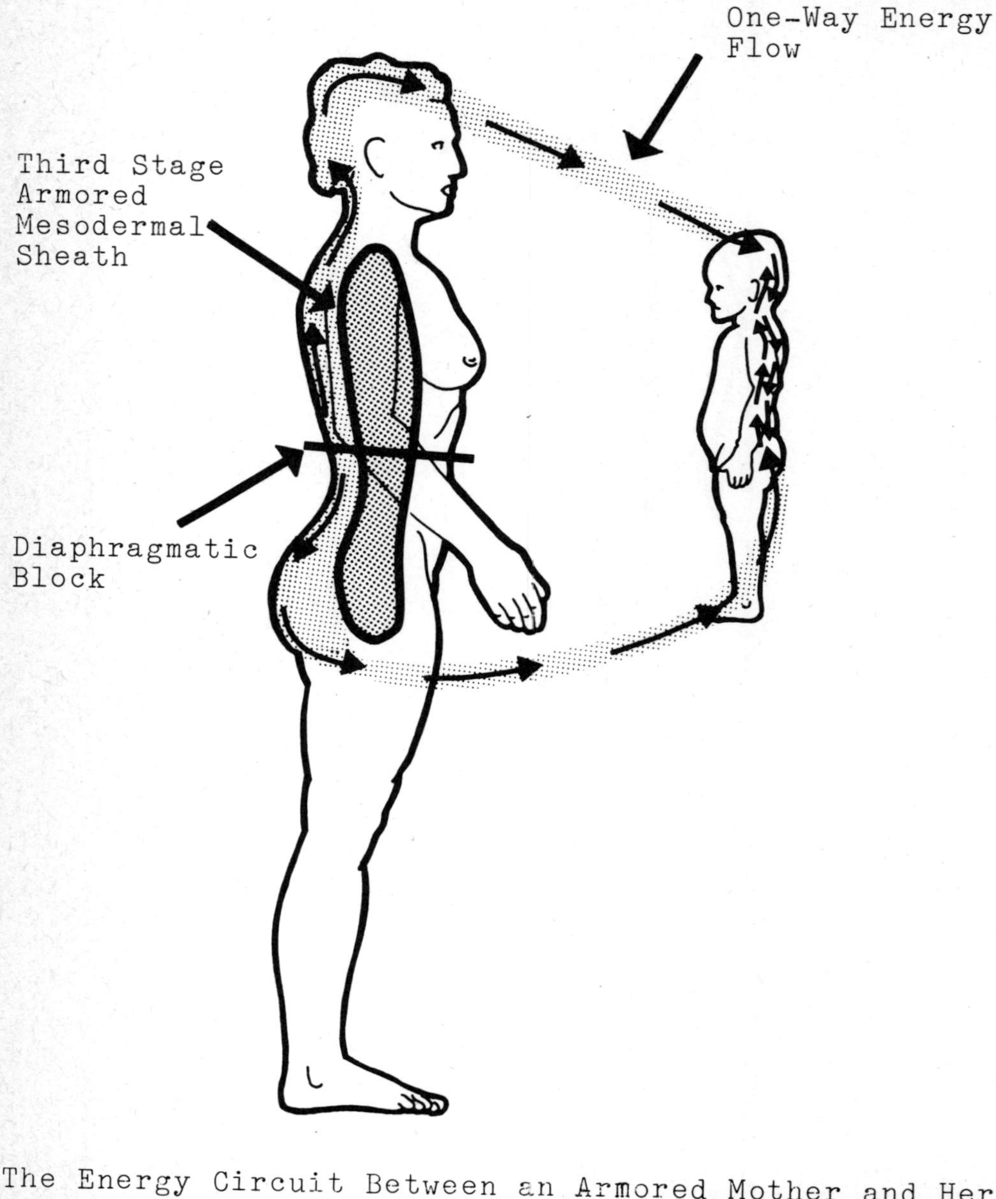

The Energy Circuit Between an Armored Mother and Her Infant During the Period of Absolute Dependency

To the contrary, either a vital preverbal energetic-feeling field emanating from her chest and belly regions is non-existent, or else it is weak, intermittent, erratic and unpredictable. And in the worst cases, it is altogether contradictory and mixed, and lacking in dynamic depth of feeling.

We are thus led to the fundamental bioenergetic postulate that the energy patterns of the human organism can best be perceived in terms of their movements between and through three embryological layers of vital tissue: the ectodermal, mesodermal, and endodermal layers. The ectodermal or outermost layer includes the skin, the cerebral cortex, and the senses. Its general function is sensory-cognitive orientation to the outer world. The mesodermal or middle layer comprises the voluntary muscles of the body. Its general function is locomotion and active motoric adjustment to the outer world. The endodermal or innermost layer comprises all the internal organs of the body that are responsible for the channeling of contact and communication between the various physiological systems.

The endodermal layer of the armor-free mother is dynamically alive. It regulates the functioning of her other two layers by an integrated vegetative longitudinal energy flow which moves up and down as well as centrifugally between the core and the periphery in her front half. The presence of armoring weakens if not completely strangles this pattern. Armoring replaces it with a cortex-dominated ectodermal and a cerebrospinal nerve-and-muscle-dominated mesodermal pattern of energy that moves across and against the centrifugal movement from the endodermal depths. This short-circuits the expansive endodermal currents so that they never reach the vital surface to find contact with the dependent child.

The armored mother is largely incapable of resonating to her child's undifferentiated energy fields and bodily needs directly from her endodermal depths. She is too narrowly defined by her false egoic self-image mediated by the head-and-cortex. Having little or no direct internal contact with her front half Being centers, she unknowingly relates to her helplessly dependent child primarily from her rational will and cerebrospinal voluntary nervous system. Instead of acting from spontaneous impulse and feeling resonance, she acts from her deliberately coping ego-observer and her unconscious need to dominate the child with her calculating will-to-struggle-and-to-survive. In other words, the last thing she is capable of meeting is the child's natural needs for a tender, containing symbiotic fusion with her two dynamic front half Being centers.

Such an armored mother cannot believe that the ideal relationship to her child is an instinct-regulated one. The concept of a transpersonal or archetypal rather than a personalized relationship is too threatening to the armored mother's egoic self-image. Archetypal means instinctual — the primal relationship between mother and child is more predetermined at birth by one's uniquely human instinctual-cultural heritage than it is willed. Only the armor-free, endodermally determined mother knows that her baby is not a primitive, instinct-driven, wild, cannibalistic and asocial animal. Her dynamic front half Being centers enable her to both instinctually and intuitively resonate to her child as emotionally and psychologically dependent upon her deepest life centers below the head. She can accurately sense her infant's psychological neediness for a primal but nevertheless human-centered relationship to her that makes her all-knowing and all-powerful, like an absolute divinity, a Great Positive Mother Archetypal Figure. She knows intuitively that it is wrong to superimpose her highly individuated needs and desires upon her absolutely dependent baby. Intuitively, she knows how to be there instinctually for her child from her embodied sympathetic Being centers in her chest and belly. Furthermore, she knows how to hold in total submission her back half will centers out of allegiance to her child's need for fusion with her front half.

Erich Neumann expresses this beautifully :

> The fusion of the child with the mother in the primal relationship and the cosmic character of the field in which the primal relationship operates have special consequences for the development of the child's personality as an individual. The primal relationship has as its field a system of relatedness with mother and child as its poles; but in the pre-ego phase of child development (the first year of

extrauterine existence) this field is also a reality independent of the poles. The primal relationship, as a specifically archetypal constellation, embraces both individuals in its transparent reality, each pole - mother and child - appearing to the other and acting upon it as an archetype. (*)

Given such archetypal fusion, it is no wonder that the child synchronizes with and imprints its energy currents upon those currents issuing from the front half of the mother's organism. This same archetypally given field of fusion between mother and infant provides a prototype for adult experiences of mystical union with the natural universe. Adult experiences of oceanic ecstasy involve some form of end-state sacred fusion with the natural universe both within and without. Their essential ingredients are a regressive return to the dual union, or participation mystique, first experienced in the loving mother-child relationship during the first year of life.

Subsequent chapters will elaborate the four stages of creatively divergent disintegration which can dissolve barriers within the personality structure, both psychodynamic and bioenergetic, which prevent us from having creatively regressive experiences of cosmic fusion. Such experiences are one of the earmarks of individuated functioning. They are one of the gifts of dearmoring. They contribute to the evolution of a core self of enduring wholeness. To be sure, adult mystical experiences of fusion cannot be reduced to the highly pragmatic, primitive, and selflessly primary-process experience of fusion which characterizes the good mother-child relationship during the first year of life. But they do have in common some of the more positive aspects of this fusion, interpenetrated with the psychodynamic polarities of the two Being centers of the back half.

Individuated adulthood presupposes a constant balancing between the two Being centers of the front half and the two Being centers of the back half. The gradual differentiation of the two Being centers of the back half constitutes the ego-building process

---

(*) Erich Neumann, Ibid, p. 22.

during the first half of life, and the higher individuation process during the second half. The gradual differentiation begins around the start of the second year of post-uterine existence, when the child begins to show signs of forming boundaries of separateness between itself and its mother. The masculine, father-polarized tendencies towards greater autonomy and the differentiation of firmly established subject-object, organism-environment relationships begin to assume increasing importance. By late adolescence, the Will centers of Beingness in the upper and lower back regions have undergone several stages of metamorphosis. They become sufficiently stable to allow the adolescent to totally surpass the earlier symbiotic fusion with the mother. The dominant needs at this point are the phallic need to be adequate in one's behavioral performances, the integrated egoic tendencies towards adaptation to the social group, and the conquest of the outer world.

Subsequently, these phallic tendencies to conquer are in turn transformed and refined into the more richly differentiated and internally centered intuitive faculties of Logos as mediated by the upper back and of the Spiritual Warrior as mediated by the lower back. This refinement usually begins from the age of thirty to thirty-five onwards. This process is more invested in inner world phenomena rather than adjustment to the outer world. It entails the emergence of needs for higher individuation that are propelled by the higher synthesis between the transcendental psyche and the embodied soul. The emergence of Logos and the Spiritual Warrior are paralleled in the self-actualizing adult by the gradual differentiation in both consciousness and unconsciousness of the intuitive faculties of Agape-Eros as mediated by the chest region and of Hara as mediated by the belly region.

II. The Interpersonal Wellsprings of Armoring

A. Introduction

The four dynamic Being Centers of the embodied soul postulated in the previous section are more unconscious than conscious and continue to remain so for the most part throughout our personal experience. However, somewhat paradoxically, they become easily accessible to consciousness simply by directing our attention inwards to our embodied feelings and the energy flow connected with the feelings, especially when we are free of chronic armoring. For the larger part of the time most of us do not allow ourselves to be aware of our embodied soul's dynamic polarities except in the most diffusely undifferentiated way, being content to leave the feeling currents and vibrations in the background of awareness as an ongoing part of our Ground of Being.

My own favorite prejudice is to believe that the four Being Centers constitute the four hidden cornerstones of what other theorists have called the collective or creative unconscious networks. I shall even be so presumptuous to declare in chapter eleven that they constitute the ontological essence of what Carl Jung has uncovered to be the Sacred Quarternity of wholeness as defined by medieval alchemy.

When character-muscular armoring is present, the four dynamic Being Centers become totally cut off from conscious awareness. Then they remain embedded in a dungeon-like prison of chronic repression, denial, and distortion. According to the portrayal in this book, character-muscular armoring amounts to a massive psychoorganismic defense against and alienation from the natural, original foundations of our embodied soul - to wit, the four dynamic Being Centers. In summary, the more armored an individual is, the more massively substantial the barrier there exists between his consciousness of self-identity and the rootedness of the latter in the four dynamic Being Centers. This is for me an accurate way to define the defended ego in a person: what the ego is defended against eventually distils back down to the feeling capacities for relatedness mediated by the unarmored four dynamic Being Centers.

It follows that armoring is not primarily an alienation from our sexual drive but from those complicated inner communications between the feeling capacities for relatedness that become aroused with intense sexual involvement with another. Both Freud and Reich's rendering of the human sexual drive as the ultimate primary psychological inner reality around which the entire personality structure hovers like a pale hulk of less important influences and powers is a most unfortunate one from the point of view to be presented here. Their rendering overidolizes the more mechanical aspects of sexual orgasm and at the same time disguises the intrinsic delicateness and weakness of our sexual instinct to maintain its own integrity with any kind of natural, original authority unless a complex set of preconditions is first fulfilled, including the awakening and full functioning of our embodied soul's multidimensional capacities for I-Thou feeling relatedness to one's beloved.

The theory of character-muscular armoring being presented here represents an alternative to Reich's for this very reason. Our raw primitive sexual instinct is almost a complete illusion when examined within the context of healthy adult functioning. It is almost never preserved into adulthood as an isolated instinctual impulse except in the most severely disordered cases of psychopathology. Our sexual libido is always subject to infinite modifications and even complete extinguishing and obliteration from the earliest years onwards. Even its glandular energy resources when viewed from a mechanistic bioenergetic perspective are capable of being diverted and recanalized into any different number of neuronal, muscular, chemical-glandular, and other metabolic pathways to form alternative circuits of psycho-organismic functioning. To give but one example, I am convinced that the mind-brain has the capacity to so thoroughly subjugate the libidinal energies as to recanalize them and funnel them up into its own vortex of synergistic activity in the region of the head under certain developmental conditions in the prepubertal child. It is this same funneling of libido up into the synergizing cerebral cortex by way of the spinal column that distinguishes one of the steps in the formation of armoring to be presented later in the chapter. In my experience it has been a rare adult among us today who has not had his primordial libidinal impulses utterly destroyed through deflection and sublimation into other channels and circuits of the psyche and organism, so much so that it is a highly significant and fortunate and even rare dearmoring-producing achievement whenever a man or a woman can discover his or her natural sexuality as an adult and affirm it with the sacred-profane dynamic Dionysian fullness it deserves. Our instinctual heritage is far, far weaker than either Freud or Reich supposed.

I believe that we must postulate the existence of at least three intrinsic sources of organismic energy upon which the individual psyche depends for its existence. All three sources are interdependent upon each other, to be sure, but also intrinsic in the sense that they cannot be reduced to the other two. They function more or less autonomously. First there is the capacity of the mind-brain to function much like a condenser and generate or synergize energy by virtue of its interaction with the five senses of outer world orientation, the voluntary motor system, and the coordinating role of the central nervous system. Secondly there is the capacity of the sexual genitals to also function like a condenser and generate or synergize energy by virtue of libidinal magnetic forces operating between two separate organisms before but more fully after puberty. Thirdly there is the capacity of the autonomic or involuntary nervous system, in alliance with the visceral effector organ network in the abdominal cavity, to function much like a harmonizer that integrates and maintains continuous currents of fluid vegetative energy flow that circulate throughout the total organism in devilishly elusive ways.

It is more the alienation from the latter energy source that character-muscular armoring is related to than from the sexual libido, I shall argue throughout this book. This is not to deny the fact that one of the consequences of this alienation is also an alienation from one's natural, original sexual drive. Armoring serves to keep both energy sources in check and impoverished and at such low levels of self-regulative dominance that it's almost as if neither exists autonomously. But it can do this partly by virtue of a secret alliance executed before puberty between the energy synergist of the upper half of the body, the cerebral cortex, and the more delicate synergist of the lower half, the sexual genitals. As a result of this secret alliance there is brought to fruition a complex and insidiously gradual tyranny on the part of the cerebralized will over and against the fluid vegetative energy flow. The antagonistic marshalling of energetic forces that then ensues unconsciously within the prepubertal organism makes possible the more or less total cutting off of the child's self-identity from the natural feeling capacities and needs for relatedness that he was born with, and particularly a total alienation from his front half sympathetic needs for love.

B. <u>Ruth</u>

Reich was right to postulate that the origins of armoring center on the matrix of interpersonal interactions. He brilliantly uncovered many of the sociological prejudices and cultural traditions of Western societies which are in part responsible for the creation of character-muscular armoring. He also gave fresh impetus to a phenomenological approach to the origins of psychopathology. Moving away from the Freudian emphasis on intrapsychic metapsychological superstructures and instincts, Reich focused on human interactions, particularly those between parents and children. He demonstrated to my satisfaction that armoring is transmitted unconsciously from generation to generation by the manner in which the parent immediately responds to the life-affirmative needs and impulses of the young child.

As stated already in the opening section of this chapter, I am convinced that armoring originates not so much from how parents attempt to gradually civilize a young child through words and actions as from how the parental organisms express themselves at a primitive level of energy field vibrations set up in the form of feeling exchange circuits with the unformed organism of the young child. For example, a mother inclined towards intermittent depression will exhibit extremely inconsistent spontaneous reactions to her child's overtures for contact. However, if such a mother loves her child deeply, she will manage to disguise her more neutral, indifferent reactions to her child which are engendered by her own depressed state. By so doing, she will be able to keep fairly alive and intact positive energy vibrations and circuits of direct spontaneous interaction between her front half and the front half of her child's organism, both in the chest and belly regions.

But such depressed and adequately loving mothers cannot always keep up pretences. Rather than jeopardize the feeling life and emotional well-being of their child, they often remove themselves physically from their child for frequent or long periods of time during the earliest stages of absolute and relative dependency. They easily contract some physical weakness which requires medical care, isolation, or even hospitalization, so as to free themselves from chronic worry. Once they have recovered their energy resources, they return to give unconditionally to their child, until exhaustion from worry and a chronic lack of energy force another collapse into depression, emotional exhaustion or physical sickness.

Ruth had such a mother. Ruth's mother was never overtly cruel, hostile or indifferent. Although somewhat ambivalent about bearing Ruth, she was an extremely responsible mother who tried to compensate as best she could. Struggling to find work whenever the alcoholic father was on a binge, her mother responsibly raised Ruth and her two brothers in the midst of economic deprivation. But not long after Ruth's birth, her mother developed a slight case of tuberculosis from all of the anxiety. She was forced to enter a sanitorium for several months, while Ruth lived with an aunt. After that, for the rest of her life, Ruth's mother was frequently bed-ridden for weeks at a time, given her chronic predisposition to anemia.

Ruth had to adjust to an insensitive, self-isolating alcoholic father and a mother who was there for her totally and adequately only less than half of the time. The feeling vibrations and energy exchanges stimulated by a warm, responsible, but sickly and depressed mother alternated with periods of almost total feeling deprivation.

From the start, such an intermittently available mother must have caused Ruth's natural dynamic feeling centers to partially withdraw their spontaneous expansiveness outwards towards the figure of the mother. Certainly there could be no strong sense of enduring emotional security and feeling of continuous containment. Ruth's young organism had no choice but to withdraw its instinctual inclination to reach out and actively seek her mother for warmth and love. Instead, it had to learn to wait patiently until her sickly mother could once again reach out to her with tender love. In order to preserve her own intact feeling vitality, Ruth's young organism needed to desensitize its ungratified need for love and affectionate containment by shrinking the very boundaries of its alive beingness away from the periphery of the body's surface. During the earliest years, this massive shrinking process is usually concentrated in the blood-vascular tubular network of the skin. It takes the form of a massive hyperconstriction of the arterioles, capillaries, and venules. (This process was reversed during Ruth's birth primal in Katherine's arms.)

Ruth's oral-depressive character-muscular armoring originated from a feeling exchange circuit established unconsciously between her mother and herself: an introjected identification with her mother's energy field as it unevenly distributed itself between an undercharged, hyperconstricted ectodermal layer and an intermittently expansive and contractive, anxiety-filled endodermal layer. Ruth must have tuned into the message conveyed by her mother organismically in a thousand different ways, beginning with the actual birth experience, that Ruth's coming was not a pure joy, but something of an unwanted and burdensome responsibility. Her natural dynamic feeling capacities for relatedness repeatedly received this message loud and clear, only to be repressed from consciousness when her mother was available for Ruth in a grimly determined but nevertheless authentically invested manner.

Ruth's own battleground of emotions in the regions of her belly, diaphragm, and outer extremities, which were constantly shifting between impulsive expansive leaps from the endodermal depths and a massive contraction and withdrawal of vital energy charge from the surface of her body, was the offspring of her mother's own underdeveloped energy flow emanating from her primordial dynamic feeling centers. Ruth's mother had a very similar pattern of underdeveloped energy flow circulating through her ectomorphic skin tissues and mesomorphic muscle tissues, and a highly labile alternating rhythm of expansion and contraction throughout her endodermal tissues. (see page 79)

Like osmosis, Ruth's young organism managed to open its sympathetic antennae in its front half to the energy patterns within her mother's organism to primitively sense the anxieties and tensions which crippled her mother's well-being.

Thereafter, Ruth had no choice but to learn to repress her own emotional needs as well as her aggressions against her mother. This repression required further anesthetization of Ruth's entire mesodermal

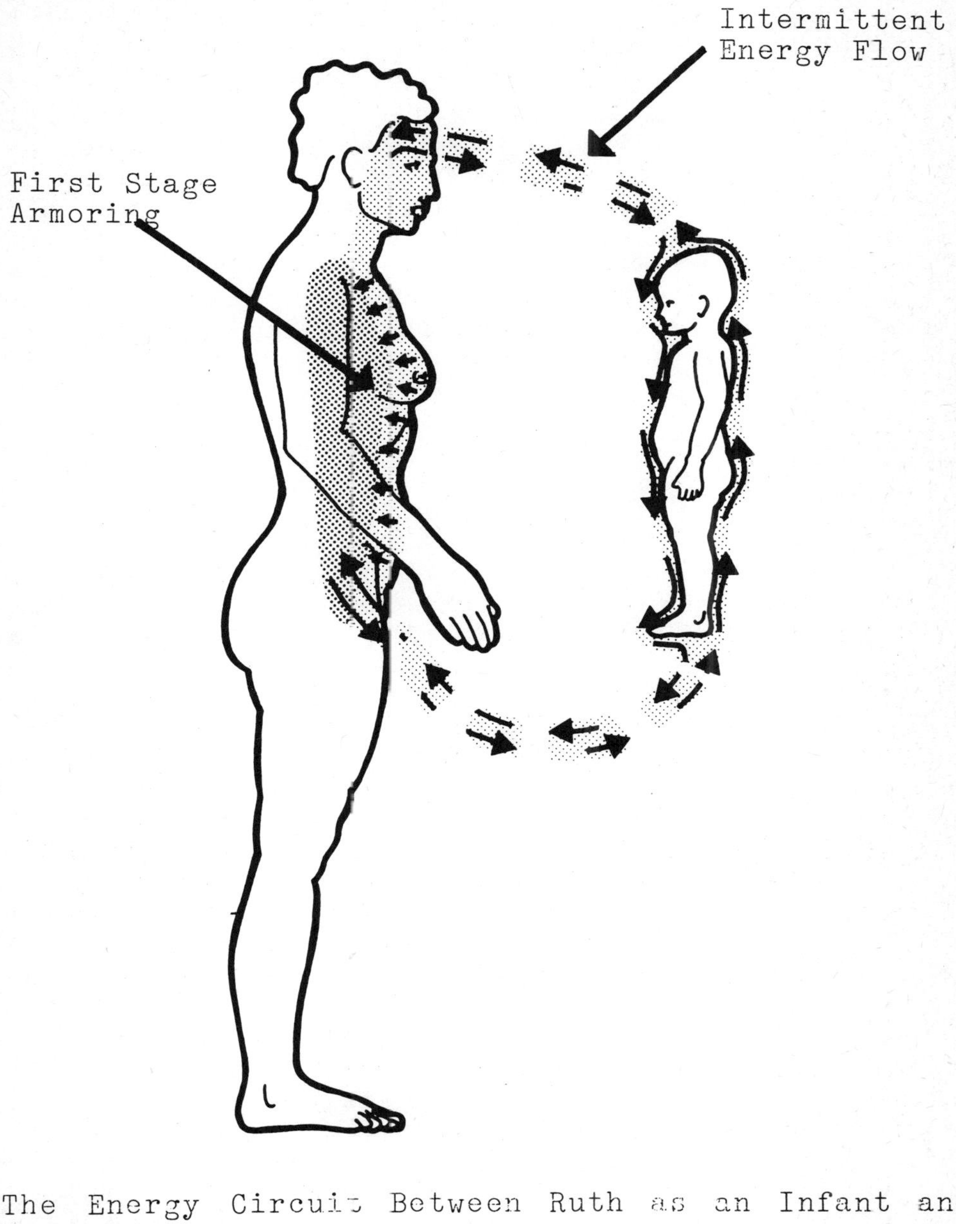

The Energy Circuit Between Ruth as an Infant and Her Mother

layer in her upper and lower back regions, and in her chest region. Psychodynamically, the end result was a total repression from consciousness of both her longing for more loving contact and her need to assert herself aggressively. Bioenergetically, the end result was a massive diminishment of vital impulses. The massive anesthetization of her metabolism in all areas and tissue layers kept her vital impulses from reaching the surface and finding fruition as actualized expressions of feelings. Rather than develop a rigid muscular armoring in her mesodermal tissue, Ruth was able to learn to constrict her involuntary muscles deep inside her viscera in the regions of her belly, diaphragm and throat. This constriction almost entirely curtailed the core longitudinal energy currents and their expansive movement towards the body's surface. In effect, her survival mechanism almost annihilated any of her natural dynamic need tendencies for relatedness.

C. Eldridge

When there is a lack of direct feeling interchange and positive resonance and affirmation of each other in the region of the back, both in the parent and the child, then the groundwork is conclusively laid for the later emergence of an armored mesodermal muscular sheath. In a healthy interchange between parent and child, the dominant parent, whether father or mother, sends a clear and simple message of approval or disapproval to the child which is communicated in a non-threatening manner. The message emanates as much from the Logos center of the upper back as from the Warrior center of the lower back. Its quality of detachment allows a child sufficient distance to feel free from any unjust superimposition of parental will. A child respects a message which rings with disinterested authority. He welcomes definite limits if they are defined and imposed with love.

But when a dominant parent is alienated from his own intuitive-feeling capacities and needs, and overfixated to his will-to-survive and will-to-dominate, he becomes incapable of expressing his own will to the child without the child feeling intruded upon. Then the message conveyed unconsciously to the child is always tinged with an unknown threat. The child feels bullied into acquiescence to the will of the parent out of fear of punishment and humiliation.

The dominant parent may never carry out such humiliating punishment, but the child still senses the overinvested will-to-control within the parent. Out of sheer fear, the child chooses either to submit totally or to inwardly rebel and deviously defy. The choice depends upon the emotional health and age of the particular child. The healthier and older the child is, the more likely he will adopt an attitude of passive aggressiveness or even open defiance, rather than passive submission.

Eldridge's father was almost totally alienated from his sympathetic feeling centers in his front half, and totally underdeveloped in his Logos and Warrior intuitive capacities in his back half. In most respects, he was unresponsive to sympathetic feelings both in himself and in others. He was at continual loggerheads with Eldridge's mother, whose chronic submissiveness to his will only served to exacerbate his anger and tyranny. This anger and tyranny particularly affected Eldridge because he was his mother's obvious favorite and personal confidant. His mother continually complained to young Eldridge about the difficulty and sorrow of life, urging him to avoid life's suffering by cloistering himself as a Catholic priest.

The first chapter reveals how insensitively and brutally Eldridge's father stepped upon his son's young budding will, literally crushing it. Not only was he indifferent to Eldridge's feelings, he was ruthlessly willful and vindictive in the way he exercised his authority over every member of the family. In all probability, he was more cruel to Eldridge because of strong ambivalent feelings towards his wife's favorite son. The situation was compounded by the fact that with Eldridge's birth, the two parents stopped sexually relating to each other for many years.

In spite of such brutality, Eldridge never did tune in to his father's need to bully and absolutely control everyone in the family. This myopia was made possible because Eldridge's mother, a zealous Christian, loved Eldridge in an enormously protective manner which was almost the antithesis of what he received from his father. She filled him with Christian ideals of love and submissiveness as the highest virtues in the face of a suffering life upon earth which would only cease in heaven after death. Her combination of Christian ethos and logos and a very real sympathetic containment of Eldridge's young budding soul enabled her to exert a very different and equally questionable but powerful influence over Eldridge's development of his dynamic feeling centers in his back. The most questionable positive feature of this influence was to seal off from consciousness any prolonged receptivity to his father's savagely vindictive will. She served to mitigate considerably any open-ended competitive struggle of wills between father and son by instilling Eldridge's consciousness with ideals of acceptance and forgiveness in the face of inevitable suffering.

Such a constellation of contrasting attitudes extended by two parents to the same child is prototypical of the masochistic character-muscular armoring. The upper and lower ends of the masochist's back are burdened by powerful clamp-like rings of armoring whose rigidity is so severe that it holds both self-surrendering and self-assertive need-tendencies in chronic deadlock. Their formation originates from a parental circuit of feeling exchanges which are heavily ambivalent and overloaded with contradictory, double-binding messages.

In Eldridge's case, his mother subtly superimposed her will upon and overloaded Eldridge's upper back volitional center with double-binding messages of Christian love which cloaked her own emotional neediness for Eldridge's feeling investment in her. And at the same time, his father superimposed his phallic will-to-dominate from his volitional center in his lower back with sufficient force to cause Eldridge to completely suppress his own lower back center from ever freely expressing itself contactfully in the relationship to his father. His mother bullied him with ideals and his father bullied him in a more primitively overwhelming manner. Neither type of bullying could Eldridge feel directly or face cognitively when he was a child because the heavy will-against-will circuit was established between Eldridge and both parents before he was three years old. (see page 83). Therefore, he never had a chance to find enough distance from either parent to feel his own primordial volitional feeling reactions to their overtures when he was still a child. He had no choice but to bury his own alive soulfulness deep inside the

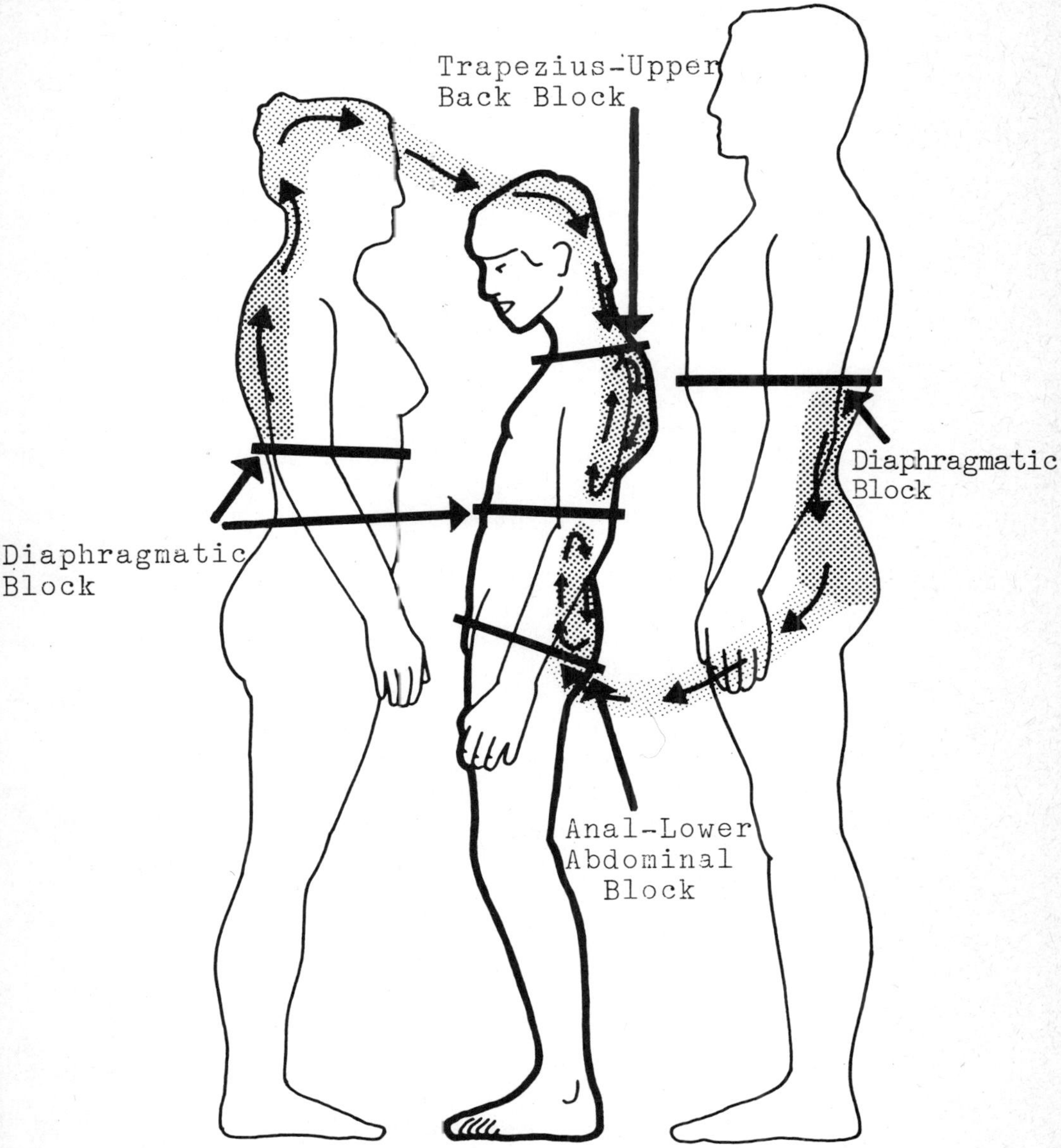

The Energy Circuit Between Eldridge and His Armored Parents at Puberty

bowels of his belly.

On the principle first clearly enunciated by Reich, that the exposed child has no other defense against the restrictive will of his parents except to introject the latter unconsciously, we see how Eldridge identified his own dynamic volitional centers unconsciously with both the will of his mother and the will of his father. This process of introjected identification of their wills overloaded Eldridge's back regions with great quantities of internalized pressure at the premature age of three to five years old. The pressure itself was the product of a rising deadening within Eldridge's back half as a consequence of his succumbing to the willed pressures of his parents from without.

Eldridge's introjection of his parents' wills paralyzed any continuing vital expression of his own will. This paralysis gradually produces a short-circuiting of fluid energy flow emanating from the visceral endodermal depths which gets abruptly throttled as it reaches the voluntary musculature near the surface of the back. This process lays the foundation for a progressive deadening of his boyish feelings of omnipotence and a progressive strengthening of his own mentally overloaded will to be a model example to his mother of Christian forbearance and self-effacement. The end result bioenergetically is the premature twisting and compressing of the cerebrospinal nerve tracts and longitudinal muscle groupings on both sides of the spinal column. The twisting is designed to seal off any vital feeling flow rising from the lower half, either from the belly or the lower back. Here is the beginning of the progressive sealing off of the entire lower half of the body which is peculiar to severely armored masochists.

D. Ronald

Ronald's mother also used her will to subtly bully her son into doing what she wanted, rather than permitting him to act freely from his own initiative. But she superimposed her will much more cleverly and subtly than Eldridge's mother. Rather than bombarding him with platitudinous moralistic ideals, Ronald's mother appealed to his evolving phallic sense of his own adequacy by presenting herself as much weaker, emotionally confused and indecisive, and more in need of sympathy and protection that she really was. She played the role of a helpless woman who adored her son and needed him intensely to make her life more agreeable. In fact, she was suffering unconsciously from an insatiable need for love and tender caring which her husband, Ronald's father, had never been able to gratify. She was unconsciously hoping to satisfy this need through her relationship with her beautiful, manly, aggressive young son.

Her perception of her son as "Golden Boy" was never a total manipulation in the sense that it was devoid of love. To the contrary, she loved her son very much, but as a woman loves a man spiritually from her heart, not as a mother loves her son wisely from her Logos and Hara faculties as much as from her heart. She loved her son from her heart so intensely that she related to him more as an older sister relates to an adored younger brother. She cultivated a quality of easy companionship with Ronald which unquestionably stimulated and polarized the phallic maleness in him as much as his tender heart. She knew that he found her very attractive physically, as she indeed was, and she permitted him to manifest as much admiration for her as she felt towards him.

Precisely because this was the case, and because she had never found sexual fulfillment with any man, she was always somewhat careful about what she revealed about her innermost feelings to Ronald. She never told him explicitly how deeply disappointed and heart-broken she felt about her whole relationship, both sexual and spiritual, with Ronald's father. And she was too underdeveloped in her own phallic feeling capacities or intuitive Spiritual Warrior capacities to believe she could change the emotional situation with her husband. She saw him as the dominant, strong male, and herself as the weak-willed, indecisive one, which she was essentially, but not in her relationship to Ronald. She had no idea how subtly she controlled Ronald. She thought she was cultivating in her beautiful son a sense of higher values and appreciation of the finer things in life, such as the pursuit of truth, beauty, and goodness, that Ronald's father in her opinion never had appreciated in herself or in himself.

On first appearance, this mother-son relationship does not appear especially imbalanced psychologically. Yet it is imbalanced because the mother has seduced the son through various devices of flattery and other adult-to-adult transactions into becoming her devoted lover, both emotionally and psychologically. A relationship of sophisticated intimacy is set up in which the mother becomes the conqueror and the child the unconscious victim of extreme frustration, both in terms of his sexuality and his inhibited aggressive instinct. By virtue of her strong needs both to sublimate her own unsatisfied sexual drive and her unsatisfied need for an intensely alive mental and emotionally tender connection with a man, she pours her adult consciousness as well as her heart into the relationship with Ronald. She unwittingly manages so excessively to overignite his dawning self-awareness of his own male sense of competency that he comes to feel like a hero in his own and his mother's eyes before he even reaches puberty.

Ronald's mother manipulates him into doing everything he can to please her, even to the point of sacrificing his own childish needs to be taken care of and genuinely mothered. The roles have been reversed very subtly, however, because she has made him into her hero and rescuer from her own unfulfilled longings. A kind of spiritual incest has been created. Ronald feels a slavish sense of devotion towards his mother and the personal responsibility to make her life as happy as possible by doing whatever she asks, and more.

Although Ronald does not develop conscious sexual longings for his mother, he does become over-sexed in other ways. He becomes increasingly aggressive with girls his own age, much to his mother's encouragement and delight, until he reaches middle adolescence and is now ready for real sexual involvement. (see page 87). Now his mother becomes mysteriously lukewarm and even cold towards his real girlfriends. If they are fortunate, mother and son may both discover how intensely exclusive and possessive a feeling bond has been generated between them. If not, the romance between mother and son will blindly continue. The son's real sexual frustration will grow and grow until in sheer desperation, he will find himself one day seeking out every woman he can find to copulate with as often as he can. He enters such relationships with minimal investment of his tender heart feelings and maximal investment of his badly frustrated phallic-narcissistic need to prove himself superior

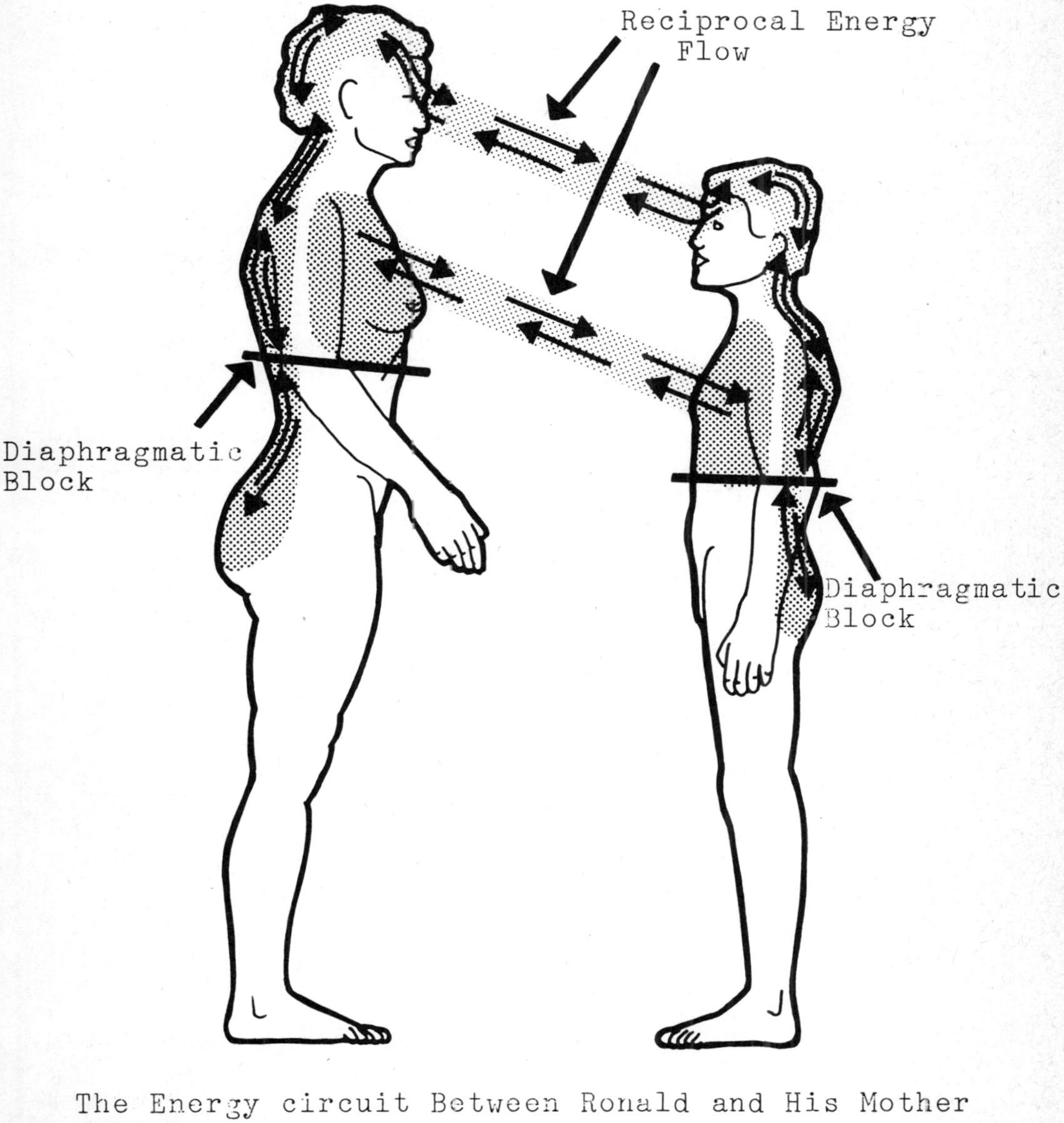

The Energy circuit Between Ronald and His Mother at Puberty

to and independent of any deep feeling need for any particular love relationship with a woman.

By introjectingly identifying with his mother's overcharged cortex and spiritual will, as well as her intensely burning but chronically frustrated heart, Ronald is deprived of a more natural and slower flowering of his dark, sensual sexual desire for a real woman. This normal psychobiological process begins with actual puberty. But in Ronald's case, his sexuality has been prematurely awakened, totally sublimated in his relationship with his mother, and ultimately frustrated. The identification process entails an osmosis of his mother's overcharged cortex and repressed but overcharged genitals, whose tyrannical possession over his mother, and then later over Ronald, prevent them both from opening themselves to their self-surrendering need-tendencies of their front half when Eros is the guiding force. Then, and only then, in my opinion, can sublimated tenderness and primitively phallic sexuality be effortlessly harmonized and interpenetrated with each other. By contrast, both Ronald and his mother are under the spell of an overcharged back whose basic function is to serve as an overheated, charge-discharge-obsessed pipeline between the cortex and the genitals. Both are caught in a vortex of back half activity which comprises volitional forces and unreleased excesses of metabolic energy. The result is a huge restlessness, a longing for discharge, but very little peace and equalization even when discharge is achieved. Ronald finally acquires his mother's basically hysterical-narcissistic pattern of chronic character-muscular armoring. Both now feel extremely lonely, sexually unsatisfied, overcerebrally controlled, latently hostile towards and suspicious of deep love, and sickly locked in a chronic impasse between dependency and independency in all their close relationships.

III. The Three Formative Stages of Armoring

The biological transformation of the metabolism which is at the nucleus of character-muscular armoring follows the interpersonal short-circuiting of contact depicted in the previous section. The physiological rigidification process always follows in the wake of the psychological short-circuiting of interpersonal feeling contact. This is because physiological formations usually change more slowly than psychological formative processes. It follows that the dearmoring process, the topic of the next chapter, proceeds no faster than the gradual unwinding and annihilation at the physiological level of the same formative processes, but in the reverse direction. All psychopathology is as rooted in physiological phenomena as it is in psychodynamic phenomena. Both levels of phenomena must be squarely dealt with before there can be any authentic and irreversible change and growth in the personality structure, whether at conscious or unconscious levels.

A. <u>The First Stage</u>

The first stage in the formation of armor consists of an undifferentiated but nevertheless real diminution of the primitive core vegetative energy currents. When healthy, these currents are forever in constant flow, moving in an uncontrolled, willy-nilly fashion in all directions, much like the pseudopodia of an amoeba. Their basic direction of movement is from the center to the periphery of the body in response to outer stimuli, and back again to form circular channels of flow. And so, when a partial arrestment of flow begins, it is the peripheral regions of the metabolism which are most affected negatively by increasingly reduced amounts of vital energy flow. The blood flow is primarily affected at first, but this is accompanied by a subtle upgrading of the importance of the parasympathetic division of the autonomic nervous system as an agent of containment against excessive secretions of adrenalin. The young child's organism tends to become increasingly retarded in its metabolic flow because of the parasympathetic action, an action which is triggered by the shrinkage of the metabolism at the periphery, or which perhaps is integral to it.

This first stage of armoring runs parallel to the maintenance of an open-ended, reciprocal circuit of immediate feeling and energetic interaction between the child's front half and the field-like vibrations emanating from the front half feeling centers of the mother's organism. Like the positive and negative poles of an electromagnetic field, the two front halves of the two organisms resonate sympathetically or antipathetically in relation to each other. We saw this magnetic circuit of feeling and energetic interaction at work between Ruth and her mother.

Ruth remained open-ended and hence totally field-dependent upon her mother's transmission of positive feeling vibrations. In the end it was not so much the intrinsic quality of these vibrations themselves, but their rarity and continual intermittency, that caused Ruth's tiny organism to initiate a self-protective shrinkage of its autonomic and blood-vascular antennae at the surface.

During the stages of total dependency and partial dependency upon the mother figure, the child's organism is hooked up to a primordial circuit of immediate field exchange with his mother's organism which must be kept open as long as possible. There is a powerful instinctual urgency operating behind this need to maintain as active an open-ended magnetic circuit of contact with the mother's front half as is practically possible. This instinct is nature's way of prescriptively dictating the most rudimentary wellsprings of love and dependency upon other human beings.

When the mother is emotionally crippled in her front half, the child usually learns in time how to positively resonate to his mother's spoken or unspoken fears and anxieties. The healthy child will then try to meet the underlying unconscious needs of the mother by doing whatever he can to please the mother and thereby mitigate her pain. But this very urge to please generates within the depths of the child's metabolism a gradual constriction of the vital wellsprings of spontaneous growth, the child's core vegetative energy currents. This is because the child begins to give up his own natural feeling needs and their spontaneous gratification -- especially the needs of the lower back half, or the needs for omnipotence and blindly narcissistic self-assertiveness -- and to overidentify with the unsatisfied unconscious needs of the mother. It was precisely at this juncture that Ruth became emotionally fixated, and hence sacrificed parts of herself in order to adjust to her mother's inadequacies. She learned how to become extremely responsive to and overconsiderate of other people's feelings at a premature age, at the price of starving her own soul's needs.

B. The Second Stage

The second stage in the formation of armor consists of the emergence of a differentiated circuit of excessively charged voluntary muscles and cerebrospinal nerve fibres which become permanently imbedded in the region of the upper back, the neck, and the head. The permanent imbedding is accompanied by a progressive intermeshing, twisting, and binding of the voluntary muscles and nerve fibres to form a relatively closed circuit of energy flow whose synergist is the cerebral cortex.

This closed circuit becomes a reservoir for whatever emotional conflicts and nervous tensions that become more than the psyche or the fluid vegetative energy currents can handle in the moment. The more emotional conflicts and nervous tensions which become accumulated and retained in this cortical-cerebrospinal circuit, the greater the twisting of the voluntary nerves and muscles, and the greater their overloading with chronic tension. The twisting and binding process is a product of the overloading since it is designed to better retain and hold in stasis larger and larger quantities of undischarged accumulated tension.

Let us examine in some detail the intricate step-by-step formation of this cortical-cerebrospinal circuit. The second stage is critical to the whole armoring process because it reveals what lies at the foundation of character-muscular armoring: the misappropriation of the two energy synergists under the dominance of the cerebral cortex to form a special and additional circuit of energy flow which functions in chronic conflict with the core longitudinal visceral currents. Armoring represents, in the last analysis, not an inhibition of the sexual libido, but a misappropriation of vital energy flow under the tyrannical control of the cerebral cortex, in alliance with the survival-motivated will, to form a wall of alienation in the mesodermal layer against experiencing the instinctual-feeling-intuitive capacities mediated by the front half of the body. The armorer is the cerebral cortex, and its antagonist is not the sexual drive, but the feeling capacities in the front half, the intuitive faculties of Agape-Eros and Hara.

The second stage is determined by and runs parallel to a definite interpersonal condition at the psychological level: some kind of bullying of the child by the back half volitional centers of the parents. Parental bullying represents an act of violence against the natural flowering of the child's dynamic primordial feeling capacities. The violence can be intuitively assessed by the extent to which the parental bullying forces the premature awakening of a survival-motivated will within the child. This awakening occurs automatically during the course of the child's growing distancing of himself from the organismic feeling and energy fields of his parents, especially from those vibrations emanating from the volitional back centers of one or both parents which threaten the child's spontaneous integrity. If the parental bullying is truly gentle, the child will not be forced to prematurely develop a survival-motivated will. But if the bullying stems from parents who are essentially armored and to some extent rigidly alienated from their core feeling capacities in their front half, the child will be forced to acquire an overdeveloped capacity to perceive himself and others as totally separate and non-contacting beings who struggle with each other for supremacy.

We saw in the previous section how different kinds of bullying produce different kinds of character-muscular armoring. The double-barrelled onslaught upon Eldridge's budding volitional centers, one from the chariot of Logos, the other from the war horse of Phallos, was so heavy that it weighed Eldridge's back down with two stationary marble pillars. The bullying was so severe, began at so early an age, and had such simultaneously opposite qualities, that his cerebral cortex took many years to catch up with the premature awakening of his will-to-survive. He was so inundated with the bullying will of both his parents that he never found the ego strength to withstand their intrusions with any differentiated perceptual awareness of what was really happening to him.

With Ronald, on the other hand, the bullying circuit was much subtler and lighter, giving Ronald's front half time to breathe. For the most part, it was directed to the volitional center of his upper back and to the sympathetic center of his upper front half. Ronald's mother bullied his heart with her intense love, and bombarded his cortex with spiritual ideals. She superimposed her will exclusively upon his upper half, both front and back. This gave Ronald ample opportunity to prematurely awaken his consciousness of himself to his back half capacities and dawning strengths, but the premature consciousness awakened both energy synergists prior to puberty.

The premature awakening of the cortico-cerebrospinal circuit of excessively charged voluntary muscles and cerebrospinal nerve fibres also tends to prematurely awaken the energy synergist in the lower back half, the sexual libido. This occurs particularly when the parent figure of the opposite sex, whether it be the father or the mother, has poured a good deal of Eros as well as Agape into the relationship with his young child. Ronald's mother was such a parent, whereas Eldridge's mother was almost her polar opposite. Ronald's mother generated a tremendous amount of cerebral contact with her son which functioned in part as a substitute for genital-erotic contact for her. She had no conscious awareness that she was pouring Eros into her relationship with her son because of her own alienation from the two feeling-intuitive centers of her own front half. She had no conscious idea that her subtle, intense, possessively seductive circuit of feeling vibrations should have been directed toward her husband rather than her son.

At an unconscious psychological level as well as at an unconscious metabolic level, Ronald's young psyche and organism had to identify itself with his mother's overcharged and overloaded cortex and libido. This identification enabled him to adjust to them during the course of opening himself to a reciprocal bond of contact with her. His cortico-cerebrospinal circuit is dominantly polarized around the cortex itself, in contrast to Eldridge's, which is more polarized around his primordial will-to-survive. Because Ronald's cortico-cerebrospinal circuit is more polarized around the cortex itself, the energy synergist in his lower half has been more stimulated and prematurely awakened than Eldridge's. If anything, Eldridge's genitals have been almost totally buried and cut off from his upper cerebral cortex because his overloaded back prevents any form of spontaneous energetic flow to move freely up and down his spinal column.

The premature awakening of the cerebral cortex will simultaneously awaken the sexual libido of the child when the bullying parent affirms rather than crushes the volitional centers in the back, particularly the one in the lower back. This happened between

Ronald and his mother. She always affirmed his narcissistic sense of omnipotence, so much so, that his phallic need to be a hero in his mother's and his own eyes, was fully awakened at a prepubertal age. Bioenergetically, this was not desireable, because it provided an additional energy source for the premature differentiation of a cortico-cerebrospinal closed circuit. This circuit acted as a retaining reservoir for uncompleted feelings and accumulated nervous tension. The more tension that becomes stored in this circuit, the more energy required from both synergists to maintain it. And the more overloaded the voluntary nerves and muscles become, the more they become twisted and bound into self-encapsulated units. Eventually, the twisting and binding action overflows and radiates downwards into the voluntary muscles and cerebrospinal nerves extending along the entire back, until a veritable hotline of excessive secondary-process activity mobilized by the synergistic interaction of the two energy synergists is chronically intact. When this happens, the third stage of armor formation has fully begun.

The bullied child needs to develop prematurely some kind of cortico-cerebrospinal closed circuit in order to build from within a self-preservative set of defenses against the bullying parent. He prematurely tightens his entire back region at the ectodermal and mesodermal layers to form a substantial wall of protection against the feeling pressures emanating from the bullying parent or parents. Once he has established an intact cortico-cerebrospinal closed circuit of energy currents, he has a better chance to neutralize and even to petrify the direct feeling impact of the anti-life feeling and energy vibrations issuing from the organism and psyche of the bullying parent. Then he becomes able to prematurely differentiate a will-to-struggle-and-to-survive which is more secondary-process than primary-process. He acquires prematurely, in other words, the internal means to play somewhat sophisticated games with the head and will of the bullying parent. He learns how to parry with their heads and wills through increasingly subtle maneuvers designed to outwit them so that they become the victims.

The more the child is prematurely forced to differentiate a mobile cortico-cerebrospinal-based capacity for defensively exercizing his own will-to-survive against the parental will, the weaker and less spontaneously dominant become the healthy visceral longitudinal energy currents in the ectodermal and mesodermal layers of the back. In fact, the longitudinal currents become progressively confined to the endodermal depths as the cortico-cerebrospinal currents become increasingly overloaded, twisted and power-polarizing. Eventually, internal territories become defined and solidified under the dominant influence of one of the two antagonistic energy currents. The no-man's-land between these two clearly defined territories becomes the region of increasingly clear-cut collisions of energy flow, or what are hereafter called internal energy blocks. The energy blocks do not crystallize until the third stage of armoring has started. Until that time, the cortico-cerebrospinal closed circuit increases its range and tenacious influence by developing more and more vortexes of twisted muscles and nerves. Picture an octopus spreading and multiplying its strangulating tentacles over its intrinsic antagonist, the visceral, blood-synergized fluid longitudinal energy flow which radiates outwards and upwards from the endodermal layers of the abdominal cavity.

C. The Third Stage

The third stage of armoring is distinguished by a rapid hardening and thickening of the mesodermal layer around the entire perimeter of the organism to form an impervious, rigid muscular sheath. This sheath functions as a barrier between the ectodermal layer on the outside and the endodermal layer on the inside. Stimuli impinging from both directions, from without and within, are effectively barricaded. Simultaneously, an imploded stalemate occurs in the interaction between the cortex-dominated currents in the upper back, neck, and head and the viscera-regulated currents in the lower and upper front halves.

Because it usually does not emerge until late childhood and early adolescence, and in some cases does not become fully crystallized until late adolescence and young adulthood, the third stage of armoring represents an intermeshing of several different kinds of processes, both psychological and physiological. At the psychological level, we have already postulated that the premature awakening of the will-to-survive is one of the fundamental cornerstones of armor formation, especially during the second stage. A premature will-to-survive introduces a more advanced psychological process which I call a cerebralized false self-system.

The totally repressed reason that this false system exists is to sustain the illusion that one's personal identity is synonymous with one's rational will. Implicit is the hidden preconception that one's personal identity has little or nothing to do with one's natural inclinations, needs or feelings, and still less to do with one's immediate feeling response and vibratory resonance with the essential 'isness' of outer or inner realities. Both kinds of phenomena are experienced as irrelevant or emotionally threatening to one's organized rational capacities. Intellectualized consciousness dismisses one's natural needs and feelings as illusory or else dangerous manifestations of one's animal instincts. This same rational consciousness judges resonance with what is as an indulgence in idle fancy, mysticism, irrational whimsy or dissociated daydreaming. In reality, such a resonance is an intrinsic and valuable exchange between soul and body.

A cerebralized false self-system is a more academic term for what is usually called a defended ego. Two kinds of ingredients comprise the defended ego: abstract ideas and principles of proper behavior derived from others, and highly structured, rationally clear and distinct perceptions and sensations mediated by the intact cortico-cerebrospinal circuit. Both kinds of ingredients are believed useful to an organized mental image of oneself and to exist omnipresently in the background of awareness. Yet in actuality, when what is defined as actual is seen from a soul perspective which is ontologically rooted in the intuitive faculties of the creative unconscious, the defended ego amounts to a counterfeit network of self-perceptions designed to repress and deny the existence of the sympathetic feeling centers in the front half of the body.

Third-stage armored persons usually cannot tolerate any kind of direct identification of themselves with circuits of feeling and energy interaction which establish immediate concrete, primary-process contact with objective realities, either within or without. They cannot tolerate falling out of their mind-brain into mindlessly empty subjective feeling states characterized by non-striving and a total surrender of the will. They tend to interpret such subjective states as a total negation of their personal identity, and they very rapidly panic if they find themselves beginning to fall into such a state. They are totally unaware that they must actively avoid experiencing such subjective feeling states primarily in order to continually render impotent their fluid energetic visceral flow which constantly circulates between their endodermal depths and their ectodermal senses in the front half of their torsos. And such impotence allows the false self-system to remain in control.

Third-stage armoring functions psychodynamically to seal off the natural dynamic feeling capacities for relatedness, especially those of the front half of the body. But this is utterly outside of the armored person's conscious awareness. Armoring is largely unconscious because its function is precisely to provide a screen against conscious awareness of the natural body and soul dimensions of real selfhood. Armoring is like a gigantic gray blanket which neuters the energetic and feeling realities of the endodermal depths and breadths, especially those of the front half. It kills the realm of concrete spontaneous immediate contact which only a fluidly blood-synergized front half can mediate.

One could argue with eloquence that the third stage of armoring unfolds primarily because of the emergence of a mentalized, survival-driven self-system. One could then postulate that the chronic hardening of the mesodermal layer to form a peripheral muscular sheath around the entire circumference of the body fulfills a psychodynamic function: to serve the ego-defense network and its compulsive need to repress, deny, and distort the existence of the natural dynamic feeling capacities for relatedness localized in the endodermal depths of the front half.

But such an explanation still does not account for the physiological characteristics peculiar to the third stage of armoring. Foremost among these characteristics is a chronically hyper-active back. The entire back half, comprising the two energy synergists at both ends of the spinal column as well as the lower and upper back regions, is overenergized and chronically restless. This restlessness is so great that the third-stage armored individual is constantly trying to reduce the energy-charge by engaging in various pursuits which provide at least some temporary relief from tension.

I am personally convinced that this condition of chronic excess energy-charge is the antithesis of real energetic vitality and fullness of vital functioning. Vital functioning is made possible exclusively by the dominant flowing of the visceral longitudinal energy currents operating in the core or endodermal depths of the organism. It has been my consistent clinical observation that clients and trainees who manifest a condition of chronic excess energy-charge are the most alienated of all from their endodermal longitudinal energy currents. Their intact peripheral muscular sheath insures this. But their chronic excess energy-charge cannot be explained simply by the fact that they possess a mental false self-system. It can only be fully explained by what happens physiologically after the premature will-to-survive-and-struggle has solidified in the older child and adolescent. It is related to the impact of physiological puberty upon an already overloaded, overtwisted, and overcompressed cortico-cerebrospinal closed neuromuscular energy circuit.

We hypothesize that the onset of sexual puberty increases to the point of intolerable exacerbation the filling up of the cortico-cerebrospinal energy reservoir with excess quantities of unreleased energy. (This is only true, of course, when this reservoir has been prematurely formed prior to the onset of puberty.) The reservoir's very existence necessitates a different deployment of libidinal energy than when no such circuit has crystallized prior to puberty. I suggest that there is a mutational leap in the quantities of vital energy which are made available by the coming of puberty, because of the catalytic impact of the glandular reconstituting process upon the whole energy economy. This additional source of energy, however, is funnelled into the synergistic orbit of activity already operating between the two energy synergists up and down the back, rather than channeled into the normal internal reservoir, the visceral vegetative energy currents. This deflection and mischanneling of normal libidinal energy flow directly into the service of the will-and-cortex-dominated voluntary neuromuscular networks in the back provide a fresh impetus to the gradual overloading of the closed cerebrospinal energy circuit.

The inordinately greater quantity of energy generated by the two energy synergists during armor formation is caused by the necessity to feed and to preserve a cortex-dominant energy circuit which is essentially closed and self-isolating, in the midst of an organismic totality whose more natural inclination is to remain world-open and regulated by an equalization law. But the natural inclination presupposes a biological harmony and stability of functioning which can only be actualized if the energy economy functions in unity. This is impossible when the energy economy is divided into a cortex-dominated voluntary circuit and a viscera-regulated involuntary longitudinal circuit. The kind of head-centered unity, harmony, and stability of functioning which the one system is striving to preserve is utterly antagonistic to the kind of equalization process which governs the other system.

The concept of a natural governing equalization process was first formulated by Kurt Goldstein. He states that any stimulus fully received by an organism elicits at first an excitation process -- whether the mode be sensory, motoric, thinking, or feeling. But the stimulus also elicits a subsequent equalization of the excitation. For Goldstein, this equalization process means a dedifferentiation of the patterning of the neural substratum: any figure-background pattern of differentiation had to be completely erased and the organism had to return to an undifferentiated mean level of stimulation before it could fully receive a new stimulus, or the same stimulus again.

For our purposes, the law of equalization refers less to the neural substratum than to the entire fluid or non-arrested energy economy, comprising every physiological metabolic system of the body. For us, the law of equalization states that there can be no real unity, harmony, and stability of core Beingness, whether at a psychological or physiological level, unless a single, unitary circulation of energy flow constantly functions between the endodermal depths and the ectodermal surfaces. Unless the excitation or synergistic process of energy mobilization, induced by some stimulus coming from the inner or outer world, is succeeded by a massive process of equalization or dedifferentiation of the overexcited and underexcited parts of the energy economy, there can be no unity, harmony, or stability of enduring Beingness. Unless, that is, there is a return of the fluid energy flow to a state of relative homogeneity throughout the total organism, there can be no return to a centering of one's being within the core regions of the metabolism. The law of equalization runs parallel to, and is the guardian of, a self-actualizing mode of functioning centered in the core longitudinal vegetative currents.

From the perspective of the law of equalization, it becomes clearer how the formation of the cortico-cerebrospinal closed energy circuit is responsible for a system of organismic functioning which is internally divided and doomed to chronic internal conflict, tension, and disorder. This is because the cortex-dominant energy network can never allow itself to become dedifferentiated, to become subservient to the core longitudinal vegetative currents. Instead, the cortex and survival-oriented will are compulsively driven to assume a greater and greater tyranny over the metabolic depths of both the soul and the body. And if the third stage of armoring occurs, they will do so ruthlessly, without the slightest sense of loss, struggle or pain, for the sake of an ordered universe which is centered in the mind-brain rather than the body and soul. The armoring is the tool which deadens the natural dynamic feeling capacities for relatedness, without the subject becoming aware of the enormous price paid.

Returning to the unique physiological characteristics peculiar to the third stage of armoring, I submit that there are significantly greater quantities of energy funneled into the closed cortico-cerebrospinal neuromuscular network with the onset of puberty. It is as if the cortex-dominated networks of voluntary nerves and muscles are compelled to expand their boundaries of tyrannical control over the rest of the organism, without ever yielding to the organism as a whole. The awakening of the powerful sexual instinct must be subverted by the rational will: essentially, it steals the vital energy flow emanating from the genitals and diverts it into the active service of the ego-defense network before it can become spontaneously directed towards the more id-like, primary-process feeling capacities for relatedness of the front half.

The upward thrust of a new source of energy which comes with biological puberty notably intensifies the interaction already occurring between the two energy synergists. This intensification produces the rather rapid hardening and insidious spreading of a hypertonic, overloaded chronic tension into every voluntary muscle grouping of the body. The hitherto rather narrow boundaries defining the cortico-cerebrospinal neuromuscular circuits spread and expand themselves throughout the entire voluntary musculature, like a Spanish moss spreads its paralyzing tendrils to slowly suck the life-giving energy flow from a vital tree. When reinforced by the prematurely awakened will-to-survive and the cerebralized self, the human mind-brain kills the fluid blood-flow of the core vegetative energy currents wherever armoring has infiltrated.

In place of a spontaneous and freely self-regulative energy flow nourished by the blood, the brain superimposes a mechanical network of mentally originated neural impulses and signals, much like the communication of logically clear and distinct messages from a computer. This computer-like control pattern is made possible by the continual twisting and compressing of voluntary nerves and muscles around and against one another into progressively tighter knots. The knots isolate the nerves and muscles from any direct, osmotic interaction with the involuntary metabolic networks of the total organism. Once the isolation is complete, all that moves inside the cortico-cerebrospinal circuit are self-reverberating cerebral messages and sensations endlessly repeating themselves along the same closed, self-contained neuromuscular pathways.

Inside such a closed computer-like circuit of congealed neuromuscular pathways, there is relative calm. But outside, at the boundaries of contact with the rest of the metabolism, there is chronic collision and potential explosiveness. It is this no-man's-land outside of the closed cortical circuit of dominance which all our energy-mobilization techniques deal with, directly or indirectly. The more the boundaries between the two opposed energy currents are congealed, the more effectively is a redeployment of metabolic energy induced by direct touch methods rather than do-it-yourself exercises. This is because when a third-stage armored client uses a prescribed exercise, he invariably calls upon the cortico-cerebrospinal circuit of control more than the core vegetative energy currents. Nothing less than a total suspension and deactivation of the cortico-cerebrospinal circuits makes possible the mobilization of the region between the two antagonistic energy currents. This particular mobilization is the only one that truly matters during initial treatment with a third-stage-armored client.

Chapter III

SOME OF THE ENERGY CHANGES OF THE DEARMORING PROCESS

I. General Introduction

In this chapter I shall attempt to bring together what I consider to be the more important healthy energy changes that everyone goes through during the course of dearmoring. My goal is to present a generalized outline of the fundamental biodynamic changes that happen when anyone who has been divided within becomes more fully functioning. I will use the cases from the opening chapter as examples of these generalized principles rather than focus upon specific types of character-muscular armoring and their dissolution.

There is no doubt in my mind that the healing and growth process consists basically of soulbuilding and transformation of the personality structure. An aspect of this process that is so intrinsic that without it there can be no real soulbuilding are the definite psychobiological changes in the fluid energy flow that underlie the psychic superstructure. All psychopathology, whether psychological or biodynamic, involves some species of arrestment of the fluid energy flow of the organism.

Objectively and scientifically we still do not know a great deal about the fluid energy flow. Orthodox medicine, physiology and anatomy teach more about congealed structures in the human organism than about its fluid energy flow. Our concern here in describing the more important features of the fluid energy flow are more in sympathy with Chinese medicine rather than with Western medicine. The patterns of change and flow to be presented are macroscopic in the sense that they treat of the organism as a holistic entity, much akin to Chinese medicine. I do not attempt to even touch upon atomistic microscopic changes at the physiological or anatomical levels. In this regard my ultimate authority remains Kurt Goldstein, the German neurologist, whose approach to the human organism comes closest to describing my clinical experience of the organismic changes in my patients.

The rather generalized and abstract presentation of phenomena and ideas that follows may be difficult for the reader to grasp cognitively. However, in the succeeding nine chapters these same phenomena and ideas will be presented again and again in the context of more precise applications to the experiences and behavior of Christa and others. This chapter represents a synthesis of the psychobiological changes that will emerge more clearly at a phenomenological level when linked to the description of other case examples throughout the book.

There are four generalized patterns of healthy energy change that I think are important. Each is sufficiently complex to understand to warrant a separate treatment.

II. The First Pattern of Energy Change.

The pattern: When there is isolation of the energy flow in parts of the organism, the psyche tends to respond to most novel situations by becoming either rigidly fixated on the objective stimuli or by responding with rapidly alternating, largely unconscious feeling and perceptual reactions which are antagonistic to each other. The greater the amount of isolation of the energy flow, the greater is the fixation or rapidity of alternation of the psychic reaction. As the dearmoring process unfolds, the rapidly alternating opposite reactions and tendency to fixation become less intensely loaded, slower and slower, until they become graspable in consciousness. Eventually there emerges at the embodied soul level a psychobiological system that can sustain internally balanced polarities of response to the same novel stimulus.

It is essential to convey that the abnormal psychic reactions of stimulus perseveration or rapidly alternating responses are mechanical, automatic, and crazy-making. They happen outside of the subject's own awareness, making them extremely difficult to bring them into the realm of the person's conscious claim of ownership. Their double-binding contradictory character makes them a nemesis to treat directly at the psychic level or at the organismic level. They have to be noticed and quietly endured by the psychotherapist for periods of treatment that last for months before the melting of the character-muscular armor permits their autonomous, self-encapsulated quality to begin to break down.

As psychotherapists, it is important that we become increasingly aware of these double-binding abnormal psychic reactions and the extent to which they dominate the patient's experience before proceeding with the use of body methods. They constitute for me the essence of all psychopathological formations, and their presence indicates some form of severe splitting at both the psychodynamic and biodynamic levels. Catalytic styles of body work are contraindicated as long as these abnormal psychic reactions prevail. This is because it is too disruptive to the patient's stability to have such patients polarize their energy circuits, whether through do-it-yourself exercises or direct touch methods, and afterwards witness them undergo totally opposite and disjunctive responses to the energy mobilization.

It was not until I had reread Kurt Goldstein's masterpiece, The Organism, many times over a period of ten years that I began to grasp the organismic foundations of my client's tendencies to manifest labile or fixated perceptual and feeling responses to body work. It then took another ten years of clinical experience to make the connections between the organismic processes and the psychodynamic processes. The latter was especially true when working with schizoid and borderline patients, whose propensity to manifest outside of their own consciousness sudden shifts of perception and feeling whose bizarreness could be assessed in terms primarily of a fragmented leaping from one reaction to its extreme opposite. I intuitively was predisposed to think for years that while the conventional psychiatric principle of ambivalence afforded us with a substantial understanding of neurotic functioning, it was not suitable to explaining the sudden total shifts of feeling and perception that I experienced clinically with my schizoid and borderline and psychotic clients. From Goldstein I learned that the neurotic's fluid energy flow is less isolated off and fragmented from the totality, and hence the tendencies to stimulus perseveration and extreme oscillation between opposite feeling reactions are somewhat slower and more quickly graspable in consciousness than in a person with a schizoid, borderline, or psychotic pattern where the isolation of parts is far more complete.

According to Goldstein pathology of any kind

entails some type of chronic seclusion and segregation off of parts of the neural substratum from the remainder of the nervous system. The larger the size of the segregated parts, the greater is the likelihood that the figure-background excitation process throughout the neural substratum is forced to become circumscribed and confined to less than the whole substratum. It is this reality that explains the gross instability and confusion between what is figure and what is background within the organism, and it is this same instability and confusion that produces at the psychic level lability and fixation at different occasions to the same objective stimulus. To quote Goldstein :

> ". . . . if we appreciate the effect of isolation properly: the phenomenon of alternation between opposite reactions. Under certain circumstances, we have an abnormal perseveration and under other circumstances a great lability, i. e. the reaction alternates between opposite extremes." (*)

> ". . . . under normal conditions, any figure formation determined by a stimulus has the whole of the organism as its background. Excitation and equalization, as well as the utilization of other stimuli required by the task in their functional significance for the particular figure - all this takes place in a manner adequate to the total organism. If the figure formation loses its stability, through a defective articulation of the figure ground relation in the whole, then the outer stimuli become abnormally effective, in an inadequate, 'random' fashion. If they are very strong, an abnormal fixation of one figure results. If such a stable figure cannot be formed, either a disturbance or disorder sets in; or the 'ground' processes will press forward, become figure, and consequently performances will occur which correspond to the ground process. This second alternative may take place when the effective stimuli are more adequate to the ground process, and therefore influence it directly so that the ground process undergoes a stimulus increase in an abnormal way. Thus we may find a permanent and abnormal perseverance

(*) The Organism, P. 133, Beacon Paperback, Boston, 1963.

of the ground, or an alternation between figure and ground . . . . " (*)

These concepts of Goldstein must be translated into the ideas introduced in the previous chapter. What I depicted there as the closed cortico-cerebrospinal circuits are here a part of the neural substratum which has become isolated off from the totality. The degree of isolation regarding our fluid energy flow varies with the severity of the armoring. With neurotics the isolation is only partial, but with those who possess cerebral armoring, schizoids, paranoids, and psychctics, the isolation is far more total, and with them what Goldstein says fully applies. It also applies relatively when the chronic twisting and compressing of the mesodermal voluntary muscles and nerves or the visceral involuntary muscles and nerves produces a condition of partial or relative functional isolation.

We see the effects of the latter in neurotics without cerebral armoring when at the beginning of treatment they will suddenly break off from doing a do-it-yourself energy mobilization movement and retreat out of their bodies back into their heads as they stand immobile, looking lost and somewhat dumbfounded. After a few seconds of silence, during which time they usually manage to recover their habitual mentalized self-identity, they will begin to ridicule and condemn the exercise they have just terminated with such judgments as: "stupid", "silly", "senseless", "painful", "horrible", "sadistic", "animal", "sexual", "mechanistic", and "exhausting". They then often refuse to go on with any form of body work for the remainder of the session, and assume some sort of defiant stance towards the psychotherapist. But if allowed to collapse on the mattress and recover their equilibrium, the administering of a nurturing direct touch will often plunge them into loaded and conflictful psychic material with lesser egoic controls than normally, so much so that they might suddenly stop the emotional cartharsis they are enmeshed in and of their own volition stand back up on their feet and start mobilizing again in the vertical position!

Such extreme alternation between opposite feeling reactions and perceptual judgments towards the

(*) Ibid, pp. 145 - 146

same energy mobilization exercise during the same session attests to considerable relative functional isolation of their armored parts from their organism as a unitary whole. This is further evidenced when they then might proceed to mobilize their energy with such willful determination that they overcharge their armored mesodermal sheath and eventually sky-rocket a discharge of energy that does nothing more than really exhaust them because of the enormous secretion of adrenalin and other emergency operations set going in the face of excessive stress created by their head-directed manner of mobilization. They have no idea or feeling for the reality that they are reinforcing their armoring more than loosening it because they are quite incapable of forming a figure background excitation gestalt that focuses with any objectivity on their armored parts or fluid energy parts. They have no idea how false and counterfeit their discharge of tensions remains, nor how they have used their exhibiting of their overmobilized bodies to avoid and escape from real feelings. They have no idea how will-perseverative their energy mobilization is.

Often when this contradictory and exhausting behavior occurs, what follows is quite predictable. They go through a sequence of rapidly shifting attitudes towards the psychotherapy and the psychotherapist, but hide this for the most part from the psychotherapist while the session continues. The extreme oscillation of attitudes might go on for hours and even days after the session is over, especially if anxiety appears, which it often does when an armored neurotic has severely overmobilized his intact armoring. The more anxiety is aroused, the greater the mechanical alternation between totally disjunctive and conflicting perceptions of the previous session and the psychotherapist. Negative feelings surface against the psychotherapist, and distrust of his judgment as well, but these negative feelings eventually subside into a fixed neutrality and ambivalence. When the client returns a week later for his next session he might not even mention the struggle he has been submerged in for days following the last session. To even mention it would mean risking more self-disclosure of his underlying emotional neediness than he is ready to permit.

Lacking a stable figure formation towards their

own body, and remaining divided within, half in their mesodermal rigidities and half in their spectator cerebralized ego, it is inevitable that a great many ground processes, to use Goldstein's terminology, will press forward and temporarily sieze the foreground of consciousness of these neurotics, but then subsequently be replaced by absolutely opposite feeling contents. Their ground processes are essentially repressed negative feelings, and the overmobilization of their energy economy that they have willed themselves to achieve has indeed undermined their usual egoic controls. However, given their tendency to remain fixated within their cerebralized self-system, the latter will struggle to maintain dominance until the energy economy itself spontaneously mobilizes a sequence of partial rebellions in the wake of the session. The delayed rebellions, consisting of a combination of swelling ground processes in the form of aching muscles, relaxing nerves, and vegetative currents seeking some tenuous sort of equilibrium together with the surfacing of repressed negative affects, cannot help but produce a chaotic see-sawing between the most disconnected and contradictory psychic material.

In the example of Gayle from the first chapter there is present a great deal of this rapid, mechanical oscillation between different parts of the psyche siezing brief dominance in consciousness. It was already happening in an excessively hypermanic rate of change between her previous session, her tenth, and the session from which the clinical excerpt was taken. The speed with which she swung between feelings of love and feelings of hate towards her two children was almost unbearably frenzied. Her positive transference towards me and Katherine must have helped her to tolerate these rapid swings, which we actively encouraged her to allow.

During her eleventh session of treatment she seemed especially well primed, partly because of these very same rapid swings between opposite feeling attitudes, to go beyond her familiar egoic boundaries into still further stages of creative disintegration regarding her irrational anger towards her two children. At the moment when she said: "I don't know how to be a mother", she lost whatever stable figure formation, or object-related structuring of herself, that she had been maintaining. Thereafter she plunged, almost helplessly and mechanically, into a random swinging between background and foreground parts of her psyche and soul. It was then that we saw unleashed hitherto repressed feelings of the most intense destructive hostility towards her two children, whom we knew for sure she really did love. To declare: "I want to take you by your feet and just throw you against the wall. I want to hurt you", could only have originated from the unfinished distant feeling past, from the period of her life when she was the child. She needed to say and feel this destructive hostility with sufficient carthartic intensity of release in order to begin to face in consciousness more squarely than she could before that she did not know how to be a good, adequately loving mother.

In actual fact she had been a very good mother to her two children. She had willed herself to be the rationally perfect mother, unfortunately. This was the real problem. She had tried too hard to be always loving and considerate towards them. Such a rationally willed and mentally idealized species of love often has feet of clay, stemming as it does from a cerebralized self-image of perfection. It is oftentimes, as in the case of Gayle, ungrounded in the dynamic being centers of her embodied soul. Gayle came to us originally because of feelings of hopelessness and anxiety centered around her realization that she was not really being the perfect mother. She could not understand or confront her growing irrational negative feelings towards her two children, whom she also knew she really loved.

Gayle's drivenness to be the perfect mother was in part a defensive reaction formation against the total inadequacy and phoniness of her mother's love for her. To maintain this reaction formation syndrome of being the perfect mother Gayle had to armor her whole body, harnessing its vitality and subjugating its instincts in the service of her mentalized will. Consequently, as soon as she lost her egoic controls, she became possessed by the unexpressed rage and hostility that she had harbored within herself for years against her own mother, and projected this on to her own children. To say it in Golsteinian terms, once she gave up her habitually rational focusing of her attention upon either herself in the role of a mother or upon her actual mother, she was split into several warring parts of her psyche and soul and swayed helplessly between the rational foreground and the subcortical feeling background. The result was an enormous overflooding of archaic negative emotions which proved to be too overloaded and explosive for her to handle productively. Too much negative raw emotion towards her actual mother began to break through from the regions of her soul that had been chronically held in stasis as forming the ground of her vitality, such that the ground became too potent, and her conservative energy economy and armoring could not stand this for very long, causing a complete shutdown of consciousness.

Gayle's loss of her egoic controls during her eleventh session was too sudden, too total, and excessively disintegrative. It could have been avoided if I in particular had been more patient and less pushy and catalytic in the way I encouraged her creative disintegration process to exceed her natural organismic and psychological limits. I shall return shortly to a critique of the way in which I colluded with Gayle's overflooding of herself with repressed feelings she could not handle.

Here I want to point out that it is not until Gayle would have arrived at the second stage of treatment that she would have stood a better chance not to have become overflooded with negative emotions. She would then be able to establish a more organismically grounded balance between raw emotion breaking through from below and a cognitive awareness of that emotion that meets, accepts, and joins with it. She would be able, in other words, to maintain a figure-background excitation gestalt rather than collapse into the chaos of rapidly alternating feelings and perceptions that remained isolated and disconnected from each other.

It is not until the second stage of treatment, when there has been established a weak but steady fluid vegetative energy flow circulating between the center and the periphery of the organism, that it becomes a realistic possibility for a general deceleration in the tempo of rapid see-sawings between opposite psychodynamic reactions to the same stimulus. This has to do with the emergence of an authentic convergence-equalization patterning of the energy economy. Such a patterning we will deal with in the next section, but here it can be said that it is the only patterning of healthy energy I believe has the power to erode and eventually dissolve from within the muscular armoring. It does this by engaging increasingly larger and larger regions of the total organism in a unitary but integrated participation when responding to novel situations. The greater the participation of the total organism, the more retarded becomes the formation of a figure-background excitation gestalt that extends throughout the organism and endures until a creative adjustment to the objective novelty has been completed. Critical to such creative adjustments is an interior synthesis and matching between cortical and subcortical psychic activities that allows for whatever polarities of feeling or intuitive response might develop.

It is not until the third stage of treatment, following the stressful upheavals and chaos attending the dearmoring process during second stage, that the embodied soul finally has the opportunity to come into its core endodermal rhythms of self-actualization. Pivotal to the latter is the crystallization of the Hara-Logos intuitive polarity and the mediation by this polarity of rhythms of alternation between periods of creative differentiation of objective novelty and periods of dedifferentiation and mindless integration. These particular rhythms of alternation can be so slow that it takes many weeks and months to achieve one's long-term creative objective and see it finally actualized by the core self. The Hara-Logos polarity keeps the internal world of the psyche and soul centered for the most part on the regular, periodic maintenance of periods of dedifferentiation and mindless integration, thereby providing over very long periods of time from its nucleus deep within the abdominal cavity a primary-process-regulated continuity, peace, and eternal natural harmony within.

III. The Second Pattern of Energy Change.

The pattern: The greater the degree of intact character-muscular armoring, the more desperately and unconsciously driven is both psyche and organism to charge up and discharge externally manifest amounts of adrenalin-sustained stasis energy. As the armoring dissolves, the need to charge up and discharge externally is vastly diminished and replaced by an organismic patterning of energy convergence-equalization, which makes possible the release of internal tension, both chronic and transient, through internal channels of energy discharge.

The phenomenon of emotional cartharsis is bound up with a desperate, unconscious drive to charge up and discharge large amounts of chronically damned up energy at the body's surface. Taking such a position, it should be apparent to the reader that I do not believe that cartharsis in itself represents a cure for neurosis. But it surely helps people with rigid types of character structure to begin the dearmoring process. And at more advanced stages of the dearmoring process it is a great help to the vertically undergrounded types, but for very different reasons than how it helps the rigid types during the first stage of treatment.

The need for emotional cartharsis presupposes a chronic inner split between the cortico-cerebro-spinal circuits and the endodermal vegetative flow. To maintain this chronic inner splitting there must be synergized tremendous quantities of energy whose basic function is that of feeding both energy systems simultaneously. This means that tremendous quantities of energy are required for a extremely negative, self-invalidating purpose: namely, the perpetuation of chronic unconscious conflict and an ongoing battle for survival and competition between the two antagonists. Reich called this energy stasis energy, and correctly hypothesized that stasis energy is the product of a binding and damning up of instinctual libidinal impulses by rational inhibitions.

But Reich, following in his teacher's footsteps, Sigmund Freud, arrived at some fundamentally wrong conclusions regarding the sexual libido. As already suggested in the previous chapter, I believe that Reich overendowed the sexual instinct with a power over the psyche and soul that it does not objectively merit except in the sphere of the intimate primary man-woman relationship when the pagan Gods and Goddesses of Eros reign. Apart from this very singular category of interpersonal relationship, our sexual libido is too easily susceptible to being undermined, stolen from, subjugated, and generally reduced to such a weak force within the energy economy that it is as if extinguished and non-existent.

Reich was led astray and lured into the same deadend street of his teacher Freud when he swallowed whole the latter's incarnation of the sexual libido as the daemonically driven tyrant of the psyche and soul. Reich thereafter was never able to disentangle the sexual libido from his valid empirical observations regarding the organismic need to charge up and discharge large quantities of damned-up stasis energy. Reich never could possibly comprehend thereafter how charge-discharge-driven behavior has only an indirect connection with damned-up libidinal impulses. (see pages 115 + 116). Reich never did recognize the tyrannical power of the closed cortico-cerebrospinal circuits and their capacity to appropriate the sexual libido entirely in the service of their own self-perpetuating orbit of influence. He therefore could not possibly recognize how it is the stress-engendered emergency functions of the energy economy, including the chronic lowgrade secretion of adrenalin, together with the chronic splitting of the energy economy into two separate and competitively operating energy networks that is the basic cause for the existence of stasis energy. Reich could never appreciate how much all manifestations of emotional cartharsis, including those that appeared during sexual orgasm, usually represented a pathological, abnormal need to periodically discharge at the surface excessively high levels of stasis energy whose functional use had little to do with the inhibition of sexual impulses.

When the charge-discharge drive of the psyche and organism is high, this is a sure indication of the existence of character-muscular armoring. It is the repressed negative affects associated with the primary dynamic feeling capacities for relatedness that are then pressuring from within unconsciously for temporary discharge and relief of tension, not sexual libido. To say it more precisely, it is the subjugation of our primary dynamic instinctual needs for feeling relatedness by the cerebralizing egoic system that has set up inside the organism a condition of chronic impasse and conflict between the armored mesodermal wall and the endodermal flow. This condition of chronic impasse and conflict causes there to accumulate larger and larger quantities of adrenalin-sustained stasis energy, so that eventu-

The Charge Phase

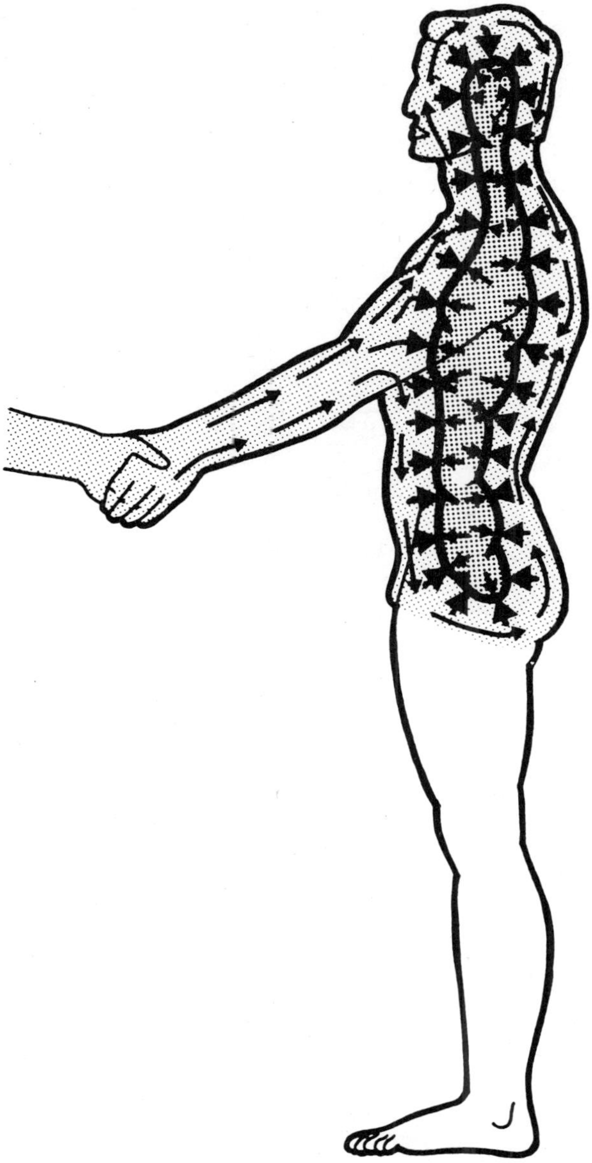

The Charge-Discharge Patterning of Energy Flow Within an Armored Receiver

The Discharge Phase

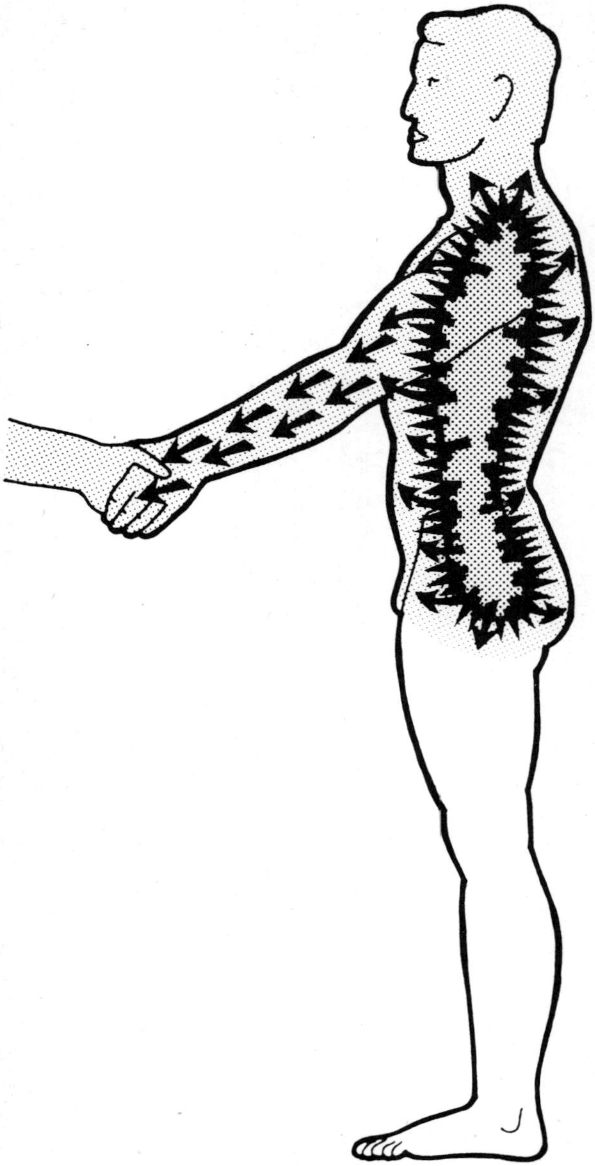

The Charge-Discharge Patterning of Energy Flow Within An Armored Receiver

ally something must explode if only to provide a temporary diminution of the energy overload.

A good deal of what is popularly known as 'primaling' is nothing more than a dramatically regressed explosion of damned-up stasis energy carried over from the distant, infantile past. What matters is the release of chronic tension at a largely primary-process biodynamic level during most primaling. It's more of a here-and-now event than any kind of authentically realistic reexperiencing of the infantile past. Primaling is a dramatic instance of energy discharge and getting rid of internal stasis pressure in the here and now more than an opening of a differentiated cognition to past objective realities in and for themselves. This happens to be the biggest weakness of every kind of emotional cartharsis, namely, its hidden motivation is not to confront objective reality so much as to primitively obliterate it.

For reality confrontation to be growth-enhancing and facilitative of interior changes in the psyche and soul there must have first occurred a dissolution of at least half to three-quarters of the internal stasis energy pressuring for discharge. Another way of saying the same thing is to assert that until there has been established a relatively free and direct energy flow across the no man's land regions of the armored neurotic that unites the endodermal, mesodermal, and ectodermal layers, the psyche is incapable of any convergence of its multi-dimensional faculties upon some objective reality with sufficient fullness to assimilate it interiorly. Reality confrontation and assimilation presupposes the capacity for sustained focal attention, and a precondition of the latter is the emergence of a patterning of the energy flow that is ordered and inclusive enough to maintain a figure-background excitation gestalt again and again and again directed towards the same objectified reality. From my point of view the convergence-equalization patterning of the energy flow as formulated by Goldstein alone guarantees the possibility for subject-world experiences of creative encounter in which the psyche and soul fully participate in congruent synchrony with the objective data.

A highly diminished quantity of internal stasis energy pressuring for externalized explosive discharge also permits the far more refined and subtler processes of internal energy discharge to make their appearance during the second stage of treatment. The latter are bound up with the opening of the front half being centers so that stasis energy can begin discharging upwards and downwards inside the endodermally located gastro-intestinal tract. The latter, however, from my point of view is always linked with Goldstein's law of equalization. That is to say, when a client begins to react to body work with nausea, vomiting, dizziness, and coughing, this indicates that not only has the gastro-intestinal tract expanded as a consequence of a fluid vegetative flow being established between the endodermal, mesodermal, and ectodermal layers. (see pages 119 + 120). It further indicates a capacity for the entire endodermal vegetative flow to assume the role of an interior channel of evacuation and discharge of stasis energy following a convergent mobilization of a figure-background excitation gestalt. The discharge of stasis energy seldom occurs spontaneously in a vaccuum, and with further and further dearmoring it occurs increasingly as the consequence of a full subject-world creative encounter. As the dearmoring process progresses, increasingly we are transformed into field-related and here-and-now subject-object agents of feeling-sentient contacting, whether during an id-affirmative mode of being-in-the-world when a figure-background excitation gestalt is non-existent, or during ego-affirmative modes of being-in-the-world when it is.

To return to the example of Gayle, we have an excellent opportunity to witness how effectively charge-discharge-driven emotional cartharsis is more motivated to obliterate the novel objective reality than meet it. Our hand-squeeze catalytic technique helped her surpass her hitherto strong egoic defenses against permitting a charge-discharge-driven externalization of chronic stasis energy. Her subsequent expression of extremely sadistic feelings towards her two children made possible her opening of her consciousness to her very ambivalent and unresolved feelings towards herself in the role of a mother. This very development would seem to contradict what was stated in the opening sentence of this paragraph, so we must review Gayle's session in greater detail.

It was not until later on in the session when I in particular continued to catalyze a creative dis-

The Convergent Phase

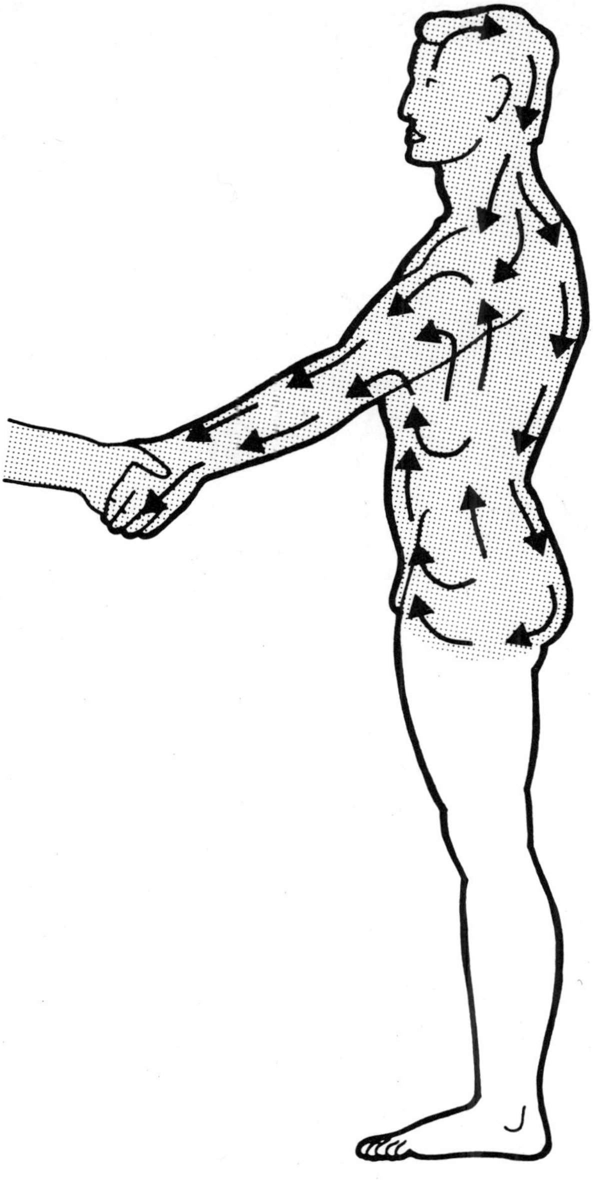

The Convergent-Equalization Patterning of Energy Within An Unarmored Receiver

The Equalization Phase

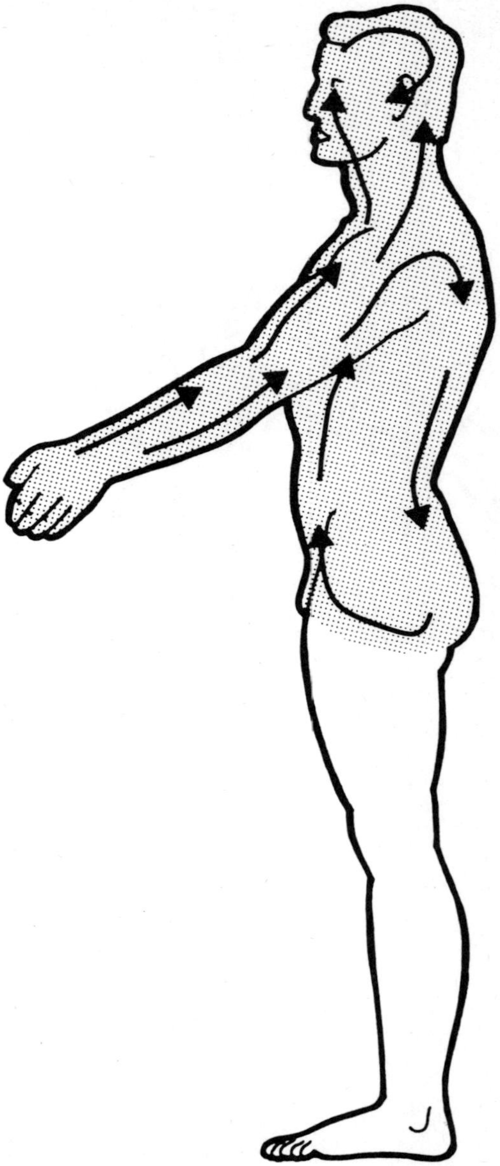

The Convergent-Equalization Patterning of Energy Flow Within An Unarmored Receiver

integration process that she was forced to obliterate the novel objective reality of her uncompleted negative feelings towards her actual mother. A lesson is to be learned here that I had myself not yet learned back in 1974 when this session occurred, namely, that one should never catalyze a creative disintegration process beyond the total organism's thresholds of convergent-equalization toleration. One of the limits of creative disintegration is when an excessive breakthrough of repressed negative affect proves to be so threatening to the ego-defense network that it arrests completely any further processing in conscicusness of the freshly released feeling content.

Let us review the later developments in her session, starting from the place where I clearly overstepped my directive, therapist-centered orientation towards her and catalyzed a disintegration process that was not creative because it happened too quickly and went tco deeply into her soul prematurely. This place was when she herself had arrived at the insight that she didn't want to push herself anymore to be an all-wise and perfectly loving mother. Instead of allowing her the client-centered freedom to explore this important insight at her own independent pace, I bulldozed her into a new series of charge-discharge-oriented encounters directly with her mother by structuring a first-person, subject-centered addressing of her mother. Furthermore, by continuing to maintain direct hand to hand contact with her body, Katherine grasping one of her hands and I the other, we had an additional device for further catalyzation of her repressed negative affects.

But even this did not satisfy me, so I insisted that she address her mother with the same feeling intensity and lack of inhibitions with which she had just shortly before addressed her children. Riding high on an already undermined control on the part of her cortico-cerebrospinal circuits, she was able to muster with a certain amount of will power a relatively well-charged amount of negative affect directed against her mother, combined with a fair amount of bioenergetic discharge of stasis energy through violent kicking movements with both legs. Given the already excessive bulldozing on my part, and her desire to please me, it is not surprising that immediately following this last exercise, she withdrew inside far enough to distance herself from her own expression of affect and judge it somewhat critically but accurately to be vaguely unreal. Such a partial withdrawal was totally called for, giving her the interior space to permit her closed cortico-çerebrospinal circuits to partially reassert their dominance. They needed to somewhat detach themselves both from her own release of repressed affect as well as from me in the role of catalyzer.

Now, some eight years later, six of which have been spent living and working mostly in Europe rather than America, I am firmly committed to the principle that following every instance of charge-discharge-driven emotional cartharsis, the psychotherapist is obligated to the client to permit the time and the freedom during the session for the latter's egoic controls and defenses to reassert themselves as much as they need to. Emotional cartharsis, or primaling, especially when combined with catalytic styles of energy mobilization, is always most stress-inducing and disruptive to the conservative energy economy as well as the ego-defense network. And unless the humanistically oriented body psychotherapist fully appreciates this, he/she will be tempted to over-mobilize and overcatalyze the creative disintegration process to the point of depriving the client of any ongoing sense of security of self-identity and feeling safety in relationship to the psychotherapist. The client needs to be affirmed in these needs for safety and emotional security during every session, or otherwise the pain, anxiety, and chaos of the dearmoring process will become too much to tolerate for the intact character-muscular armoring. In brief, the armoring must always be respected as an indispensable part, however undesireable, of the client's present personality structure.

Above and beyond this, I am now more firmly committed than when practicing in California to a more consistently client-centered approach to the client throughout all stages of the treatment. This means that I am ethically obligated to extend to the client an unconditional positive regard and trust that he/she can and will find his own tempo and mode of dearmoring, even during the first stage of treatment. The greatest hazard of the body psychotherapist is to think that he does know what the patient needs so well that he also knows how to bring the patient out of his armoring. This is a quality of arrogance on the psychotherapist's part that has been especially prevalent in the practice of body psychotherapy, given the models of Reich and Lowen, the leading innovators. Both have relied upon an arrogant medical style of treatment which has superimposed upon the patient an imperative towards charge-discharge-driven emotional cartharsis almost at any cost. The same can be said for primal therapy, except more so.

I am guilty of not extending to Gayle sufficient unconditional trust to find her own route and tempo of self-exploration during the session under discussion. I was far too one-dimensionally goal-directed to make the defenses collapse and precipitate a disintegration process. During 1974 I also did not know how easy it is to do this, and to overcatalyze a patient with a compulsive-hysteric character structure. I blinded my eyes and feeling antennae of my front half being centers to her already overstressed condition, and refused to give her the space to explore reflectively her ambivalent feelings towards her mother. I aggressively interrupted the latter and asked her once again to directly address her mother from a feeling-centered, subjective frame of reference, knowing full well that this would affirm her subcortical feeling activity more than her reflective consciousness. Then precisely at the moment when she began to give up addressing her mother and turning her attention backwards upon herself and the problem of how she could become a whole person independently of mother, I administer an extremely severe catalytic pressure to the back of her neck at the base of the skull in the very middle.

I have no doubt that there is a direct cause and effect relation between the applying of this catalytic direct touch technique and her statement a few minutes later, "I don't want to feel my feelings". My catalytic touch to this area of her body at this particular time was intended to weaken her tenacious super-ego tyranny, the attribute of every compulsive structure. Indeed it must have succeeded - but too well, because it was but a few minutes later when everything shut down inside of Gayle as she began to contort her facial expressions into the ugliest grimaces, and her psyche and soul became as if paralyzed. This total shutting down I now see to be a spontaneous self-protection against my drivenness of will as well as against her own drivenness to comply with my requests. She had to stop the creative disintegration process that I had been programming her into, even if it required an almost desperate flight from the here and now into an extremely regressed, closed off, and fragmented psychic space.

There are three things to be learned from this session with Gayle in the light of the present topic of the virtues and limitations of emotional cartharsis. The first is that each psychotherapeutic session should contain some sort of balance between ego-disintegrative and ego-affirmative methods structured by the psychotherapist. This is especially true when the psychotherapist has available a sack of catalytic direct touch as well as do-it-yourself energy mobilization exercises. If he practiced an exclusively nurturing style of body psychotherapy, much like orthodox Reichians do, this would be a less delicate matter. When catalytic body methods are available, the greatest hazard to their creative use is the therapist's own impatience and mistaken belief that he knows better than the patient's own dynamic feeling capacities for relatedness how to further the de-armoring process.

The second learning to be gained from Gayle's session is that there are always two modes of affirming the creatively id-affirmative forces operating in the client, even during the first stage of treatment. The one is to catalyze the repressed primary dynamic feeling needs for relatedness directly, as I did with Gayle during the session. The other mode, the one I did not employ but should have part of the time, is to simply structure or suggest nothing to the client, giving the latter a total freedom to initiate whatever happens at whatever level. If the first mode is pursued one-dimensionally this might polarize the stasis energy locked inside the organism to unconsciously press from within for charge-discharge-driven cartharsis. If the second mode is pursued with sufficient affirmation on the part of the psychotherapist, given enough time there will usually begin to unfold a subtler, finer species of energy release coming from the endodermal depths. I refer to the phenomenon of spontaneous vegetative release reactions that almost always occur in the wake of charge-discharge-driven cartharsis. These reactions have no chance of emerging during the session itself without the therapist permitting generous amounts of time in which neither he nor the patient does anything. The permitting of such do-nothing time is always integrative, facilitating the equalization of energy processes that follow inevitably after charge-discharge-driven activity. The heart of the opening up of new internal channels of energy discharge consists in affirming the integrative equalization process and its spokesmen in the moment: the spontaneous vegetative release reactions.

The third learning from Gayle's session is that the explosive discharge of damned up stasis energy and repressed negative affects at the surface has healing potential only to the extent that it facilitates afterwards a convergence-equalization patterning of the energy economy. It is precisely the latter development that was sabotaged during Gayle's session by her and my collusion of wills to overcatalyze the ego-disintegrative process. The reality is that if the psychotherapist lets the client be and stops making any kind of interventions following emotional cartharsis of almost any degree of intensity, a convergence-equalization patterning of both the psyche and the organism will eventually flower during the session. Both spontaneous self-explorations initiated by the psyche and soul of the patient and spontaneous vegetative release reactions will eventually flower, and between the two levels of flowering a great deal will happen within the patient without the psychotherapist doing anything except receiving where the patient is.

Anyone who is still in the first stage of the dearmoring and treatment process, as Gayle was, can permit incipient, short-lived, and partial spontaneous vegetative release reactions at best. This relates to the fact that most rigid types still in first stage have hardly any direct experience of a fluid energy flow circulating longitudinally in their endodermal depths or centrifugally between their endodermal, mesodermal, and ectodermal layers. This brings us to the next pattern of healthy energy change.

IV. <u>The Third Pattern of Healthy Energy Change</u>
<u>The pattern :</u> <u>The loosening and melting of the</u>

mesodermal wall, whether as a whole or at its more severely blocked muscle-nerve complexes, permits the increased appearance of spontaneous vegetative release reactions. With further dearmoring these reactions tend to undermine, at first only briefly, larger and larger regions of the mesodermal wall, moving usually in a circular fashion from center to periphery and longitudinally as well within the endodermal depths. This energetic change is one of the fundamental causes behind the psyche's progressive ease in creatively regressing to feeling states dominated by an original natural harmony of fluid energy flow during periods of non-engagement with objective novelty.

Most spontaneous energetic release reactions towards the beginning of treatment remain localized in a circumscribed part of the body, usually confined to a specific voluntary muscle complex within the armored mesodermal layer. The energy release originates and usually terminates within the mesodermal layer, and hence has nothing directly to do with the vegetative fluid flow and its origins in the endodermal depths. As long as the mesodermal armored sheath is chronically intact and dominant, whatever energy release reactions happen take the form of the novel stretching and spasming of voluntary muscles hitherto held rigid within a chronically hypertense web of imploded stasis energy. The release is usually painful, but also limited in space and time, and quickly passed beyond without the slightest investment of unsatisfied primary feeling needs or repressed affects. The patterning of the energy release remains confined to the outermost edges of the mesodermal sheath and discharges at the ectodermal surface directly adjacent to the specific muscle complex that is having the release. With further mobilization of the mesodermal sheath, it also becomes possible to trigger off a muscle spasm in those muscle groupings that form the antagonist network to the particular muscles at the opposite end of the body or joint that are being actively mobilized through body work.

For example, if a person with a rigid, third-stage pattern of armor does some really powerful and authentic charging up and discharging of stasis energy in the region of his overloaded and thickly muscled spinal column, and even manages to ventilate some repressed archaic aggression lodged in the muscles of the spinal column with the help of the kicking of the legs, the pounding of the arms, and the spontaneous thrusting of the pelvis, when he/she lays out horizontally on the mattress and does nothing for several minutes afterwards, there may suddenly appear an acute attack of muscle spasms. The spasms might be localized along the back, in the arms, in the legs, but oftentimes in the antagonistic muscles in the area of the diaphragm. After severe pain lasting a couple of minutes, the pain will completely vanish with the yielding of the spasming.

It is quite another state of affairs when with further loosening of the armored mesodermal wall incipient, short-lived, and partial spontaneous vegetative release reactions begin to appear. They always have a quality of streaming movement about them, of sensing that something is moving from one point to another point within the body. They usually appear between sessions at first rather than during sessions. This is because it takes many hours after a session containing charge-discharge-driven relief of stasis energy before equalization of the energy economy has fully terminated. Spontaneous vegetative release reactions never happen until the equalization process has fully or almost fully completed itself. Usually during the first stage of treatment it is very rare for a patient to experience spontaneous vegetative release reactions during the session because the mobilization of some amounts of adrenalin is almost unavoidable as an accompanyment to charge-discharge-driven cartharsis or even stasis energy relief exclusively.

Another important feature about spontaneous vegetative release reactions when they first start to occur is their strangeness and tendency to frighten the subject. The patient usually thinks that something is fundamentally wrong with his body, something bizarrely wrong, so much so that he begins to phantasy all kinds of horrible possibilities, such as coming down with cancer or malaria or jaundice or whatever. The patient will run off to his physician for a checkup, so great is his expectation of catastrophe, but even when he is reassured that the medical tests prove that nothing is organically wrong, he will still continue to have pathological phantasies about his body's growing deterioration and weakening. In spite of the psychotherapist's repeated reassurance that all he is having are probably spontaneous vegetative release reactions having to do with certain energy blocks beginning to melt, he will continue to ruminate until one day the intensity of the spontaneous vegetative release reaction will be so great that it will carry with it hitherto forgotten memories and feelings from the uncompleted past. Then the patient may begin to realize for the first time that his armoring is indeed beginning to melt and bringing with it feelings from within that he associates with former injustices that were superimposed upon him by others. There then unfolds in subsequent treatment sessions the resurrection of forgotten incidents in which the patient felt clearly victimized by his tormentors and persecutory authority figures, and the more he processes in consciousness these particular incidents, the more overwhelming become subsequent experiences of spontaneous vegetative release reactions.

Ronald from the first chapter provides us with a good example of how the psyche and organism increasingly interpenetrate and polarize each other the further strengthened becomes the endodermal flow and the emergence of spontaneous vegetative release reactions. Even from his first session Ronald was in the second stage of treatment by virtue of his absence of an armored mesodermal sheath and his capacity for sustaining a vital vegetative flow between his endodermal, mesodermal, and ectodermal layers. Nevertheless, he did still possess some amount of armoring, and it necessitated placing him in a standing vertical position of the highest stress for an indefinite period of time before the chronic tensions in his pelvis could loosen sufficiently to permit authentic energetic and emotional release.

The slowness with which his fluid endodermal vegetative flow was mobilized is itself one unmistakable earmark of how relatively free from armoring he essentially was. To have sustained this flow without skyrocketing his energy on account of the mobilization of a counter energy force within confirms his capacity for forming a figure-background excitation gestalt involving both cortical and subcortical processes. What Ronald exhibited in terms of mobilizing an endodermal vegetative flow within a period of twentysix minutes normally takes between six to eighteen months to emerge in a third-stage rigid type of armored neurotic.

One striking feature of Ronald's mobilization of his vegetative flow which increasingly served to integrate his total organism are the changes his vocal tone production went through. His vocal production was transformed from a state of total withholding of any sound to a loud but resonant bellowing that had the richness and fullness of an opera singer in a rage. People scream out of extreme anxiety and desperation, but they roar and bellow when there exists a fertile, robust vital vegetative flow longitudinally up and down across their diaphragm which extends into their four limbs and upwards into their head. Every organ of Ronald's organism stood squarely and unifiedly behind his externalization of sounds whose ferocity overfilled my consulting room. He looked like a roaring lion, and also sounded like one.

Another aspect of his performance that attests to a rather remarkable mobilization of his endodermal vegetative currents is the manner in which his breathing deepened and expanded his front half energy fields so that a peristaltic wave-like movement was observable between his throat and his genitals. His diaphragm evidenced not the slightest resistance or contraction against this peristaltic movement. With a rising polarization of all the voluntary muscles in his lower half on account of the severe stress generated by his position on his feet, he required larger and larger quantities of breath to sustain the position. This he managed to do splendidly, gradually mobilizing his entire pelvic floor both by means of rhythmically powerful voluntary thrusting movements and involuntary tremors. The latter in particular, when sufficiently slow-paced and unmistakably pleasureable, are one kind of spontaneous vegetative release reaction that consist of a dynamicization of the mesodermal musculature in its entirety by the endodermal vegetative flow moving centrifugally outwards against it.

Perhaps the most striking feature about Ronald's experience that attests to the mobilization of his endodermal vegetative currents is the relative ease with which he managed to creatively regress to childhood. He was able to process both his positive love feelings and his negative feelings of frustration and rage towards his mother with such fullness of investment on the part of his embodied soul that the latter participated in his regressive metamorphosis to childhood as much as his rational consciousness. He really did become transformed in his outward appearance into either a grotesquely defiant and rageful boy or a severely needy, hurt, and helpless child whose tears bespoke more pain than relief. He reexperienced both categories of feelings, the anger and the needy helplessness, with an abandonment worthy of a vital child.

The fact also that after laying out following the vertical standing stress position he manifested great ease processing in consciousness the connections between his repressed rage at the way his mother spiritually seduced and manipulated him and his present adult need to take revenge on all women upon whom he felt dependent for sex and/or love testifies to the genuineness of his fluid vegetative flow. The latter was all-pervasive, infiltrating the very citadel of his hitherto defended cerebral cortex and opening the latter by way of his Logos intuitive faculty to the chronic ambivalence that had always existed in his front half feeling centers towards all women - especially in his heart center. To be able to convergently focus with both his cognitive Logos faculty and his subcortical dynamic feeling capacities upon mother's double-binding of him and his unconscious need to similarly double-bind the ladies he fell in love with during the course of a two-hour session was most admirable.

Much the same admiration can be extended to the example of Ruth and her achievements during the course of her two week intensive. Like Ronald, from her initial session onwards she exhibited evidence for not possessing much armoring in her mesodermal layer. However, she did have a lot of armoring deeper down throughout large regions of her endodermal depths, as is usually the case with the oral-depressive character-muscular armoring. Given her lack of mesodermal armoring, it was quite easy to awaken her capacities for spontaneous vegetative release reactions if the endodermal depths were directly polarized through nurturing direct touch to her skin. I did not realize this during my first two three-hour sessions with her, mistakenly believing that she was more of a rigid hysteric than an oral, and so consequently I needlessly catalyzed semi-willed charge-discharge-driven expressions of aggression in her. The tender - consistently tender and nurturing - kind of direct touch she received from Katherine during a straight massage had a more catalytic impact upon her enbodied soul than any of my efforts to catalyze her back regions through do-it-yourself energy mobilization work.

Katherine's nurturing direct touch facilitated with almost a magic-like ease in Ruth an altered state of consciousness in which she was both regressed and felt like a child and Katherine the mother as well as an adult woman in touch with her longing need for direct loving touch from another adult woman. This altered state of consciousness triggered off inside Ruth a maelstrom of memories from the first seven years of her life the night after her massage. The very fact that these memories had remained inaccessible to consciousness through repression or denial until that night indicates how awakened had become her endodermal vegetative release reactions. The resurrection of long buried memories in consciousness is for me correlated quite directly with the circulation of longitudinal endodermal flow upwards into the primitive brain stem and cerebral cortex combined. Ruth's spontaneously impulsive outpourings of cries of anguish during the night when remembering these long-buried memories would seem to confirm the degree to which her endodermal vegetative flow had been mobilized because the most healing consequence of this mobilization is the emergence of the unfinished and unsatisfied primary dynamic feeling needs for relatedness.

The pains associated with the latter are distinct in kind from the pains associated with muscular spasming. The emergence of the unsatisfied primary feeling needs brings with it the pathos and suffering of a soul hitherto bound in chains and a body divided against itself. With the arrival of such suffering there begins a more total disorganization and reconstituting of the very foundations of the psyche and souls' centers. Mother nature, being ultimately a benign source of guidance within us, sees to it that such a total reconstituting of the very foundations and axis of our souls does not begin until there first flows within our endodermal depths enough vegetative currents to be able to support and adjust to the interior changes in the soul's foundation that must be tolerated. In Ruth's case, for example, there was sufficient opening of her vegetative endodermal currents from Katherine's massage to permit her psyche and soul to also open themselves to her unsatisfied feeling needs of her front half in relationship to her mother. Ruth's mesodermal wall as well as hardened and anesthetized endodermal regions were melting so rapidly that her whole upper front half, from her diaphragm upwards across her chest to her throat and mouth, were in all probability in expansive movement and disorganization during the night while she was remembering the first seven years of her life.

Ruth's fourth session of her intensive, which also happens to be the first session that Katherine and I worked together as a man-woman treatment team, provides us with a vivid account of how it is seldom possible for armoring to melt and with the melting usher us into feeling states of an original natural harmony of fluid energy flow without first traversing a pathway of pain and suffering. The more embodied the pain and suffering, to be sure, the quicker and fuller is the passage through.

The first bodywork of the session involved Katherine and Ruth lying on their sides on the mattress embracing each other chest-to-chest and belly-to-belly. It felt like coming home to mother for Ruth - not just her actual mother, but to a Positive Great Mother Figure in the form of Katherine. Ruth creatively regressed to a fuller feeling state than during her massage with Katherine in which an original natural harmony of fluid energy flow prevailed. The women, and particularly Ruth, were free to decide when and how to terminate this direct touch exercise, and after twenty-two minutes of soft tears and sobbing, Ruth terminated and at once launched of her own initiative into a set of standing do-it-yourself exercises designed to polarize her anger towards her actual mother. It was no accident that she mobilized a more spontaneously vital charge-discharge-driven venting of aggression on this occasion than she had with me alone during the first three sessions of her intensive. Once the endodermal vegetative currents are fully mobilized, they are prone increasingly to satisfy all four categories of unsatisfied primary feeling needs, and not be content with the satisfying of only one.

Ruth did not feel satisfied enough with the beating of the mattress violently with a tennis racket. She therefore invented her own original energy-mobilization exercise, which consisted of having Katherine hold her two arms pinned down behind her back while she descended to her knees and then struggled with Katherine actively to free herself while at the same time she addressed her mother angrily. The exercise ended with Ruth collapsing on the mattress, sobbing heavily. The sobbing was deeper than hitherto because the primitive phallic anger she had just succeeded in mobilizing was probably the most charged she had ever experienced in her life to date.

We see here an example of what characteristically happens to clients in the second stage of treatment regarding the phenomenon of alternation between opposite primary feeling needs and capacities for relatedness. The tempo and rhythm of alternation is much slower than during the first stage of treatment, and, as in the case of Ruth, unfolds spontaneously from within the endodermal depths at its own pace of oscillation. We see how Ruth oscillates in a manner and pace mysteriously and absolutely right between satisfying her front half and back half feeling needs. There clearly seems to be functioning some intuitive sensibilities emanating directly from her body - her embodied soul - that tell her how to satisfy her unsatisfied feeling needs. For instance, when I proposed that she return to a chest-to-chest embracing of Katherine a second time during the session, her intuitive sensibilities told her to refuse to do as I suggested. She chose instead to have Katherine place her back half against her front half as they laid adjacent to one another.

The deep wisdom of her preferred choice soon was confirmed. After about three minutes she began to experience periodic contractions in her diaphragm that caused her to harden herself against receiving the nurturing warmth of Katherine's back. Katherine encourages her to intensify the contractions by deliberately squeezing her muscles, with the result that shortly thereafter her entire lower half from her diaphragm down begins to freeze into a massively hardened contraction of her voluntary musculature.

The contracting is so extreme and total that a few moments later she starts to scream in sheer desperation and panic. This evokes a bout of violent coughing which threatens to cut off her breathing, so she suddenly is forced to take a vertical position resting on her knees and go through a sequence of catastrophically aggressive thrusting movements with her pelvis and lower back in order to break the paralyzing impact of the massive contracting upon her respiratory tract.

It is prototypical to second stage dearmoring for there to occur again and again and again a reversal between a melting of the armoring and a reassertion of the armoring such as we see here with Ruth. This particular cycle perhaps is the most upsetting and anxiety-making alternation phenomenon of second stage. There is a catastrophic quality to it almost everytime it happens, pushing the conservative energy economy to the extreme limits of its toleration. Accompanying this reversal is a retrogression from a convergence-equalization patterning of the energy to a charge-discharge-driven externalization of stasis energy patterning, such as happened here with Ruth.

If the patient can rise to the emergency-like, catastrophe-threatening nature of these sudden transitions from melting to freezing-up again, but freezing-up in the most exaggeratedly extreme way, the rewards on the further side of the experience are enormous, both biodynamically and psychodynamically. Let us briefly recall Ruth's rewards as an illustration. First, biodynamically. After laying horizontally immobile on the mattress for several minutes in silence, during which time Katherine and I did and said nothing, she rolled over on her back very, very slowly, as if she were drugged, and after another minute said: "I feel full, like I'm gaining weight. Does that make any sense?" She then proceeded to describe how positively marvellous she felt being more fully in her body than she had ever known before. Following the massive reassertion of her mesodermal and endodermal armoring and its extreme recontracting, she obviously let go more fully and subsided into an equally extreme state of armor-free fluid vegetative flow whose circulation between her central and peripheral regions of her organism included the blood flow in its embrace. She was able to directly sense the blood flow streaming through her total organism unimpededly. The latter feature is one of the more important characteristics of having experiences of feeling states which presuppose the capacity for full horizontal groundedness, the subject-matter of the next section.

Secondly, let us review the psychodynamic rewards of her fourth session's dramatic reversal of energy patternings, but briefly because they have already been dealt with at length in chapter one. These psychodynamic rewards can be summed up as the emergence of her Logos dynamic feeling capacity throughout the week-end following her fourth session. I refer to her initial discovery of how to allow waking phantasies to guide her with extraordinary intuitive accuracy into confronting her night dreams as well as her body's pattern of chronic muscular armoring. Both achievements were beyond her capacity previous to her fourth session because of the dominance of her closed cortico-cerebrospinal circuits and their paralyzing effect upon her psyche's intuitive potentialities.

An essential prerequisite to the emergence of logos was a deeper equalization of her entire energy economy than she had ever experienced as an adult. She needed to spend several hours alone in her hotel room resting quietly and living exclusively in the here and now from moment to moment before logos could appear in the form of an imaginal consciousness that could penetrate appearances and go to the inner essences of her embodied soul. The emergence of logos is usually the last of the four dynamic feeling needs to flower during the dearmoring process of the second stage of treatment. It cannot emerge, even for a brief period, until there has been established a fairly substantial longitudinal vegetative energy flow in the regions of the upper back, the neck, and the head itself. It was the latter biodynamic development during the fourth session that opened the gates to the more subtle revelations that happened to Ruth in consciousness over the week-end, permitting her to acquire an almost visionary X-ray-like capacity to visualize the truth - the objective truth - of her embodied soul's internal battlefields. She was able to bring to bear upon her battered and still actively suffering interior Being centers a higher synthesis between perceptual-cortical and sensory-motor-affective subcortical modes of cognition, which is precisely the distinguishing virtue of the logos feeling-mediated need. She finally understood what it meant to be armored and deprived of her mother's love since early childhood. This newly acquired knowledge contributed decisively to the further polarization of her back half feeling centers during the sixth session of her intensive.

V. <u>The Fourth Pattern of Healthy Energy Change</u>

<u>The pattern:</u> <u>Once the hardened mesodermal or endodermal layers have been softened from within by a center-to-periphery circulation of fluid energy flow, it then becomes possible for the energy currents to slowly crystallize three very unique formations. In the first formation, that of full vertical grounding, or pattern A, the predominating energy current flows up and down the back in the region of the spinal column from the feet to the cortex. This energy current is highly channeled as well as rapid in its tempo of flow, being circumscribed by the mesodermal and ectodermal tissues adjacent to the spinal column. Such an energy current facilitates the volitional Being centers of the back half to function congruently with the cerebral cortex in the service of making subject-object creative encounters with the outer world. In the second formation, that of full horizontal grounding, or energy pattern B, there is established an energy current that is predominatingly four-directional. There is a horizontal movement from front to back at both ends of the spinal column and simultaneously a longitudinal movement upwards and downwards. Both directions of movements are primarily endodermal in their orbit of localization with the currents remaining confined to an expanded front half region that temporarily obliterates the functioning of the mesodermal musculature. In the third formation, that of full embodied soul grounding, or energy pattern C, there is established an energy current that is also predominatingly four-directional. However, this current does not remain confined either to the mesodermal and ectodermal layers, as in full vertical grounding, or to the endodermal layer, as in full horizontal grounding, but by moving from front to back at both ends of the spinal column and diagonally across the diaphragm in the middle of the torso simultaneously, integrates the three layers into a predominantly endodermal fluid flow. These three distinct energy patterns make possible three distinct modes of being-in-the-</u>

world and being-for-oneself respectively: egoic coping, oceanically undifferentiated, and integrative middle-in-mode modes. (see pages 138, 139 and 140).

The clinical basis for attributing to these three styles of grounding an equal significance as preconditions to self-actualizing functioning arises from my recognition of the fundamental polarity between the front half and the back half primary dynamic Being centers. Although the final objective is clearly a reconciliation of these opposite polarities, the crystallization of four distinct feeling circuits and energy fields rests first upon the emergence of energy patterns of full vertical and full horizontal grounding. The polarity between the front half and the back half dynamic Being centers is so powerful that either energy pattern A or energy pattern B usually must prevail throughout the long second stage of dearmoring. It should be obvious to the reader how there is a direct correlation, or cause-and-effect relationship, between becoming vertically grounded fully and the deployment of energy flow that happens when the self-assertive volitional centers are affirmed or strengthened, as well as a direct correlation between becoming horizontally grounded fully and the deployment of the energy flow that happens when the self-surrendering centers of the front half are affirmed and strengthened. Both sets of polarities need enormous amounts of reaffirmation and strengthening throughout the long second stage of dearmoring before there can be any realistic possibility of full embodied soul grounding.

I feel deeply indebted to the thinking of David Smith in a series of articles written by him for the neo-Reichian Journal Energy and Character. Smith was the first thinker to postulate the fundamental importance of both horizontal grounding and vertical grounding as indispensable to self-actualizing functioning. He helped me greatly to appreciate the fundamental differences between the two types of grounding and to evolve the theory of healthy energy change being formulated here. Although I had known it intuitively for many, many years, I could not formulate in clear theoretical constructs how the basis of my original style of body psychotherapy rested upon an affirming of both horizontal and vertical styles of grounding with equal emphasis. I fully agree with Smith that to be vertically grounded only does not

Self-Actualizing Energy Pattern A

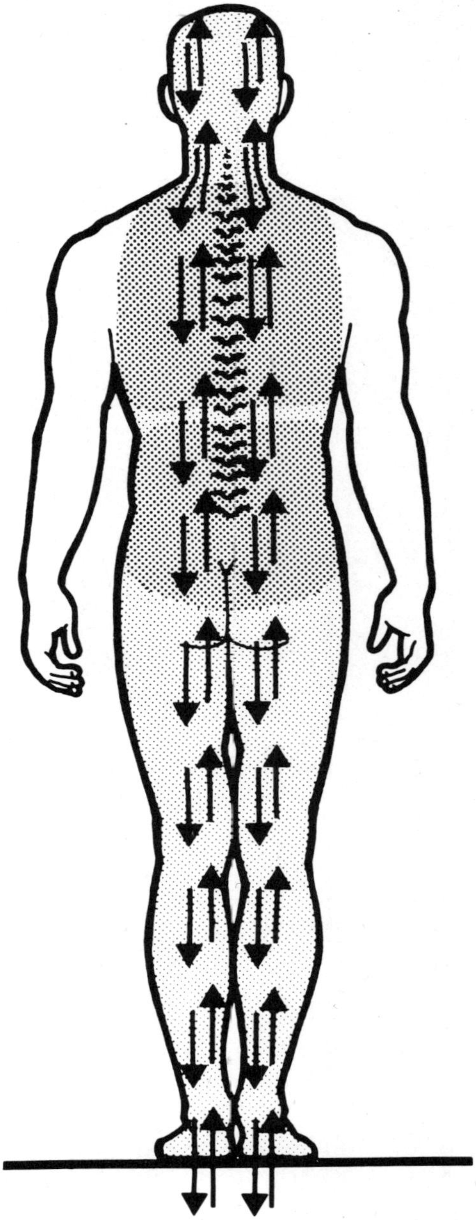

Full Vertical Grounding

Self-Actualizing Energy Pattern B

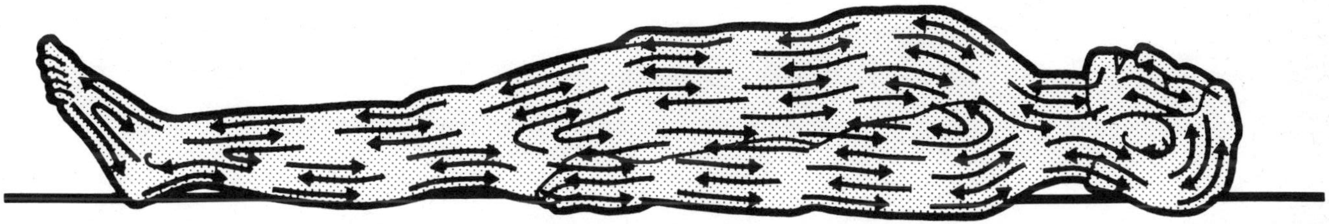

Full Horizontal Grounding

Self-Actualizing Energy Pattern C

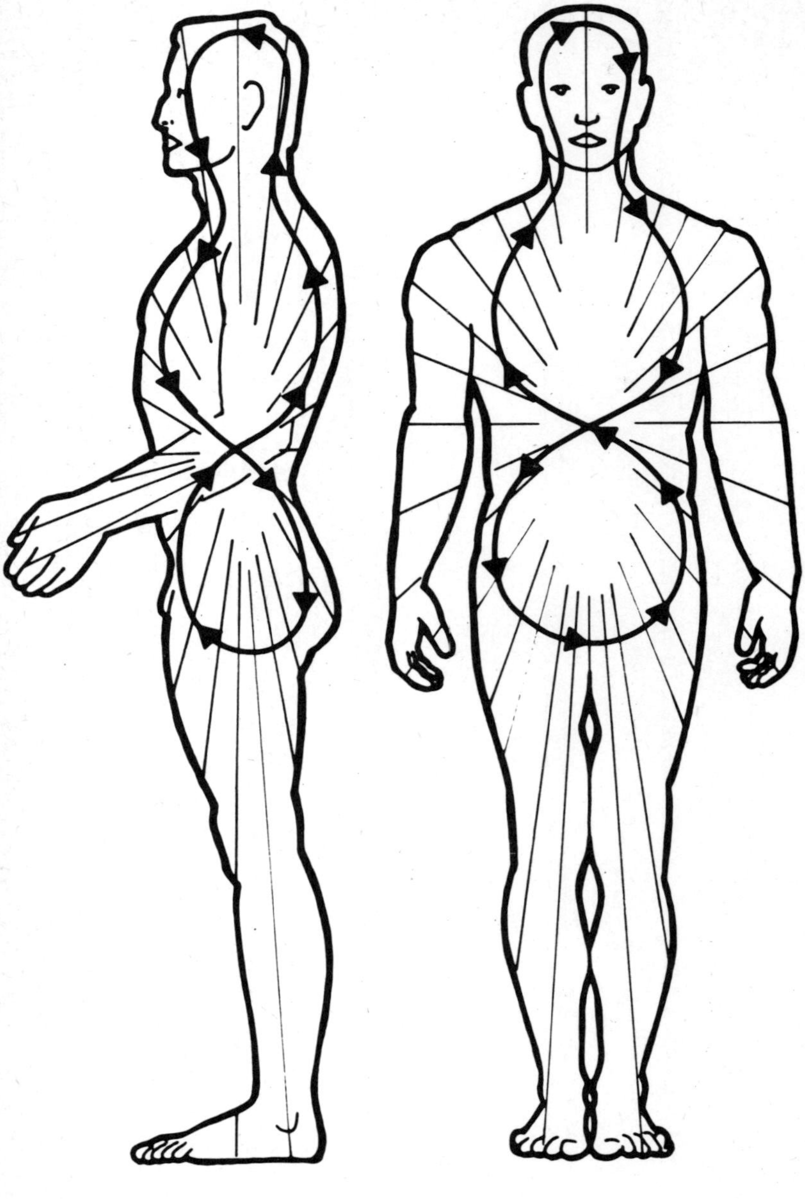

Full Embodied Soul Grounding

constitute armorfree functioning, and in this respect I must part company with the orthodox Lowenian position which makes precisely this presupposition the cornerstone of both its metaphysics and its methods. To quote Smith :

> "Neither overgrounded nor undergrounded characters are able to ground adequately in either a horizontal or vertical way; they are incapable of both full orgasmic surrender, oceanic fusion, 'letting go' (horizontal grounding) and a real feeling of their own separateness, individuality, boundedness (vertical grounding). An individual who is inadequately grounded is not able to engage fully in either self-transcendence (horizontal grounding) or self-assertion (vertical grounding)." (*)

Smith arrived at this psychodynamic hypothesis as a way of unifying the biodynamic thinking of Wilhelm Reich with the object-relations thinking of the Scottish psychoanalyst Donald Fairbairn, and as elaborated upon subsequently by the British psychoanalysts, Winnicott and Guntrip. In his efforts to articulate a comprehensive and coherent theory of psychodynamic individual development, Smith arrived at the conclusion that all psychopathology consists becoming stuck between the mode of being-in-the-world described by Fairbairn as infantile dependence, which at the biodynamic level resembles in most respects being horizontally grounded according to energy pattern B, and the mode of being-in-the-world described by Fairbairn as mature dependency, which is functionally identical at the biodynamic level to energy pattern C. According to Smith the neurotic fears both full horizontal grounding and full vertical grounding, and consequently clings to various psychodynamic patterns of quasi-independence. The latter amount to the various constellations of the false self system referred to in the previous chapters, all of which are characterized by remaining arrested at some point in the various transitional developmental periods between infancy and adult maturity.

My own clinical observations regarding the changing patterns of healthy energy flow during the dearmoring process have brought me to a theoretical

(*) "Birth and Submergence", p. 22, Energy and Character, Voluma II, No. 1, 1980.

position very akin to David Smith's. I have observed again and again how each type of rigid character-muscular structure - the phallic-narcissist, the obsessional, the hysteric, the passive-feminine - has displayed, each in his own stuck way, a clinging to a chronically overgrounded vertical set of defenses, or egoic cerebralized mode of being-in-the-world, in order to deny or distort an underlying fear of falling into a state of being-in-the-world that reflects full horizontal groundedness at the biodynamic level. The fear of fully affirming their self-surrendering feeling capacities for relatedness towards their primary love relationships is too enormous even to be faced by the majority of rigid types until advanced second stage of dearmoring, and even then it takes on the quality of a demonic struggle between opposing forces within the psyche. Vertically overgrounded character structures have far more than their stuckness in an Aedipal fixation to the parent of the opposite sex to work through. They have further to work through letting go the smoothly coordinated controls of their back half mesodermal and ectodermal energy flow and falling forwards and downwards into the nebulous vastnesses and boundarylessness of themselves when they become energetically fused with their beloved during sexual intercourse. Vertically overgrounded character structures cling defensively to their identification of their embodied parts with their back half voluntary musculature, and continue to cling even after as much as two thirds of their mesodermal armoring has melted out of sheer terror at falling into a primal, foetal, floating-like state of full horizontal groundedness. David Smith is absolutely right.

I am personally convinced that consummatory sexual lovemaking is distinguished less by the fear of the high excitation and charging up that accompanies orgasm than by the greater fear of losing one's familiar vertical boundaries in the four-directional energy currents of the endodermal front half flow. In this respect I once again challenge Reich and Lowen in their tendency to overestimate the primary importance of energy charge and energy discharge in relation to healthy sexuality. The latter is one among many determining biodynamic factors, to be sure, but certainly not the most important one to fulfilling adult sexuality. The psychodynamic movement out of convergency into increasing divergency presented in subsequent chapters - or what I also call the creative disintegration process - is a movement ultimately towards a species of fulfilling sexuality in which full horizontal groundedness of the fluid energy flow opens us all to the cosmic transpersonal instinctual sources within. Reich would tend to dismiss such a portrayal of healthy sexuality as mystical, and Lowen similarly. Neither thinker can appreciate the primary importance of full horizontal grounding of the energy currents to healthy sexuality, given their own bias towards perceiving sexuality in terms of back-half-dominant, orgasm-obsessed, primitive phallic performance. And the same can be said for Masters and Johnson.

An important corollary of the fourth pattern of healthy energy change is that it is the gradual crystallization of the two absolutely opposite constellations of the energy flow in terms of vertical and horizontal grounding that is the reason for the tremendous upheaval and chaos at all levels throughout the long second stage. Not only is there at stake the undermining and eventual dissolution of the closed and charge-discharge-imploded cortico-cerebrospinal circuits, together with the armored mesodermal and endodermal layers. There is also the unpredictable and revolution-making business of a gradual polarization and filling in and affirming of the more underevolved of the four primary dynamic feeling capacities for relatedness. For instance, with vertically overgrounded types of character structure it is usually the two front half feeling centers that are the most underevolved, and consequently it is an extremely see-saw-like business of oscillation between extreme opposite reactions to gradually facilitate the patient's approaching of full biodynamic horizontal groundedness. With vertically undergrounded types of character structure - orals, schizoids, true paranoids, and masochists - it is usually the back half feeling centers that are the most underevolved. And it takes even longer to affirm, polarize and fill in the holes of the vertically undergrounded character's energy fields than it does to open the vertically overgrounded to their front half feeling capacities.

Perhaps the one most essential reason behind the chaos and upheaval of second stage is the impact that the affirming of both vertical and horizontal groundedness has upon the psyche and soul, tossing the latter about like twigs and broken branches in a vast sea of unknown and always changing energy currents. The more stasis energy is freed from its anchored embeddedness in maintaining stable boundaries between the antagonistic energy networks within the no-man's-land regions, the more unpredictable and heavier becomes the sea of fluid energy flow newly released to travel along new underwater channels. It is precisely the latter development that unleashes new kinds of anxiety and insecurity within the psyche and soul, and unless the psychotherapist knows what he is releasing inside the patient's organism, he will eventually overflood and engulf the patient's psyche and soul. This is especially the case when using catalytic energy-mobilization methods that focus too one-sidedly upon the more underevolved energy fields and shadow soul centers of the patient. Gayle was a good example of the psychotherapist's blindness to the impact of energy-mobilization techniques upon the patient's psyche and soul, and this during the first stage of treatment.

A much happier outcome in the use of catalytic rather than exclusively nurturing energy-mobilization methods is to be found in Ruth's sixth intensive session. Ruth was able during the course of this single session to move away from her neurotic mechanisms of pseudo-independence towards fuller vertical grounding and then swing over towards affirming a fuller horizontal grounding. She was able to move in both directions during the same session with minimal upheaval and anxiety on account of the relative lightness of her muscular armoring and her relatively well-evolved intuitive Being centers of her front half. The latter virtue often is one of the secret strengths of vertically undergrounded types.

She was well-prepared for her dramatic achievements and energy metamorphoses of her sixth session. Her week-end self-initiated guided phantasy trip through her body had opened her intuitive Logos faculty to new horizons regarding the extent to which her hitherto severely Christianized soul resided in her body more than in her mind-brain. She was ready for launching herself into the kind of energy-mobilization of her back half energy fields that normally threatens vertically undergrounded types. Her initial work in the vertical position on her feet rapidly deanesthetized the paralysis generated in her legs from Katherine's starting direct touch to her feet and legs. In spite of suffering the considerable physical discomforts of nausea in the belly, further paralysis in the legs, strong neck pains, and increasingly constricting pains in the chest, she persevered with the vertical grounding work without becoming overflooded with anxiety.

It was she who soon siezed the initiative after the starting of the session at structuring a progressive charging up of her back half energy fields by placing her feet against my chest when she was lying on her back. The self-assertive quality of her movements that were awakened from taking this position while using the direct touch with my body as an object to resist against provided a kind of unconsciously ingenious prelude to what was to follow. She succeeded from this one position alone to mobilize a more vital and quickened energy flow along the mesodermal and ectodermal tissue of her spinal column than any she had arrived at during previous sessions. The after-effect was totally desireable as well as fully immediate and here-and-now: namely, a creatively regressive return to an almost infantile level of screaming and wailing in anger that at the same time was endodermally rooted and hence discharged large masses of stasis energy throughout her organism internally.

The creative regression psychically did not satisfy her for some reason and she chose to return to mobilizing in the here-and-now her back half energy fields, progressively polarizing the energy flow in her lower back half near her pelvis. The latter achievement prompted a massive coughing attack that produced a further disintegration of her endodermal stasis holding by virtue of awakening a vital urge to surpass the choking and loss of breath that accompanied the coughing attack. She had obviously at this point reached her organismic threshhold of toleration towards fuller vertical grounding, and relapsed into a relatively withdrawn mode of being-in-the-world that at the same time spontaneously affirmed a tendency to swing over to further horizontal grounding again.

The subsequent unfolding of her rebirth experience could not have happened, to be sure, without Katherine's guiding presence and nurturing and catalytic touches. Nevertheless, the rebirth experience could not have occurred in such a smoothly positive and anxiety-free manner unless Ruth's internal energy currents were not fully primed and prepared for the event. Almost paradoxically, Ruth's reexperiencing of her birth, although more broadly speaking it reflected a movement towards fuller horizontal grounding, at the same time permitted her to actualize what was not permitted her in her actual childhood: an affirming of her extensor muscles in her legs and pelvis-leg joints against the interior walls of her actual mother's womb in such a manner as to further her vertical grounding up and down her back from her feet upwards. To save her mother from unnecessary anguish during her actual birth, she had inhibited her spontaneously aggressive thrusting of her legs that one associates with the natural movements of the birth reflex. This inhibiting of her extensors of her legs by her reactor muscles before she was even born had to be reexperienced and reversed in terms of the energy currents before Ruth could truly be said to begin to become vertically grounded.

The fact that Ruth's experience of her birth contains energetic components both towards fuller vertical and horizontal groundedness simultaneously stamps the event as belonging more to energy pattern C than to energy pattern B. She was having a peak experience of total characterological growth, which is the unique psychodynamic feature of energetic experiences of full embodied soul grounding, or energy pattern C. The latter type of grounding happens most frequently during the third stage of treatment, when the higher individuation needs for self-actualization regulate the energy economy. The latter needs relate explicitly, in my personal understanding, to the emergence of the intuitive faculties of the core self and the latter's establishment of a middle-in-mode balancing between the dynamic polarities of the four Being centers of the embodied soul.

Ruth's entire personality structure was altered from having this single peak experience of her birth. In other words, it amounted to something more than an evanescent shaking up of her energy economy and a loosening of her stasis energy. It was an experience of transformation, in the sense that the very boundaries of her psychological self-identity were expanded, making it possible for her to establish a fuller centering of her identity in her endodermal fluid energy flow and its greater integration with her mesodermal and ectodermal tissues from her feet upwards. The experience facilitated a further shifting of the axis of her psychological boundaries downwards out of her mind-brain into her embodied parts.

By experiencing herself in terms of an original natural harmony of being, she was regressing to early childhood and having an experience that belongs to the floating, foetal-like altered states of consciousness that energy pattern B make possible, which is always oceanically tension-free and predominantly undifferentiated and diffuse. But her experience did not remain except for a few minutes undifferentiated and diffuse, and blissfully child-like in its unity and simplicity. Otherwise she could not have actively resisted my willful efforts to get her back on her feet and back into her head. Her spiritual warrior intuitive faculty resisted me effectively, and by remaining in the horizontal position for the remainder of the session she was able to reap the many benefits of the four-directional energy flow that prevailed within her body and at the same time make creative use of her intuitive logos faculty.

The latter could not have flowered so richly unless her endodermal vegetative flow had found the vitality to penetrate from below upwards the inner, middle, and outer regions of her brain - and especially the diencephalon, which stands between the middle brain and the cerebral hemispheres and contains the hypothalamus. It is one of my subjective intuitive convictions, based on my clinical observations, that the dearmoring process is not completed until the endodermal vegetative flow has extended itself into the diencephalon area and by so doing accomplished the last major biodynamic step towards disisolating the closed cortico-cerebrospinal circuits. In Ruth's case it was the simultaneous radiation of her endodermal vegetative flow upwards into her diencephalon area and downwards into her legs and feet that permitted her intuitive faculty of logos to make many growth-enhancing cognitive-intuitive connections between her adult armoring and the events surrounding her actual birth.

It was not a freakish accident that Ruth managed

to have a peak experience of embodied soul groundedness during her sixth session following the events which preceded it, both during and prior to the session. On both of the latter occasions she displayed an increasing facility for spontaneously polarizing her back half energy fields and their inclination towards a greater vertical groundedness. In terms of her characterological patterning of tensions she was more undergrounded vertically than horizontally. This particular patterning unconsciously propelled and guided her awakening fluid vegetative flow to polarize the shadow energy fields of her back half, and particularly those from the pelvis-leg joints downwards. The latter regions had to be polarized again and again and again, being her weakest and most isolated organismic parts, before their integration into the longitudinal endodermal vegetative flow facilitated a total regression backwards in time to the event in her early development which began the stasis-building process, namely, her birth.

Ruth's case reflects what usually happens to vertically undergrounded character-muscular types once the back half energy fields from the feet upwards are awakened spontaneously from within. They then exhibit almost an uncanny astuteness at creatively regressing to those events from their early years that have held them bound in energy stasis and psychodynamic arrestment of normal development. Like Ruth, they can find the right combination of energy-mobilization exercises and bring themselves to a fuller horizontal and vertical groundedness during the most minimal time possible, and then proceed to carry through the gains made by allowing their intuitive logos faculty to arrive at higher syntheses between cortical and subcortical cognitive processes, wedding rationality with instinct.

A vastly diverse state of affairs prevails clinically when vertically overgrounded character-muscular types - that is, all rigid types - begin to awaken their shadow energy fields in their front half regions. In my experience there does not unfold a evenly progressive and continuous opening of their front half soul centers. To the contrary, a very long series of extreme alternations between falling into their unsatisfied front half feeling needs and retreating from even recognizing the priority of those needs ensues. It has much to do with the greater tenacity and intertwining of their egoic defenses with their overcharged and well-coordinated mesodermal voluntary musculature. A far greater biodynamic revolution must first occur with rigid types than with vertically undergrounded types before they can risk becoming more horizontally grounded. Christa, the case example which occupies the clinical subject-matter of the next seven chapters, will demonstrate this vividly.

Another implication of this fourth pattern of energy change is the growth in the range of potential modes of being-in-the-world and being-for-oneself that become available to the person who becomes adept at feeling at ease in a position of vertical groundedness, horizontal groundedness, or embodied soul groundedness. Modes of being characteristic of full horizontal groundedness have a pure primary-process, pleasure-oriented floating quality to them. Since they are mediated by the front half Being centers exclusively, and in particular the Hara center of the abdominal cavity, they remain oceanic and subterranean in nature, essentially undifferentiated in the sense that they remain passively non-engaged with the outer world. These are the modes of the life-sustaining positive id, full of boundaryless reverie and innocent absorption in disconnected sensations and feelings that come and go from moment to moment. Modes of being characteristic of full embodied soul groundedness are more core-self-centered, and hence always more individuated and subject-object-relationship-oriented while at the same time mediated through the here-and-now vegetative energy circuits of the front half Being centers. In chapter twelve there will be presented five distinct categories of such 'higher' pleasures, involving in every case a middle-in-mode balancing between the vertically grounded Being centers of the back half and the horizontally grounded Being centers of the front half. Modes of being characteristic of full vertical groundedness have a more egoically charged, world-conquering quality to them. They come into dominance whenever there is required an active concentration and focusing of all of our energy circuits and rational consciousness upon some challenging outer world reality. They are goal-directed and volitionally achievement-oriented.

In a very loose sense one can say that the tendency towards full horizontal groundedness is synonymous with the pleasure principle, whereas the tendency towards full vertical groundedness is synonymous with the reality principle. Here I want to challenge the orthodox Lowenian bioenergetic rendering of the pleasure and reality principles. According to Lowen:

> ". . . the act of reaching out is itself the basis for the experience of pleasure. It represents an expansion of the total organism, a flow of feeling and energy to the periphery of the organism and the world."

Such a rendering is for me far too outer-world-directed, far too action-performance-oriented, and far too Western-World-Americanized mesodermal-ectodermal in nature to describe the essence of pleasure in any of its many manifestations. My understanding of pleasure is that its biodynamic essence can best be distilled into the law of equalization and naturally preferred behavior in the sphere of immediacy as postulated by Goldstein, or into what Gerde Boyesen calls endodermally centered vegetative peristalsis. It is a far more passive, actionless, non-reaching-out kind of engagement than that which Lowen portrays, and has nothing to do with the outer world. It amounts to a kind of choiceless receptivity to and fused submergence in the inner world of fluid energy flow and imaging which constitutes the adult psyche and soul when non-engaged with outer reality.

I also want to challenge Lowen's rendering of the reality principle as consisting of a very literal and mechanistically reductive mobilization of one's vital energy in one's feet in the vertical position and how this grounding to the earth generates a high tension electrical circuit of charge and discharge constantly throughout the organism. Such a rendering reflects Lowen's fixation to a extroverted, vertically overgrounded, and phallically overcharged presentation of what reality is really about. My understanding of the reality principle is that its biodynamic essence can best be distilled into the centered organism's capacity for maintaining differentiated figure-background excitation gestalts that enable a person to convergently focus upon and creatively adjust to outer realities adequately during the earlier decades of life. However, once the individuated core self assumes increasing dominance, the reality principle and the pleasure principle cease to exist as separate or contrasting entities. Thereafter it is the evolution of the spiritual intuitive faculties of the core self and their perpetually changing balancing of the energy fields and instinctual inclinations of the four dynamic Being centers that define the pleasure and reality principles equally. Objective reality and subjective pleasure become inseparably interwoven to the extent that both become agents and consequences of the pursuit of intrinsic universal values. When a person becomes fully grounded in his or her embodied soul and psyche, facts and values and needs become integrated into a single unitary whole.

VI. The Three Stages of Treatment

We are now ready to attempt a formulation of a sequence of events that unfold in a continuum with fairly regular occurrence during the long course of Organismic Psychotherapy. From the broadest possible perspective I divide our style of body psychotherapy into three stages. Here in this chapter I shall try to state the more important biodynamic sequence of events that happen, and leave the psychodynamic and interpersonal changes that happen uniquely during each stage to subsequent chapters.

A. The First Stage of Treatment

The gaining of the patient's respect and confidence in the therapist is perhaps omnipresent throughout first stage. We all have within us a fear of depending upon anyone else to help us change ourselves. The greater our need to change, the greater is our fear of dependency upon the other whom we seek out for help. Consequently, during the initial phases of treatment the therapist should respect this fear of himself within the patient, as well as the patient's self-defeatist, games-playing need to deny his fear. From his front half dynamic Being centers the therapist needs to emanate an unconditional positive regard and respect for the patient in the face of also sensing at the same time the patient's fear and denial of his fear and often hardly concealed negative expectations of the therapist. A positive transference towards the therapist must slowly and carefully be built by the therapist. Otherwise, the patient cannot feel secure or safe enough during the sessions to permit the therapist to begin to relate directly to his body in unavoidably intrusive ways.

The challenge of the first stage of treatment is to shake up and loosen the rigid deployment of energy circuits that have been established in order to maintain the closed cortico-cerebrospinal network without undermining the patient's ego defenses to a point where he cannot feel safe and secure in the relationship to the therapist. What this implies is that the therapist who is too one-dimensionally goal-directed towards loosening the muscular armoring will usually be over-intrusive in terms of his or her impact upon the patient's psyche. This is particularly true with vertically undergrounded patients, who need large amounts of time in the presence of the therapist during which no overt bodywork is happening. Then, even after a positive transference relationship of trust and a feeling of safety and emotional security has been established with the patient, the bodywork has to unfold slowly enough to give the patient time to recover from the shaking up and loosening of his muscular armoring that overt bodywork entails. The wise humanistic body psychotherapist will not overextend the patient's organismic or psychological threshholds of toleration even during the session following overt bodywork. He will, in other words, not push for bodywork even during first stage that threatens to overflood the patient's egoic defenses beyond very definite limits. Time for equalization following overt bodywork will be carefully estimated with each patient, and the more vertically undergrounded the patient's energy patterns are, the more time the therapist will allow during each session for the equalization process to occur.

With vertically overgrounded types one can risk pushing overt bodywork with more persistence and less fear of overextending the patient's organismic and/or psychological threshholds of toleration. This goes with their possession of an overcharged and overloaded back half and a hardened mesodermal wall over most parts of their body. Given the greater toughness of their hardened voluntary muscular wall, they can indeed tolerate a far more dramatically catalytic charge-discharge-oriented kind of body work without feeling overthreatened in terms of their intact defenses. Nevertheless, even with vertically overgrounded patterns it remains a constant temptation to the therapist to overpush catalytic charge-discharge-oriented kinds of bodywork which lead to clearly observable externalized results. Using some of our more catalytic styles of direct touch or do-it-yourself stress positions, it is relatively easy to provoke in these kinds of patients massive discharges of energy and explosions of negative affects that reach a primal level of intensity.

Such primaling, I have found, proves to be healing only to the extent that it is not externally provoked through the use of body methods instigated by the therapist. Primaling can be healing only if it erupts with absolute spontaneity from within the organismic endodermal depths of the patient. It cannot possibly erupt from the latter regions during the first stage of treatment with vertically overgrounded patterns except during the periods of energy equalization, or periods following overt catalytic bodywork during which time the therapist remains completely non-directive and does nothing except wait and watch the patient's reactions. Most primaling is counterfeit and phoney precisely because it originates in the mesodermal musculature in response to psychological messages communicated by the false cerebralized self which reigns supreme within the closed cortico - cerebrospinal circuits.

The challenge during the first stage of treatment when working with vertically overgrounded patterns is a more modest one than provoking primaling through the use of directive bodywork. It is simply to reduce the chronically high energy overload up and down the spinal column to the point where some amount of fluid vegetative flow can happen longitudinally across the diaphragm following overt catalytic bodywork. This is not as simply achieved in actuality as it can be stated in words. The project is always to undermine the closed cortico-cerebrospinal network through the diminishing of the adrenalin-sustained energy overload by virtue of loosening not only the voluntary muscles themselves but simultaneously mobilizing the fluid vegetative flow. It is a tricky, always individuated achievement to accomplish both energy changes more or less simultaneously.

The therapist has to run the risk of either overmobilizing or undermobilizing the intact mesodermal armoring while using catalytic charge-discharge-oriented methods. If he overmobilizes the armor, there will always be triggered off within the metabolism a neutralizing counter energy force of either an adrenergic or cholinergic nature, and this from my point of view is usually undesireable. If he undermobilizes the armor, there is not enough loosening of the voluntary muscles themselves brought about to shake up the no-man's-land region between the two antagonistic energy networks to permit a passage from the endodermal across to the alienated mesodermal musculature of limited amounts of fluid vegetative flow. It is much like walking a continual tightrope between too much mobilization and too little, but it must be walked, I say, in order to accomplish both a further loosening from within of the mesodermal musculature and at the same time reduce the total tension level of the energy overload up and down the back. It is this latter effect that prepares the organism of the patient for tolerating an expansion of consciousness towards facing the repressed affects from the unfinished feeling past that make their appearance with increasing spontaneity during the long second stage of treatment.

B. The Second Stage of Treatment

The second stage of treatment is ushered in as it gradually becomes possible for the energy economy to spontaneously initiate of its own accord, free from interventions by others, centrifugal surges and pulsations of fluid vegetative flow that move from the abdominal viscera outwards across the mesodermal sheath to the skin's surface and back again. With vertically overgrounded patterns these surges do have to pass through the mesodermal sheath, whereas with vertically undergrounded patterns the surges have to move longitudinally up and down the entire spinal column and back again since their exists no barrier-like mesodermal sheath.

The emergence of this spontaneous circulation of fluid energy flow from the center to the periphery of the body and back again, even when it is weak and short-lived and takes the form of incipient vegetative release reactions, cannot be ever underestimated by the practicing body psychotherapist. It signifies nothing less than that it is no longer possible for only the parts of the organism that are bound up by chronically stasis energy to be primarily mobilized with the use of energy-mobilization exercises to the relative neglect of the rest of the organism's energy economy. Hereafter unarmored parts, and the whole endodermal tissue region in particular, become capable of also being mobilized.

We are talking here about the emergence of an energy deployment that is peculiar to horizontal grounding. During the dearmoring process it is the emergence of horizontal grounding that alone guarantees, from my experience, the possibility for an authentically unitary and conflict-free participation of the total organism in the patient's here-and-now experiencing. In this regard I challenge the orthodox Lowenian metaphysics and practices and their tendency towards a blindly uni-dimensional emphasis upon facilitating vertical grounding as all that matters. The Lowenians do not appreciate the biodynamic reality that as long as the energy patterning is dominated by a charge-discharge-driven deployment of the energy flow, the total organism cannot possibly participate as a single unitary whole. For the latter to occur, especially when armoring still exists in the organism, it is only the spontaneous emergence of the longitudinal-centrifugal endodermal flow that has the power to truly integrate the total organism in the here-and-now. To be sure, such experiences of integration at the beginning of second stage must happen during periods of equalization rather than convergence of the energy economy, and hence tend to lead to a dedifferentiation of the energy flow internally. But these experiences of a simple unity of energy flow, however short-lived, are indispensable to the dearmoring process.

During the long second stage of treatment it is necessary for the humanistic body psychotherapist to affirm with equal emphasis the body's tendencies towards both a regression-inducing horizontal grounding and an ego-building vertical grounding. Affirming both organismic capacities makes in itself for great suffering, confusion, and chaos within the patient. This very fact makes it that more imperative that the therapist does not overpush the patient through the use of stress positions that in themselves generate more internal conflict between the armored and unarmored parts of the organism. Yet this is precisely what is generated by a uni-dimensional overemphasis upon vertical grounding exclusively, and why the Lowenian approach to experiences of pleasure is for me such a counterfeit one. A premature emphasis upon vertical grounding builds only the will, not the self-surrendering capacities which alone provide a path to true pleasure. Only the Eastern attitude and approach towards life grasps this truth, while the Western approach, including that of the Lowenians, remains always circumscribed and essentially trapped in a will-building metaphysics and an exclusively ego-building set of long-range clinical objectives. The emergence of the universal, transpersonal faculties of the id are completely sacrificed.

The path to the latter is through the progressive emergence of the person's awareness of his or her unsatisfied primary dynamic feeling needs for relatedness. This awareness will almost necessarily and inevitably manifest itself as the tendency towards regression-inducing horizontal grounding unfolds. If the latter tendency is overemphasized, as it tends to be among practicing orthodox Reichians whose vegetotherapeutic direct touch methods ignore altogether the importance of vertical grounding, the primary dynamic feeling needs of the back half are eclipsed and passed over in favor of the front half dynamic needs.

One of our best criteria for judging whether or not we are affirming equally the biodynamic inclinations towards both vertical and horizontal grounding is the extent to which the axis of the person's body-image moves downwards out of the head towards the diaphragm region and pelvic areas, both front and back. This gradual descent of the center of one's embodied self-identity goes hand in hand with the gradual diminishing of a chronic high tension overload generated by the closed cortico-cerebrospinal circuits up and down the spinal column between the brain and the genitals. This gradual descent out of the head also relates to the manner in which the four dynamic Being centers of the embodied soul are polarized and affirmed by the therapist in the patient. Both the back half and the front half dynamic feeling capacities for relatedness have to be affirmed alternatingly throughout the long second stage by the therapist in order to bring about the crystallization of the endodermally centered core self, which is essentially a product of the third stage of treatment.

One of our best tools for judging the extent to which the axis of the patient's body-image is moving downwards out of the head is how well the patient can permit a convergence of his focal attention to those body parts that continue to remain isolated off and resist absorption into the endodermal vegetative flow. For this focussing of consciousness to happen presupposes the formation of a figure-background excitation gestalt throughout the total organism that can maintain itself with relative stability long enough to permit an objectified body part to become centered in awareness. But this is not enough. In order to be able to focus with objective accuracy upon our subjective body parts there must also exist a fluid vegetative flow that can pass unimpededly between the endodermal, mesodermal, and ectodermal tissues, thereby providing us with a vitalized set of proprioceptive and kinaesthetic sensations which rise upwards and fuse with consciousness. Once the patient has acquired this ability to focus upon selected body parts, and particularly those that resist the fluid vegetative flow, he alone can truly know how to further his own dearmoring process, and never the therapist.

C. The Third Stage of Treatment

The third stage of treatment is the time when the process-oriented core self becomes sufficiently solidified to assume dominance over the old structure-bound cerebralized self-system. The magic "it" during third stage is pure and total process flow from moment to moment. It is the time when the embodied soul and transcendental psyche have acquired the fluidity to discover how to create one's very boundaries of self-identity from moment to moment, how to actualize, that is, different modes of beingness-for-self and beingness-for-others. It is the time when the religious dimensions of learning how to create, share, and perpetuate intrinsic universal, transpersonal values and higher pleasures becomes the primary motivation of the individual.

For such process flow from moment to moment at the psychic level to have substance, depth, continuity, and form it must be firmly rooted in the organism's naturally spontaneously self-regulative capacities. The latter are for me centered only in the endodermal layer in the form of a constantly quiet but steady circulation of the blood flow that moves diagonally, vertically, horizontally, and in every other imaginable direction. The energy flow has reached an oceanic stage of fluidity which defies any further scientific attempts to measure or observe its currents or logically dissect its structure. The living flow has finally triumphed over logical analysis.

What is important to point out about this oceanic stage of fluid energy flow is how great has become the territorial influence of the endodermal tissues and organs. It's as if the latter have expanded to actively embrace in its range and sweep of blood flow as much as ninety-five percent of the body's substance, including the head region. The entire blood-vascular network, comprising the arteries, arterioles, capillaries, venules, and veins, extends into every nerve and muscle complex of the body, permeating the thickest voluntary muscles of the back, from the neck to the pelvis-leg joints. The hitherto separated off mesodermal sheath has become incorporated, it would seem, into the instantaneous web-like functioning of the endodermal energy flow. Although there is no diagram that can be drawn that adequately depicts the patterns of the latter, one could say that it's as if there existed a chain of many different figure of eights. One huge one is located in the front half of the body with its central crossover point placed two to three inches below the diaphragm - at the precise point designated by Japanese Zen doctrine as the "Ki", or life energy center. Then there is a column of little figure of eights that sit on top of each other up and down the spinal column and resemble in many ways the chakras of Indian doctrine.

I believe the most important as well as most powerful energy center of the endodermal flow is the Hara, or "Ki", energy center. It is this center that provides a self-actualizing adult with an inner source of spontaneous self-regulation capable of balancing the spiritual opposites of the embodied soul. I also believe that it is more feminine than masculine in nature, and hence peace-giving, quiet, deep, and fundamentally earth-polarized. It is the very guardian and container of our ongoing core self, and the final product of the horizontal grounding process of second stage. It is this center whose flowering obligates the wise psychotherapist during the third stage of treatment to encourage if not demand without words that the patient is responsible for making all decisions regarding whatever body exercises are employed and when throughout the whole session.

The column of crisscrossing smaller figure of eights that weave up and down the spinal column, from the tailbone to the cerebral cortex, are more masculine than feminine in nature. It is these energy centers that provide meaning and differentiated structure to person-to-person, person-to-universe, subject-object relationships under the intuitive guidance of the logos and spiritual warrior faculties of the will. It is also the function of these masculine energy centers to assume dominance whenever some outer world threat to safety and survival requires that there be polarized a quickened, adaption-oriented response to the outer reality. Then the two energy centers of the back half, the cortex and the genitals, intermingle creatively to meet and resolve the threatening outer reality. These centers are functionally more brain-polarized and will-polarized than pleasure-oriented, and hence are polarized upwards towards heaven rather than downwards towards the earth. But the heavens in question are neither transcendental nor spiritual in nature, but purely and pragmatically ectodermal-mesodermal survival-motivated. This is because it is these centers that ignite a coordinated use of the ectodermal-mesodermal apparatus and its superior confrontative focussing upon making actively differentiated responses to outer world realities. These energy centers represent the final product of the vertical grounding process of second stage. During the third stage of treatment the wise psychotherapist affirms their intuitive embodied soul aspects and hardly ever their survival-motivated functions unless the ego of the patient is still weaker than his core self.

Chapter IV

PITFALLS OF DIRECT TOUCH

Nurturing or Catalytic Touch ?

In the first stage of treatment, a therapist must facilitate a spontaneous discharge of chronic energy overload which moves outward to penetrate the tough outer rind of armoring. There is no formula for selecting the appropriate technique to mobilize enough fluid energy flow to penetrate the armor from within: what works for one client will not work for another. The more experienced the therapist, the more possibilities he can intuitively discard. Nonetheless, even the most seasoned therapist must initiate a trial and error process before he can discover the best method to break through the peripheral armoring.

A body psychotherapist actively directs the treatment, particularly in the earliest stages when the client's desperate underlying psychophysiological condition demands attention. However, the therapist cannot focus exclusively upon the client's desperate bioenergetic condition. If he proceeds one-dimensionally to blast away at the peripheral muscular sheath, the client will become overwhelmed by emotional disruption and physical pain. Therefore, the therapist must assume the responsibility of intuitively sensing the appropriate timing and level of concentration when using body methods.

A seasoned body therapist knows how far he can undermine the client's ego defenses by mobilizing internal fluid energy currents without overtaxing the defended psyche. He knows that the desperate client is totally unaware of his compulsive psychological need to perpetuate relative emotional isolation. This urge derives from the armored organism's need to maintain as deadened an energy economy as possible. The peripheral muscular sheath prevents the client from responding dynamically or spontaneously to any kind of immediate stimuli without a sense of impending catastrophe. For these reasons, a therapist must exercise considerable caution and restraint as he gradually facilitates the internal mobilization of energy flow within a client's organism.

While maintaining caution and restraint, a body therapist must also toe a narrow line between an excessively non-directive passivity and an actively directive posture. I explicitly denounce an exclusively Rogerian, non-directive style of orientation towards a desperate client. Rogerians naively believe that an unconditional positive regard, empathic understanding and willingness to disclose one's own immediate feelings in response to the client are sufficient to loosen the character-muscular armoring of the desperate neurotic. They believe that such a constellation of attitudes will polarize the client's organismic tendency towards self-actualization. By contrast, I believe such an orientation represents clinical and moral cowardice. Moreover, it greatly extends the treatment time.

The tendency towards self-actualization simply cannot be awakened until the peripheral rigid musculature is softened to the point where it can be spontaneously penetrated from within by the release of dammed-up organismic energies. The armored neurotic cannot know what he needs or what he feels as long as the peripheral armoring remains intact. The clients's isolation within his head, when fortified by his twisted will-to-suffer-and-to-survive, is too powerfully entrenched within the protective walls of the armoring to be affected by a therapist's affirmation on a feeling level. And only this level will generate the forces which facilitate healing, not the detached understanding of the analytical mind.

The Rogerians are right that the therapist's unconditional acceptance and respect for the patient can be an efficacious healing force from the outset of treatment. But this attitude cannot be deeply, objectively, truly felt by most clients with third-stage armoring until they reach the second stage of treatment. Then the peripheral armoring has loosened enough so that the primary dynamic feeling centers become accessible to polarization by the other-affirming feeling vibrations emanating from the therapist. And, unless a therapist feels an unconditional positive regard for the client's continuing need for his ego defense network from the outset of treatment, the therapist will not possess the emotional compassion and depth of intuition necessary to modulate the de-armoring process.

Coupled with the appropriate attitude, our body and psychic methods effectively disrupt the client's psychophysiological status quo. Their greatest hazard is that they are actually too effective in this regard. They can make too many processes, both psychological and physiological, happen too quickly and too forcefully for integration. If this happens, the still intact defenses of the client will rapidly reassert themselves with a ferocity incited by the very effectiveness with which they have just been temporarily overrun. They mount a massive counterphobic movement against the continuing effectiveness of these methods. The integrated regions of the client's ego will usually respond to this movement by terminating treatment out of sheer confusion and dread of further turmoil.

Given the potential hazard, a body therapist must steer a middle course between proceeding too quickly and too catalytically, on the one hand, and too slowly and too passively, on the other hand. He selects the right course by remaining attuned with respect and compassion to the client's condition. This is perhaps the only safeguard against overusing energy-mobilization methods, whether by themselves or interwoven with structured psychological methods. The treatment of any psychopathology ultimately depends upon the richness of psychological soul contact established between client and therapist. Ultimately, it is not a matter of the right techniques, the right theoretical constructs, the right verbal interpretations, or the right attitude towards the client. What authentically treats and, if sustained, will heal is the immediate generation of a circuit of primary-process feeling vibrations between therapist and client. It is the therapist's informed passion when directed towards the client's battered soul which has the power to heal.

Only the therapist's fully alive and present functioning of his own primary dynamic Being Centers can guide in the selection of energy-mobilization methods. This is doubly true when administering direct touch techniques. They should be used sparingly at first. They can be too frightening to the armored neurotic because of their directness. And when begun, the touch must be purely nurturing so as not to threaten the defended psyche. Even then, the touch should be confined to the safest, least sexually stimulating parts of the body -- the back of the neck, the top and back of the head, the outer shoulders, the feet and the hands. And the same nurturing touch sequence should be administered session after session until the client's body begins to definitely relax under the touch.

One fundamental problem with working too directly at the bioenergetic level during first stage is that the client is totally unconscious of his muscular armoring. The client does not realize that a third to half of his vital energy resources is used exclusively to feed the chronic energy collisions. Instead of reaching out towards productive subject-world encounters with objective novelties, this energy is fixated in maintaining a chronic impasse which is as much biological as it is psychological. Consequently, if the therapist does not proceed cautiously with energy-mobilization, this precarious impasse will capsize, resulting in emotional havoc rather than any immediate sense of relief from chronic tension.

A therapist must introduce energy-mobilization methods according to how they affect the client's conscious experience of them, rather than how they succeed at loosening the psychic impasses and energy collisions at the unconscious level. This point cannot be over-emphasized. Throughout treatment, a therapist must intuitively listen to and intrinsically respect the client's conscious receptivity to any energy mobilization methods. This is important even during first stage when the therapist must risk the most in upsetting the underlying psychological and biological impasse. Only an insensitive or inexperienced body therapist will not attentively gauge the impact of each body technique upon the defended dimensions of the client's ego.

If a client has the rigid kind of peripheral armoring which characterizes the compulsive type of neurotic character structure, it is seldom advisable during first stage to administer catalytic direct touch. Catalytic direct touch deliberately polarizes a localized energy flow in the area directly touched. It is the most assertive possible touch: the therapist places his finger tips and thumb upon narrowly defined spots of the peripheral muscular sheath. Using one or both hands, he either presses straight inwards against the peripheral muscle tissue and holds, or he presses inwards at an angle of introduction and then moves slowly along the contour of the primary muscle grouping which defines the body's surface at the actual point of contact.

Such a touch can be outrageously intrusive, particularly to someone rigidly armored at the body's surface. Because of the rigidly hardened musculature, a catalytic direct touch will rapidly evoke active resistance. This resistance will manifest itself at several levels. At the bioenergetic level, as described in the previous chapter, a counter energy current will almost instantly begin to resist such an intrusive touch. This localized reaction is characteristic of an emergency-oriented response to an external stimulus -- a catalytic touch does threaten to overwhelm the enormously raised stimulus threshold of a peripherally armored compulsive neurotic.

A shock of recoil ensues. The relative isolation of both the muscles actually touched and their antagonists which set up a counter current begin to mobilize a fullscale catastrophic panic reaction throughout the rest of the body. An initial adrenalin secretion from the endocrine glands behind the abdominal viscera is followed rapidly by a spiralling of a counter energy current so intense and energy-consuming as to eradicate any semblance of a differentiated figure-background excitation pattern. Overwhelmed emotionally, the client will either flee from or fight against any continued direct touch. This is precisely what happened to Gayle as described in earlier chapters.

A third possibility which reflects an even greater severity of chronic armoring, is that the client will freeze his energy responses to the point of active desensitivization, thereby shutting down any immediate awareness of his inner panic and peripheral physical pain. This often happens with schizoid clients who are able instinctively to stiffen both their total muscular sheath and the energy flow in the joints underneath, in order not to feel painful or frightening stimuli.

Any catalytic direct touch is probably too disruptive to the psychobiological impasse when it evokes an emergency-oriented response. Rather than facilitating any yielding, such a touch causes the armor to tighten at a bioenergetic level. Furthermore, an extraordinarily complicated chaos of delayed psychic reactions usually occurs after the therapist withdraws his hands. Such reactions are so defensive in nature as to totally distort objective reality. The client loses touch with what happened to him both during and subsequent to being touched. Physical pain and emotional anxiety rapidly compound into hysteria and paranoia. The client questions not only the therapist's intensions, but the very treatment itself.

Given the dangers, a sensitive therapist will always use touch to facilitate a loosening of the peripheral muscular rigidities from within rather than from without. This usually happens if he applies a nurturing touch to the least armored parts of the peripheral muscular sheath, especially when treating a compulsive type of character armoring. A nurturing touch means that he lays his hands on the client's skin without the slightest movement or presure. Often, after several minutes, such a quiet, non-threatening touch will polarize the client's energy currents. Gradually, the no-man's land region will begin to charge, but with the desireable difference that the reaction will not mobilize the organism's survival-motivated emergency responses.

In order to ground this discussion of nurturing versus catalytic touch, we turn once again to Ruth.

In her first session, Ruth talked continuously for forty minutes while seated in an upright position. Although I had asked her to lie on the mattress fully dressed and to talk freely, she was unable to lie for more than a few minutes before she spontaneously sat up. When I mentioned this behavior, Ruth laughed and acknowledged that it signified some kind of resistance. She immediately resumed talking somewhat compulsively about her history with many previous therapists. Sensing the degree of her resistance to lying down, I directed a position which permitted her to sit on the mattress, but with enough stress to begin to mobilize her breathing and energy flow: she remained seated, but leaned her upper half back as she supported its weight on her elbows with her arms extending down to the mattress. Hanging her head straight back, she continued to talk compulsively without pause for at least another twenty-five minutes without referring to her body sensations or feelings.

Anyone who can maintain this stress position for twenty-five minutes while relating in detail her past history must be armored indeed. This position puts considerable pressure on the muscles of the arm-shoulder joints and the muscles around the neck. (see page 168). Yet Ruth remained totally unaware of any discomfort, of any tension buildup in these muscles, or of any underlying buildup of stress in her entire organism. Finally, I asked her to lie on the mattress.

After a long pause -- the first silence of the session -- I asked Ruth what she was presently experiencing. She replied :

> A pain in my head when I lay down. It came all the way down to here. (She points to the middle of her torso on one side).
>
> And it stopped right there. (The same place she just pointed to). At the point where it stopped was also the point where it felt like crying...... (Long pause.)
>
> Then I thought that it was silly to feel like crying when I didn't know what to cry about. Then I thought that it isn't so silly to feel like crying even though you don't know what it's about.

After waiting to see if she was finished, I responded, "Stay just as you are -- I am going to touch your forehead from behind you." With one hand on each side of her forehead, I touch her directly for the first time. I hold my hands gently without pressure or movement. My fingertips extend to just above her eyes while the heel of my palms rests on her scalp, just above her hairline. After two minutes of silence, I ask what she is aware of. She replies that the pain has left her head. After another minute, I withdraw my hands and sit some distance away. After three minutes of silence, Ruth says :

> There's a pressure now on the top of my head. When you put pressure on the top of my head I felt energy trying to get out and on its way. It was like when you put your hand that way (Slightly

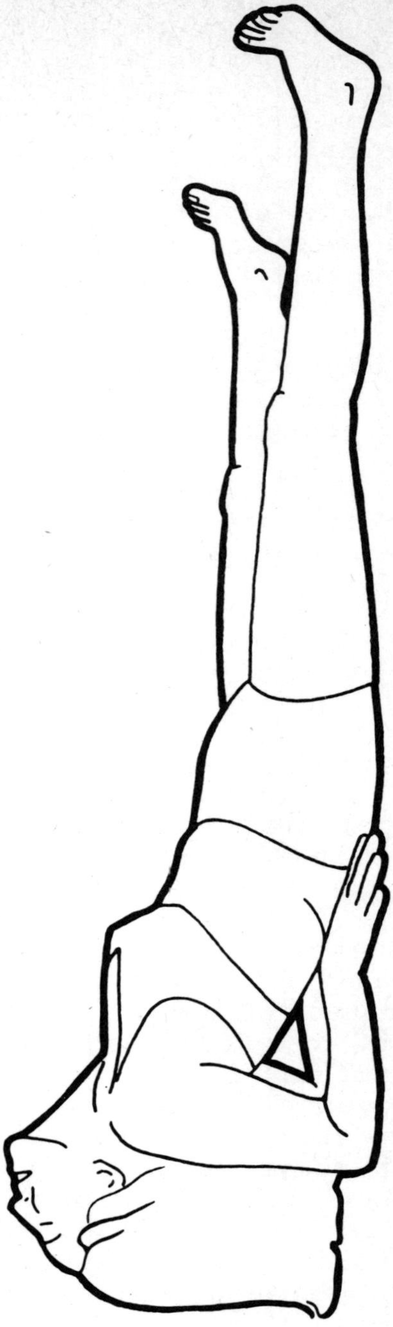

pressed downwards the heel of the palm into the top of the head so that it pushed from behind horizontally downwards into her body.) (see page 170).

I felt energy coming all the way down here. (She indicates the sides of her torso.) I then felt genital pleasure, and I didn't know if it was because of a combination...

I felt the pain going out of my head and going down this way but it wasn't painful but like energy moving. And I could hear you breathing, and your head was that close to mine, and I didn't know if my feeling of the genital arousal came from hearing you breathe or was a combination of your breathing and this energy movement.

Ruth breaks the ensuing long silence by saying :

Sadness from that touching too. I feel like I'm going to cry. Doesn't make any sense to me... doesn't make any sense to me my feeling sad and wanting to cry... don't know that well at all... I would go away if you came over here and got close to me now.

This excerpt demonstrates a successful initial application of do-it-yourself and direct touch methods to a sensitive woman moderately alienated from her body. The initial energy-mobilization exercise helped to mobilize Ruth's inner core energy currents and to facilitate the spontaneous surfacing of an unfamiliar vegetative release reaction. This reaction took the form of a pain in her head which moved down to her diaphragmatic region. The mobility of this movement indicates that Ruth is not severely armored as a whole, but that she is very armored in her neck region and that her diaphragm is blocked deep inside. If she had been severely armored as a whole, there would have been less spontaneous transference of the pain from one region of the body to the other. Ruth's mobility of transference presupposes a certain fluidity of energy flow beneath the peripheral muscular sheath, especially in response to such a low-grade stress position. Her severe neck armoring is indicated by her ability to talk for twenty-five minutes in the stress position without allowing a single body sensation to enter the foreground of consciousness.

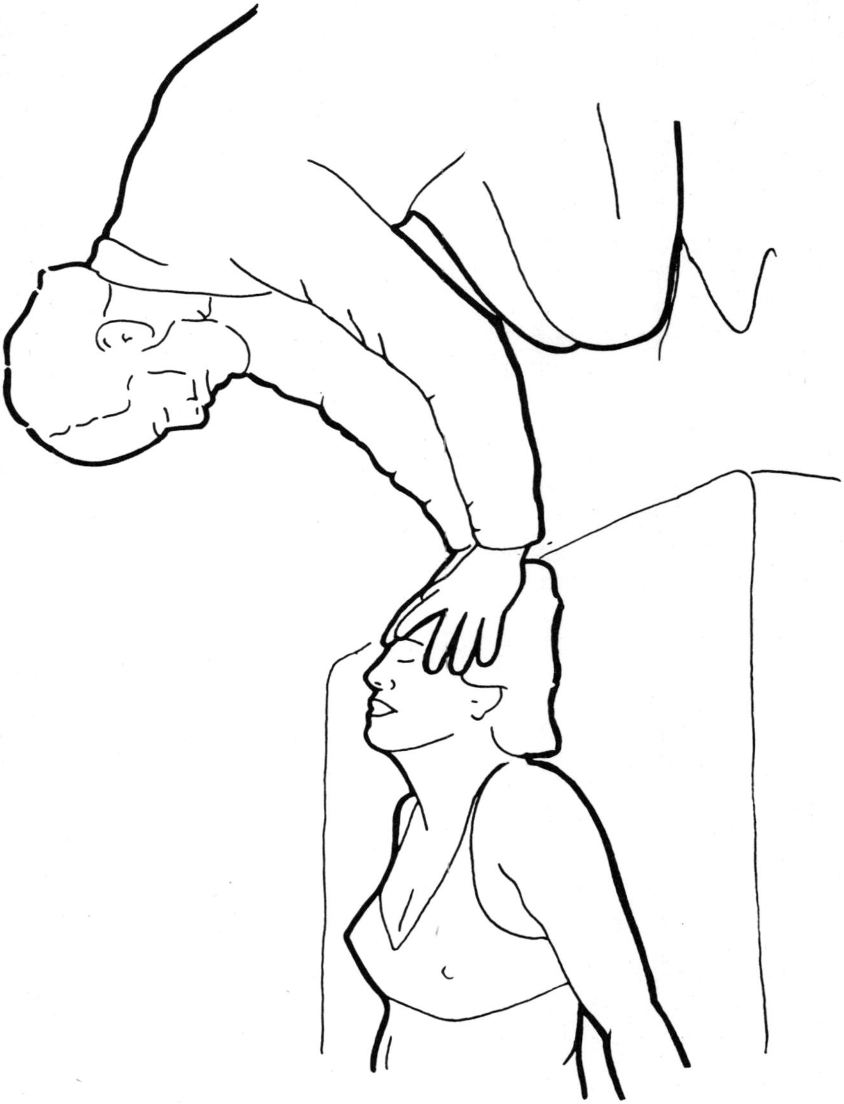

After lying down in silence, Ruth did become conscious of pain emerging in her head. Spontaneous pain in the head usually indicates a great deal of holding in the neck region. Finally, the fact that the moving pain stops in her middle torso suggests a deeper desensitivization from the middle of her torso downwards. Once a pain starts spontaneously moving at the surface, it develops momentum unless it is cut off by a more powerful deadening of energy flow from deep inside.

I deduced that Ruth was not so severely armored as to be likely to become overwhelmed by direct touch. This deduction came less from the bodily sensations themselves than from her psychological response to the sensations. Ruth was able to associate her desire to cry with the fact that the moving sensation of pain stopped in her mid torso. Furthermore, she was able to imbue her middle torso with this feeling. These responses indicate a capacity for psychic differentiation of feeling. This is confirmed by the subsequent alternation in Ruth's thought processes which enable her to articulate and fully share in the present what is actually happening. This ability indicates a fluidity of psychological awareness that is creatively alive in the sense that it functions spontaneously in response to immediate subjective novelties. Thus reassured, I could risk direct touch in spite of her armoring without fear of triggering a massive anxiety attack.

I chose to touch Ruth's forehead for two reasons: my belief that it was probably not very armored, and my understanding that it is usually productive to touch those areas which are currently the focus of some motility of vegetative discharge, unless those happen to be erogenous zones. Because a therapist does not know a new client's bodily or psychic condition, it is best to touch those areas near to where spontaneous release activity is already occurring. This practice usually facilitates further mobilization of the release. My immobile, nurturing touch did mobilize Ruth's release activity. And yet, it was not so catalytic as to induce an emergency-oriented response which would have precluded subsequent equalization of the energy economy.

It was essentially a very loose and evanescent convergence-equalization response that occurred inside

Ruth's organism. It was sufficiently non-threatening to lead to a rather incisive interpenetration of both bodily and psychic after-effects. I gave Ruth ample time and space to experience her bodily reactions without interference. I allowed her time to process experientially and cognitively after removing my hands. Leaving her alone made it more possible for Ruth to identify accurately her novel sensations and feelings even if she could not comprehend why they were happening.

I do not believe that Ruth was really aroused genitally by my hands pressing upon her upper forehead. Whenever a new client of the opposite sex manifests such a response to my direct touch, it indicates that she is more or less cut off from any real viscerally alive kinaesthetic contact with her genital area. What is really stimulated is the set of muscles which innervate the genitals rather than the genital organs themselves. These muscles are invariably hypertense and armored as well as isolated from the primary sexual mainstream of energy which flows deeper inside the organism when real sexual arousal occurs. These muscles form a protective wall around the genital region and are a part of the peripheral muscular sheath.

Ruth must have been forced at an early age to mobilize the antagonistic set of muscles in order to defend her psyche against experiencing real sexual sensations in the presence of her father or some other man. Her detached tone when reporting these genital sensations indicates that her total being is not invested in them. This is confirmed as Ruth subsequently experiences her first real feelings in response to my touch -- a deep and incomprehensible sadness which longs for but cannot find release in tears. And Ruth's sadness is coupled with a desire to flee if I were to suddenly come close to her. This complex of contradictory feelings constitutes Ruth's real psychological feeling state in response to my direct touch to her forehead.

My silence tacitly gave Ruth permission to fully crystallize her response to my touch. Without that silent reflection, she may not have finally discovered her feelings of sadness, of wanting to cry, and of needing to keep me physically distant. If I had, for instance, proposed that she resume the low-grade stress position, she would have probably done so without resistance. But I waited until later for such a proposal. I did not intrude upon her internal psychological process partly because I sensed her psychological aliveness. I knew that she needed a non-threatening space in order to fully realize her response. She would have mobilized more energy flow if I had immediately returned her to the stress position. However, she would also have become freshly invested in a new figure-background awareness gestalt, and thereby have erased the real complexity of her contradictory feelings. After each body exercise, the right timing and optimal degree of emotional and physical separation greatly influence the effectiveness of any technique used.

Chapter V

THE BEGINNING OF CHRISTA'S INTENSIVE

I. The Potency of Nurturing Touch

When working with rigid character types during first stage, it is usually most productive to alternate nurturing direct touch with some form of do-it-yourself exercise. This process of alternation is most likely to mobilize the vegetative energy currents, if only for brief moments. The more the vegetative energy currents are awakened, the greater the likelihood that negative repressed emotions can surface by penetrating the peripheral muscular sheath from within. But before such emotions can fully break through, the mesodermal sheath itself must be gradually loosened and expanded by less energetically demanding vegetative release reactions. An individual intensive will be presented fully in order to illustrate this sequence of development. Our example is called Christa.

Christa, a thirty-year-old German university teacher, came for intensive treatment with us accompanied by her closest friend, Ilse, a woman psychotherapist. Christa's armoring was so severe that it threatened to engulf her in a paranoid web of ideation which was basically schizo-affective and hysterically dissociative in nature. Except for an unusually tenacious will to struggle and survive, coupled with vital energetic and intellectual resources, Christa might well have succumbed to a full-blown paranoid psychosis at many critical junctures in her life. Her strong will to survive in the face of an unsympathetic environment stamped her as desperately neurotic with a low sense of self-esteem, and rendered her acutely alienated from her body's emotional needs.

Christa was so desperately starved for real affection and genuine emotional containment that our slightest mutual direct touch triggered a dramatic chain reaction of contradictory intellectualizations and emotionally charged pseudo-opinions about herself that are so typical of the desperate hysteric. After our first full session, I knew that nurturing direct touch would facilitate a release process more easily than do-it-yourself energy mobilization exercises. The reverse is true for clients more dominantly paranoid: they need a lot of do-it-yourself mobilization work before a therapist should risk any direct touch. A positive therapist/client rapport must clearly emerge in such cases and even then, direct touch should be used with the greatest caution. We had already established such a rapport with Christa during two previous professional training workshops.

During the second session, we continue to explore verbally Christa's situation. She reveals not only the enormity of her emotional deprivation, but also her merciless inner self-castigator. This critic has undoubtedly prevented her from ever realizing any full satisfaction of her needs for affection and tenderness.

I ask: What are you doing right now when you look at us like that ?

C : Control... I don't know, I'm just feeling I'm making something wrong. I know that it's bad. A feeling of being dependent upon your reactions... It shouldn't be so.

Me : Well, can you accept that it is ?

C : No.

Me : Right. That's one of your problems.

C : I know that no persons do not have it. I know that I have little ego. I hate me for that. You are right. I should not be so dependent, and I should not accept being so independent.

Christa speaks with a rising pitch of remorseful self-loathing -- the basic message since the session began. I decide to initiate bodywork to reduce her enormously high tension stemming from a longstanding emotional insecurity. Direct touch can be twice as effective as any kind of do-it-yourself energy mobilization technique to rapidly reduce the chronically overloaded cerebrospinal neural network. Many body practitioners fallaciously believe that by mobilizing the musculature and discharging the feelings through various physically centered means, the underlying hypertension in the neural network will be subsequently reduced. I have found this to be only relatively true at best. A dynamic motor discharge of energy through active mobilization of the voluntary musculature is not sufficient in itself to reduce cerebrospinal neural tension. The discharge must be accompanied by a spontaneous uppacing in the circulation of the fluid metabolic networks, most especially the blood-vascular network and the glandular-hormonal network. Only the renewing of an inner continuity of circulation in these networks has the power to reduce the excess and then restore the median level of excitation throughout the organism.

I ask Christa to remove her outer clothes and to lie on her belly on the mattress. Both Katherine and I sit on either side. In synchrony, we each place one hand upon Christa's upper back in the region of the twelth vertebra on either side of the spinal column and the other hand directly over the outer region of the arm-shoulder joint. We hold our hands lightly and completely immobile. (see page 178). After about twenty seconds, Christa begins to cry and sniffle quietly. She continues for about two minutes until I say:

> Stream of consciousness. That means to just say what you are experiencing and what you are aware of.

Christa begins instantly to talk :

> I was afraid that I was not adorable, not a child like the others. I was outside. Never in school did they see what I was, that I needed to take time there. At home my mother was arguing that I was crying and screaming.
>
> She said: 'Oh, I'm ashamed to have a child like you.' I felt guilty too. I was always afraid I would kill my mother with my vitality. She would say: 'I wish I didn't have a child like you. I cannot tolerate you.' And she put me away. (Referring to her being placed in a children's home on several occasions.)
>
> And she had heart attacks, and I felt guilty because I could not love her -- never. (Her voice begins to rise to a pitch of intensity that conveys anguish and pathos.)
>
> I could not love her. (She now cries openly.)

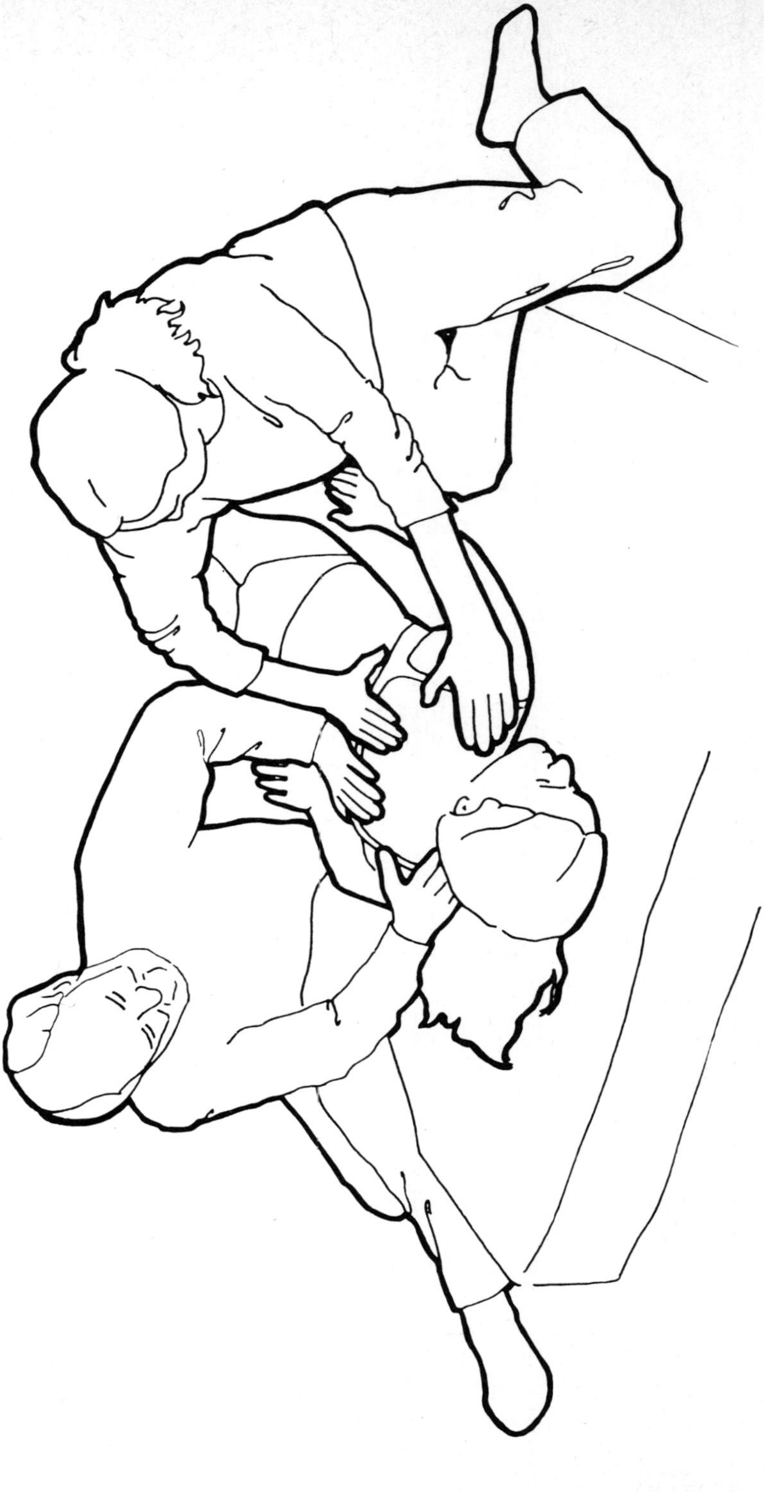

I needed her, I was dependent on her. I was afraid she could die not because I loved her but because I was nobody without her. Always I was with her.

My father was away. He worked in a hotel and I saw him little. Always I was with her. But I didn't love her. (Her voice begins to crescendo.) A good child has to love the mother. I could not. I still cannot. I have no feelings for her.

Christa begins to cry with a fullness that finally overwhelms her verbalizations. Silence follows this immense release as Katherine and I continue our direct nurturing touch. Christa continues :

I always thought that I was not her child. I hated her. When my father came home, she pushed me away. She would say, 'He needs to be quiet. Go away.' I would wait in my bed until midnight in order to see him, but she would put me back in my bedroom.

Another silence follows which is punctuated by an angry quality of throttled crying which indicates her resistance against the tears. After describing jumbled impressions of her father, Christa is again silent. After another minute, she resumes :

And I could never accept tenderness from my mother. But when she came to me, it was like I could not breathe again. It was possessive. (Her voice rises in anger.) It was not tender, it was possessive.

(Imitating her mother's voice with anger and with a surprisingly controlled venemous caricature) Mine. My child, you are mine. You are mine. Mine. M-i-i-i-i-ne...

And it was she who was married to my husband, not me. It was her marriage. Now she's so cold. So cold when I phone up. She doesn't know what it is to ask somebody if he is cold or not. She's always asking me to give her more attention. She's always thinking and looking at me to see whether I'm a good enough child for her.

I didn't love her. (Suddenly her voice assumes an hysterical intensity that whines and whirls at rapidly changing pitches.) And I think that's my guilt feeling that I can't love her. I could never love her, and I was always running to ask some tenderness from somebody. I came back and she said that nobody else except the mother would be good to the child and that all the others would go away from me.

(The hysterical inner voice continues to whirl, but at a more subdued level.) I couldn't love my mother, but I believed my mother that they would not like me. And so... I was alone again. (Her voice descends to its normal timbre.) She interfered in the relationship between my sister and me (Her voice begins to rise again), between my father and me, between my friend and me, between my husband and me.

Because this was her work. She said to me, 'You are my life's work -- (Silence of a minute) -- That's the problem. I am not normal. I am sick and perverse. I am bad. I am a monster. I hate myself, and I know that I'm always against me because I'm against my mother.

A two minute silence ensues. Christa makes no sound as she lies stuck in what appears to be a psychological impasse. Her withdrawal into a new cycle of self-loathing more or less prevents her from feeling the impact of what she has just been describing. Sensing the impasse, Katherine and I remove our hands. Each of us takes one of Christa's hands in our hands. Direct hand to hand contact is a potent way to polarize an energy flow which moves from the center to the periphery of both organisms. I direct Christa to squeeze our hands in order to increase the flow.

Almost immediately after Christa begins to squeeze our hands, she starts to cry loudly. Sensing that she is using only part of her strength, I direct her to squeeze tighter. This permits her to cry louder and more freely. Gradually, her crying turns into infantile wails -- she begins to gasp. Suddenly, she becomes silent, remaining quiet for another two minutes until I say, "Hold tight". By this time, Christa has rolled over to one side with her legs curled into her chest and belly. She makes spontaneous rocking movements with her lower half which release her total organism. Her breathing deepens as these movements subside. After a few minutes of silence, I ask her to turn on her back and then ask again for her stream of consciousness.

> I think I must be very little. I didn't know it could be so good to have two hands to go out of... I don't know what it was. It was the first time that I knew what it is to have a father and a mother -- both on each side. Every time before it has always been one person.
>
> I can't describe these feelings... It was always a mixture of security and tension that came from her, and when you were both by my side I had not this feeling of tension. It was so strange... (Deep sighs)... I don't understand it.
>
> Don't try. Just accept it if it feels real.
>
> It feels real. It's like two poles became balanced in me. I don't know how. I never had balance before. I was always turning from one side to the other. I never felt them both together. I never knew who I was in this turning from one side to the other.

Bioenergetically, our direct touch was correct. If her feeling space had been more depressed and if her core energy resources had been more thoroughly encapsulated, do-it-yourself work on her feet would have proved more effective. On this particular day, Christa's anxiety level was so high and so much a part of her self-awareness as to indicate an emotionally labile state. She did not need further energy mobilization, but the very reverse -- a sizeable diminishment of her resources, both in quantity and lability of flow.

Once the underlying tension level is reduced, hysterics especially have the capacity to channel their usually enormous quantities of undischarged energy into productive avenues of expression. They are chronically overcharged at both the bioenergetic and the psychic level because of their encasement within a rigid peripheral muscular sheath. If that sheath were directly assaulted by catalytic touch, the client would plunge into a fitful sequence of fight and flight reactions which would yield little or no emotional release in spite of a lot of screaming.

But when that sheath is touched nurturingly, enough yielding occurs to allow the client to relax the enormous internal barriers between center and periphery.

This yielding process is the outstanding bioenergetic development in our work thus far with Christa. We placed our hands softly on four places where we knew the musculature was rigidly hypertonic. This created a circuit of polarized interaction between her peripheral muscular sheath and our combined core energy flow. The polarized circuit drained off the excess charge at the surface enough to permit the deeper vegetative energy currents to partially resonate with, and even slightly penetrate from within, the peripheral muscular sheath. Our touch permitted a reduction in the force of the counter energy currents that work centripetally from the surface inwards whenever the peripheral sheath is intact.

The mesh-like resiliency of Christa's armoring was what enabled her to channel all of her psychological and biological resources into venting her frustrated negative feelings in one rapid semi-release after another. To be sure, her externalization of negative affects is erratic, somewhat contradictory, occasionally self-defeating, and sometimes totally suppressed. Nevertheless, she is able to channel a lot of energy into focusing briefly upon several past events which contain a tremendous amount of chronically repressed feeling. The whole release sequence exhibits several rapid alternations between one psychodynamic extreme and its opposite. The very rapidity of this alternation stamps the experience as a distinctly first stage dearmoring process according to the basic law of alternation between opposite reactions formulated earlier. But the interesting development is that the rapidity of the self-destructive alternation progressively slows down and eventually almost stops during the session just described. It is most rapid before Christa is touched as she harshly criticizes herself for expectations from us. She ends by condemning herself for both being dependent while wishing for independence. Her slowest alternation and greatest degree of self-acceptance emerges as she turns onto her back near the end of the sequence. Thereafter, she remains stably focused upon her totally new feeling of internal emotional security stimulated by our joint touch.

Christa's most extreme alternation between opposite tendencies occurs as she moves from infantile wailing to complete silence after she squeezes our hands more tightly. Her crying moves rapidly into an extraordinarily regressed and primordial wail. She sounds like a tiny infant wailing with absolute abandonment in an isolated room. Such a species of cries could not have emerged during our first bodywork exercise unless Christa had already formed a positive transference to both of us. And it could not have emerged until we had touched her nurturingly for about ten minutes. The immobile touch thawed the muscular sheath to permit her pent-up psychic vitality underneath to find outlets for expressing increasingly greater amounts of repressed rage. She has to throttle this anger by retroflecting it back upon herself in the form of self-hatred. However, this does not occur until she has externalized quite a lot of feeling infused with a growing differentiation of awareness. She touches upon nearly all of the nuclear chronic conflicts in her long struggle against her mother's insidious possessiveness. She touches upon them and immediately bounces off, but to something still in keeping with her growing release of repressed anger.

Christa's infantile wails could not have occurred until she reversed the movement of negative energy flow back upon herself by squeezing our hands as tightly as possible. Her ability to reciprocate our progressive hand squeezing broke up the centripetal direction of flow, transforming it into a primitive centrifugal release of tensions which peaked in the wailing. This is another example of pathological alternation between opposites: as the centrifugal vegetative energy currents find greater and greater outlet, there must subsequently occur a more severe temporary suppression produced by a tighter intensification of the centripetal energy currents in the service of the peripheral muscular sheath. In other words, the intensification of feelings, attitudes, and modes of response spiral in both directions as the armoring loosens.

Selection of the body techniques which will best facilitate this process of progressive intensification of energy movements is a highly evolved intuitive art. Sometimes, it is better to structure a technique to affirm and actively intensify a client's emerging need to disinhibit repressed impulses. At other times, it is more productive to use a technique which deliberately affirms the repressed impulse. We chose the former when we began the reciprocal hand squeezing. At this point, Christa had crushed her centrifugal venting of negative feelings -- her consciousness was realigned with her centripetal counter energy currents mediated by her peripheral muscular sheath. When I asked Christa to squeeze our hands, we merely repeated what we had been doing earlier with our nurturing touch: establishing a polarized circuit of interaction between her peripheral sheath and our core longitudinal energy flow. Because our combined flow was the more powerful and the more outward flowing, it quickly reestablished a draining off of her inward turning currents and reversed them outwards again in the form of infantile wails. The inner forces thrusting towards freedom from chronic imprisonment defeated the life-defeating forces dedicated to a neutralized status quo. Therefore, Christa was able to penetrate her armoring with a massive breaking down of the inner censors. Soon, however, the anti-life forces reasserted their dominance, silencing her crying for the remainder of the session.

Asking a client to squeeze our hands is not a nurturing style of touch. It is catalytic since it sets up a narrowly circumscribed polarization of energy flow in a localized part of the organism. Usually, such a touch induces a rapid escalation of whatever fluid energy currents are dominant at that moment. If the anti-life currents are most dominant, they form a negative counter current against the intruding energy polarization of the toucher. If the armoring is less intact and the centrifugal, impulse-affirmative currents are dominant, the metabolism builds to a massive externalization of feelings interpenetrated with cognitive significance. Neither of these possibilities prevailed in this instance with Christa.

With Christa, our touch gradually changed from a nurturing to a catalytic mode that was low-grade enough in aggressive intrusiveness so as not to launch a fullscale defensive reaction. At first, we held Christa's hands in a soft, nurturing manner. Gradually, we began to squeeze, and shortly thereafter, I asked Christa to squeeze. Finding that she was able to respond to our increasing pressure, I encouraged her to squeeze harder. The mutual collaboration enabled her centripetal energy currents to move longitudinally up towards her hands from the rest of her periphery. They finally broke outwards by a rather sudden convergence of antagonistic energy currents in the regressive wails. Such a bioenergetic situation usually happens when catalytic styles of direct touch are sagaciously administered throughout all stages of treatment. Ideally, catalytic touch is used to bring about an escalation of the process of dynamic intensification of release from within inwards or from within outwards. Its special function is its capacity to polarize enough expansive pressure internally to induce a collapse of chronic collisions, vortexes, and pockets of deadened energy flow. This is most effectively accomplished by knowing how, when, and where to administer a catalytic touch which triggers both reservoirs of energy currents which are at loggerheads. Used improperly, it can overwhelm the receiver biologically or psychologically.

With Christa, our low-grade catalytic touch was more effective than any self-mobilization technique -- her basic underlying need was to polarize and diffuse her tightly encapsulated energy impasse rather than to vitalize it. To accomplish this, she needed a little polarization and redirection of her already mobile energy currents. I may have already begun to sense that her metabolic reserves had nearly reached their threshold for change that day. Consequently, the primitive charge-discharge process could best be furthered by requiring a minimum of controlled exertion or voluntary movement initiated by her. I may have surmised this from Christa's sudden turning against herself in violent self-loathing. This was no longer a matter for conjecture, however, a few minutes later when she abruptly moved from wailing into silence. I knew that asking her to come off her belly and to go onto her back would enable her to gradually recover her familiar ego and emotional boundaries.

Christa did recover her boundaries. For the remainder of the session, Katherine and I used direct touch designed to re-equalize her energy economy and to facilitate the most conflict-free state of inner feeling harmony which she could tolerate. Our touch remained nurturing. It reinforced her sense of a greater unity and stability of energy flow. Its intention was to gradually decelerate the prior progressive intensification of alternating reactions. Harmonization of chronic internal collisions is another unique function of nurturing touch.

II. Christa's Dissociated Hands

The following day I realized that it would be premature to introduce Christa to do-it-yourself energy mobilization exercises on her feet. Arriving vulnerable in both mind and body, she reported many emotional upheavals since yesterday's session. Just talking about them was so upsetting that Christa's body began to tremor involuntarily as she sat on the edge of her chair. I asked her to remove her outer garments and to lie on the mattress on her back. Katherine and I sat on either side, but not touching her. I asked Christa to do the jelly fish exercise, a modified voluntary movement appropriated from what Reich believed is the essence of the orgasm reflex. The lower legs are brought up so that the knees form the top of a triangle with the feet firmly planted on the floor. With each exhalation, the client allows the knees to collapse outwards to both sides simultaneously. With each inhalation, the knees are drawn upwards again until they touch each other. After coordinating the breathing cycle with the two directions of movement, the client allows the head to fall backwards and the upper shoulders to rise up and forward simultaneously with the exhalation and outward collapse of the legs. Thereafter, with each inhalation the head returns to its normal position -- the back of the head is directly contiguous with the floor, and the shoulders rest flat on the floor.

I no longer use this particular exercise since I have gradually realized that it represents an unnaturally forced caricature of an orgasm reflex rather than a spontaneously graceful movement. Nevertheless, it was most effective in uncovering an underlying constriction in Christa's throat and upper chest region -- she developed a repetitive cough which assumed the intensity of a small convulsion shortly after her breathing began to deepen. Finally, she could not inhale deeply without an involuntary compulsion to hold her breath entirely. All her adult life, she prevented herself from breathing, especially during the night when she began to imagine a cherished friend deserting her. Christa describes this terror-filled experience:

> When I'm thinking that the other will go away -- that I'm too bad... that the other would not continue to stay with me. Then I see myself with a great open mouth and I can't scream a single word at all.

Christa's revelation indicates a severe fixation to an infantile fear of abandonment. Her body's defensive wisdom compels her to suppress her deep breathing entirely, so as to avoid the acute emotional pain and anxiety of fully reexperiencing this infantile fear. Recognizing this, I knew that we had to gradually guide Christa towards regressively reexperiencing this terror in its here-and-now fullness. The more nurturing our touch, the more likely we could facilitate her gradual regression. Only then could Christa tolerate the emotional pain of fully externalizing these negative constellations of affect. She needed our emotional containment of her fragmented psyche in order to descend into such a snake pit of horrors. (see page 188).

As soon as Christa spoke, I asked her to hold my hand and to return to the jellyfish exercise. She persisted until her coughing reached strangulation proportions. I commanded her to make the sound of 'Ah-h-h' with each exhalation, and to make louder and louder sounds. By superimposing my will, I was risking either that her organism would clam up altogether, or that she would break through the peripheral muscular sheath that held her encased in chronic emotional fixation. Christa rapidly regresses to the earliest period so far. Her wails are more open-throated and angrier than before. Repetitively, she begins to scream, "MA-MA, MA-MA". Suddenly, she stops, but not as abruptly as the previous day :

> I have a strange phantasy -- that my mother would kill me. I don't know why. She never did. But I couldn't live -- I had to fight against death... I don't know why... I'm so afraid... Don't go away.

She holds my hand as she asks me not to leave.

Christa struggles in silence with her feelings.

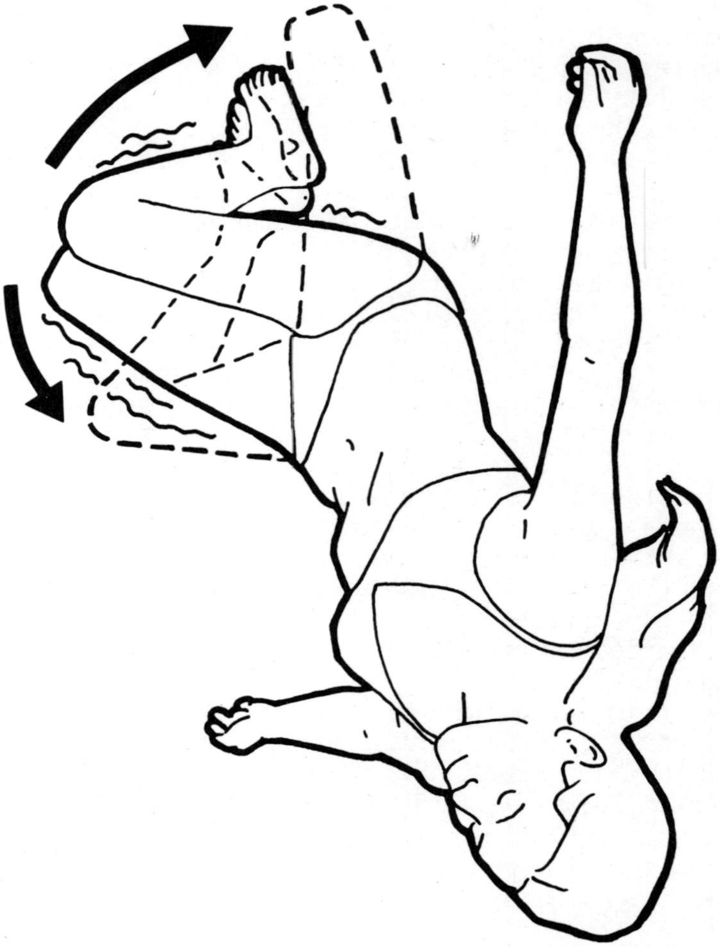

Her erratic and partly audible breathing indicates that she is remaining in a regressed state. After three minutes, Katherine asks what she is experiencing. Christa replies :

> I'm in a dark room. There is nobody... I have no hands, but the fingers of an animal... They can hold nothing... I would like to fight against something, but there's nothing... Or to get out, but there's nothing to get out of... nothing to do... I have to accept that it is so... like I am a baby who is forgotten.

Christa recalls that her mother recently told her that she spent the first four months of post-uterine existence in an oxygen tent while her mother was hospitalized. For the second four months, Christa was cared for by nurses at her aunt's home, while her mother remained bed-ridden. Christa describes the countless times her mother complained to friends about the ordeal of giving birth to her daughter. As a result, Christa began to feel that she should never have been born.

I ask Christa to resume the jellyfish. With encouragement, she begins to vomit phlegm. Somewhat relieved, Christa spontaneously begins to make unprogrammed movements. Her legs begin to move downwards, jerking as if they were pushing something away. It looks as if she is trying to shake something loose in her pelvic-leg joints. Simultaneously, her left arm rises as if fearing attack. It thrusts repetitively from the shoulder joint forwards into the air as if to ward off an attacker. After about five minutes, Christa describes the experience :

> It was so frightening... Like a spasm... first in my legs. I was so afraid of my left hand... I had no control... it begins to make like that (She makes a thrusting in the air movement). Now I have this strange feeling all over me except in my right hand... It's the only part of my body that's not cramped... I can't explain anything. I have only the impression that things go on that I absolutely do not understand... I don't know what's happening... I am afraid... Malcolm, when I did that (She thrusts her left hand) it was not like a human being anymore... It was like an animal... like a terrible bird.

Me : A Claw ?

Mm-mm. Not like a hand who can take somebody, but like a hand who can take nobody... it's so terrible.

Me : What can the claw do ?

Take the others away... because the animal is so terrible that no human being would come... I could do nothing... it was too cramped in my left hand. My right hand was the only human part, but my left hand is my dominant hand.

The session ends.

Bioenergetically, it is fairly certain that from the time Christa screams "MA-MA", she has penetrated her peripheral sheath of muscular armoring. From that point, she reexperiences the same kind of feelings she actually felt as a very young child, but with the addition of adult consciousness. Given her extremely mobile, mesh-like armoring, the penetration from within of the outer walls of rigidities at the bioenergetic level enabled her to regress to the psychological events which initially induced the armor formation.

The dearmoring process cannot really begin until the client is able to permit the psyche to surrender to the reexperiencing of those feelings that originally attended the objective realities which caused armoring to develop. Christa's ego-defense network was not strongly entrenched because she never acquired a positive belief in herself or any kind of idealized self-image built largely upon compensatory reaction formations. She was too brutally honest as well as far too intelligent to evolve an inflated and basically unrealistic false self-system. Her basic defense had been to deny in consciousness the truths she was feeling. On other occasions, she numbed her feelings bioenergetically by becoming totally paralyzed every time she approached her real feelings. These are typical defenses of the hysteric syndrome. These defenses began to crumble from the moment Christa began screaming "MA-MA" with pathos and abandonment. By surrendering to her feelings for the remainder of the session, she managed to penetrate her psychic barriers of repression as well as her peripheral muscular sheath. The dearmoring process cannot begin until the client can penetrate these two sets of barriers: the psychological barriers against feelings which have been repressed because they are too painful, and the muscular barriers of rigidity which represent the front line of the psyche's defense.

After these two barriers against feeling the painful past have finally begun to loosen, Christa's first feeling is that her mother wanted to kill her when she was a very young child. She describes this feeling in an extremely hesitant, tentative, almost incredulous manner. For the first time, Christa is confronting consciously the only subjective proof she has that her mother probably did feel murderously towards her without any literal impulse to kill. And probably her mother unconsciously attempted to kill her. Any woman who could allow her child to be cared for by another woman for the first eight months must unconsciously want to kill the child indirectly through neglect and deprivation. Christa is experiencing an inner struggle between living and dying: "But I couldn't live... I had to fight against death". We can safely conjecture that this is an authentic reexperiencing of what was both objectively and subjectively true at least during those first eight months if not much longer. As Christa becomes frightened and holds me to her, she is feeling the absolute helplessness and fear that typified much of her earliest years without a real mother to give her the emotional containment and loving touch fundamental to every child's security.

After a few minutes of uneasy silence, Christa speaks of a 'phantasy' that she is in a dark room alone and that her hands have been replaced by the useless fingers of an animal. Christa is describing an image of herself that she must have had during those first four to eight months after birth. The fact that there was no one person available to mother her would explain why she could not feel her own body schema as truly human. Christa was almost totally deprived of any constancy or adequacy of holding. Confined to an oxygen tent for the first four months, she was severely deprived of any kind of direct affirmation of her sensorimotor boundaries of contact with her immediate environment. Her mother refused to even see her child but once during this entire period. Consequently, Christa could not develop an ego-integrative sense of her own body.

Perhaps one of the primary achievements of adequate holding during the stage of absolute dependency is to provide a baby with enough sensorimotor direct touch to enable him to develop a self-image which is more human than animal. In Christa's case, it is probable that the severe absence of such physical contact forced her to fall back upon a set of phylogenetically primitivized defense reactions. She had no other choice if she were to survive the complete absence of any adequate human environment which could provide her primary dynamic feeling centers with even a rudimentary sense of continuity. She had no choice but to prematurely struggle to survive. By so doing, she had to undergo a low-grade sense of catastrophe and acute anxiety throughout her first year of life. Only by resorting to a desperately aggressive form of animal survival embodied in the form of a terrible bird of prey could she fight off real death.

Christa's identification of her left hand with the claws of a bird and the thrusting of her arm presumably express a self-protective fending off of a real attacker outside of her rather than any assertion of aggressive animal instinct. Christa's need to ward off a hostile environment did not end when she was eight months old. She was reabandoned several more times before she was ten. Her mother repeatedly sent her away to a children's boarding school for months at a time because she could not tolerate Christa's need for attention and affection. No mother could do this unless she were almost totally alienated from her own primary dynamic feeling centers, especially the two sympathetic centers.

Christa's mother was unquestionably very neurotic. Essentially a vampire mother, she unconsciously tried to suck the living vitality out of her daughter. Had she been in touch with her own primary feelings in her solar plexus, she would have found the inner strength to instinctively mother her child after birth. If she had been in touch with her own primary feelings in her lumbar ganglion in the lower back, she would have been able to affirm Christa's extreme willfulness and aggressive self-assertiveness as she grew from one to five. Instead, she persuaded Christa that she was a bad child with no consideration for her mother's delicate heart condition and low toleration for noise. She filled Christa with a strong sense of guilt and unworthiness at the conscious level. At an unconscious level, she insidiously bound Christa to her in a state of emotional dependency which intensified as her daughter matured. Throughout childhood and adolescence, Christa was plagued by such horrible nightmares that she sought relief from various psychotherapists. And until the age of twenty-three, the year of her marriage, Christa often slept in her mother's bed at least half of the night because of her deep fear of these nightmares.

Christa's experience of her claw-like left hand also represents an unconscious introjection of her mother's negative image. To borrow from both Jung and Reich, the terrible bird of prey and its mechanical gestures which Christa attributes to her own hand is an unconscious incorporation of the Terrible Mother embodied in her mother's life-destroying aspects. The symbolic significance of the Terrible Mother is her threat to take away the life of the child she has already given birth to. To the extent that Christa's identification with a menacing bird of prey reflects her mother's negative image, to that same extent she had to armor her body and psyche against receiving and feeling the full impact of her mother's feelings. As Reich would explain it, she had to identify with the dominantly aggressive parental figure in order to neutralize its dynamic force.

Thus, the peripheral armored muscular sheath serves a self-protective function. Its formation helps to preserve the vitally alive core dynamic feeling centers and whatever possible flow of the longitudinal energy currents by sealing off direct impingements from threatening objective realities. The hardening of the surface rigidifies the feeling responsiveness, to be sure. But it also neutralizes the traumatic impact of the objective stimulus itself. It partially neutralizes the stimulus by unconsciously introjecting it and setting up a counter image and energy force designed to squelch the power and terror of the outer force and image.

This process of introjecting the negative parental image and making it an active part of the character armoring is the essence of a neurotic splitting of the psyche into a true and a false self. Such a process of unconscious psychological introjection seems indispensable to every rigid type of characterological armoring. The second stage of the dearmoring process involves the gradual dismantling of the counterfeit negative image within the secret crevices of the psyche.

Before this can happen, however, the client must be able to authentically reexperience the subjective feelings generated by the impingement of anti-life vibrations emanating from the destructive parental figures during childhood. Christa is beginning this process in the sessions just presented. The fact that these anti-life vibrations have become compounded into a complex condensation of negative feelings towards herself is a later elaboration of what Christa's mother unconsciously superimposed upon her defenseless child. This is true of Christa's terrifying dreams as well. But the unravelling of these more complex forms, including the revelation of the image of the Terrible Mother, is a process that cannot happen spontaneously within Christa's psyche until there is a greater loosening of the barriers between the central and peripheral regions of her body.

Hereafter, our presentation of Christa's case will be limited to her gradual reclamation of her objective organismically defined boundaries of contact with the outer world. This goes hand in hand with her gradual giving up of her distorted body image. We have already glimpsed the gross distortion in Christa's body image: she has a cramped feeling all over, except for her right hand which she experiences as her only human part. This is a surprising discovery for Christa to make about herself. She did not know this consciously before. She could not possibly know it until the centering of her consciousness upon her concretely embodied self had shifted inwards to the mesodermal layer where she experienced her body from inside the surface of the skin. This was not possible as long as the peripheral muscular sheath remained fully intact. Then her only perspective towards her body was from the cortex looking downwards, much like an outside observer watching the responses of a foreign object. This is the universal perspective of anyone who is armored.

Christa opens her next session by describing the three day interim :

> The first night after the last session I had cramps here in this arm (left arm) and in the two legs. I don't really know where in my arm. Then I woke up again and I had no feelings and no circulation in this arm and my feet. And Saturday when I was walking I was aware that sometimes I made a movement like this (she moves her pelvis into a very slight undulated twist) -- I don't know if I did it before, but I was aware of it.

Both of these bodily reactions signify that Christa has continued to maintain the gains she achieved in the two prior sessions -- the softening of the sharp cleavage between the central and peripheral regions of her metabolism. Such irrational presentations of vegetatively unpleasant and fully embodied sensations indicate ongoing positive release reactions in her voluntary muscle and blood-vascular networks just below the surface of the skin. One can safely assume from these delayed reactions that there was a lot of alternating expansion and contraction of her fluid energy currents in these regions. The expansive periods cause the muscle cramps. The periods of contraction cause the sensations of deadness and absence of blood circulation in her feet and left arm.

It was totally new for Christa to experience these involuntary muscular sensations and to be aware of them belonging to her rather than to some foreign object such as her 'animal flesh'. The same is true of her awareness of a new freedom of flow and greater pelvic spontaneity as she walks. Hitherto, she experienced walking as a disjointed catapulting on two bean pole legs. The initial leg spasms during the prior session indicate an initial loosening of the deeper layers of muscles that encompass both of her leg-torso joints. This loosening probably triggered a similar loosening of the arm-shoulder joint of her left arm. This in turn permitted Christa's left arm to involuntarily express a primary-process impulse hitherto fully repressed.

These second session bodily reactions are localized at the outer boundaries of the loosening of the peripheral muscular sheath. However, they are experienced by Christa at the level of psychic felt sensations from just inside the sheath. After the second session Christa begins to experience organismic reactions which are localized at the inner boundaries of the freshly loosened sheath. Because they are deeper within the organism, Christa is totally unable as yet to crystallize a stable internally centered perspective towards them. She describes her reactions as follows :

> Since the last session when I lie down I have the impression (She suddenly inhales deeply with the sound of Ah and holds her breath in an inflated position) I cannot breathe any more during the night... The last two nights I couldn't sleep well. I kept waking up with this feeling of, of, not strangulation -- not here (She points to her throat) but here (She points to the middle of her chest between her throat and breasts). Such a strange feeling. I don't understand what happened the last session. I felt like a very little baby.
>
> Oh, yes, last night I woke up and I took myself like this (She cradles her own chest with her arms and hands) and sometimes I took Ilse like this and I don't know what's happening, but I realized that in this moment I feel just like a baby who is myself or somebody else who is holding me... it's not holding themselves with their own hands, but like this (She embraces her chest again with her arms).

Christa's feeling that she cannot breathe when she lies down is new. The something pushing from inside her chest is probably the rigid musculature of her peripheral sheath. The significant feature is that she can vaguely experience her sheath as it pushes inwards from all sides, keeping her imprisoned. She is not cognitively focused enough to be aware of this objectively. All that she knows is that she must hold her breath in a chronically inflated position when she lies down. This combination of events confirms that her peripheral armoring has loosened enough for her to feel the centripetal pressure imploding from both the front and the back regions of her upper half. It is unlikely as yet that her diaphragmatic muscle is pressing upwards into her chest region -- this cannot happen until the peripheral sheath has been at least half dissolved in her upper half.

Since Christa is evenly armored all over her torso, the area which manifests the greatest spontaneous vegetative and muscular activity at the inner boundaries of the sheath might well indicate the area where there is the greatest opposition of energy currents. However, it might also indicate the area where the greatest loosening has already occurred. The latter case would explain why Christa is able to become newly aware of how much her organism is accustomed to the holding of the breath in a chronic inspiratory position. Up until now, her cortico-cerebrospinal tension has masked her awareness from what was going on inside her organism from moment to moment at the sensory level. With this tension reduced, Christa can discover, from the simple act of lying down, the underlying reaction of her metabolism which has probably been the dominant pattern for years: her chronic inability to breathe deeply and regularly even when not facing an externally threatening situation.

Another indication that Christa's chest has loosened is her newly discovered need to clasp her arms tightly around her chest. It makes no difference whether she squeezes with her own arms or holds someone else's body close to her chest, as she did the preceding night with her closest friend Ilse. When Christa says that she felt 'just like a baby', she is feeling the tactile pleasure of being touched in a loving and tender manner. Whenever clients become aware of their need to be so touched in the chest region, regardless of the character type, I recognize an incipient expansion of the core longitudinal energy currents which are struggling to reach the surface of the chest from the central regions of the metabolism.

Christa's experiences following the second session indicated that she was at last ready to begin a more demanding do-it-yourself energy-mobilization exercise. Such exercises are usually not advisable until a client can experience enough spontaneous muscular release to appreciate their positive impact upon the breathing cycle. This is particularly true of exercises while standing on the feet. Energy mobilized at the periphery is not of great value unless there is enough circulation of energy flow between the center and the periphery to insure a genuine mobilization of the core longitudinal currents. Only the mobilization of core currents has the power to heal. And during the first stage of dearmoring, the mesodermal muscular sheath cannot be penetrated unless the core currents are awakened. With Christa, for example, it would have been premature to stand her on her feet until there were definite signs of loosening of her peripheral armor. Otherwise, the more demanding stress positions and movement exercises would have polarized her anti-life, centripetally organized energy currents that dominate her ectodermal layer. This would have produced an overexcitation of a highly limited and essentially isolated part of her metabolism. To support this excessive excitation of the cortico-cerebrospinal circuits, emergency-motivated adrenalin would then begin pouring into her bloodstream.

Do-it-yourself exercises cannot benefit a client until he can sense the difference between the mobilization of a manic kind of surface activity which threatens to release a neutering secretion of adrenalin, and the mobilization of a slower, quieter, but far more massively synergistic groundswell of endodermal vegetative energy currents. Otherwise, he will unconsciously use do-it-yourself methods to totally obliterate consciousness of the here-and-now subjective dimension, whether at the psychological or bioenergetic level. He will quickly drive himself into a tailspin of total oblivion, much like the desperate drinker who downs one heavy cocktail after another in order to swamp his sensibilities entirely. There are phenomenological criteria by means of which one can discern the difference between these two opposite kinds of mobilization. First and foremost is the impact upon the breathing cycle. If a client is really alienated from his body and rhythms of energy circulation, he will be unable to even listen to the impact of energy mobilization upon his breathing cycle. He will be unable to sense how his breathing becomes labored and increasingly constricted the longer he continues the exercise. And most armored clients will persevere in an exercise until they become locked into a willfully determined, neutered state, devoid of feelings and sensations. Unless there is receptivity to vegetative sensations of expansion from center to periphery in the front half of the torso, a client will be unable to sense the impact of the mobilization upon his breathing. And unless the mobilization process manages to slowly open up and deepen the natural breathing cycle, it is prematurely undertaken.

For Christa's first do-it-yourself exercise, I place her in a position I call the standing start: the two feet are placed parallel at a comfortable distance as the client closes his eyes and simply listens to his breathing. I seldom give any more verbalized structure than, "Parallel the feet.... Close the eyes.... Listen to your breathing". Minimal instructions free the client to explore any number of possible movements. This is infinitely preferable to fully structuring what they are allowed or forbidden to do, a procedure which I used to follow when influenced by Lowen's approach. Over the years, I observed that the human organism is an extremely delicate instrument which needs only the slightest but correct external stimulus to discover the internal stimuli which will correct its imbalances.

A psychotherapist is an indispensable channel and sounding board. But if he becomes an authoritarian bully and super-ego combined, he actually prolongs the time before the client can begin to trust his own immediate organismic cues in the form of sensations and feelings. When introducing do-it-yourself mobilization bodywork, a therapist has an obligation to the client to try a broad range of diverse methods and to structure them as loosely as possible. Such a procedure facilitates the client's early discovery that he can initiate his own energy-mobilization exercises. During the first stage of treatment, it is seldom possible for the client to permit himself to freely explore his capacities for spontaneous initiation of novel movements or standing stress positions. His severe armoring prevents any real trust in his own body. But if a client has not learned by second stage to improvise his own methods, this must be partly attributable to the therapist's unacknowledged need for overcontrol.

In response to the standing starting position, Christa quickly began to tremor rapidly and to cough uncontrollably. Her tremors indicate vitally alive cortico-cerebrospinal and vegetative currents. Her cough reveals a rigidly armored chest and throat region. I ask Christa to put her head as far back as possible, while keeping her pelvis consistently forward, and allowing the sound of 'Ah-h-h.' With each exhalation, she quickly moved into sounds that were so vital and loud that they had the aura of incandescent explosions. However, her repetitive coughing soon throttled the explosions. Coughing is another form of vegetative release and therefore should be encouraged because it helps to loosen the peripheral muscular sheath. With this in mind, I ask Christa to shake both of her shoulders wildly with each exhalation. Her coughing grows in intensity to assume almost the same explosive quality of her previous vocal sounds. I ask Christa to lie flat on the mattress, sensing that more bodywork on her feet would skyrocket her energy into some form of manic surface excess, thereby calling up defensive hormonal secretions.

After touching Christa around the shoulders and upper chest, I ask her to renew the jellyfish exercise. After a few breaths, she became engulfed in a sequence of striking behavior. For the next twenty five minutes, she spoke not a single word as she alternated between convulsive coughs and spasmodic jellyfish movements. Eventually, she moved into a compulsive holding of her inhalation, just short of strangulation. Then she began to gasp for new breath with desperate gulping sounds. Cries began to alternate with the coughing. As the crying rose in intensity and assumed the same infantile quality of the previous session, she simultaneously began to pound the mattress with her arms and legs.

The mobilization work on Christa's feet had loosened her core longitudinal energy currents to a new level of motility which allowed her to move spontaneously to such dramatic intensity. The greater totality of investment of both her feelings and behavior was partly due to the greater loosening of her peripheral muscular armoring generated by the do-it-yourself body work. She remained in a highly regressed externalization of her damned-up stasis energy for much longer than during the previous sessions. This too was made possible by the increased opening in her peripheral armoring. Both the extension in time and in space of the areas of her body that remained engaged in cathartic self-expression indicate a greater expansiveness and fluidity of bioenergetic flow throughout Christa's organism.

During fifteen minutes of verbal self-exploration following this cathartic release, Christa returns to the same themes explored in the first two sessions. Because of her fruitful response to do-it-yourself work, I intervene upon her psychic space to ask her to get on the Lowen stool. I place her so that her nipples are directly above the center of the stool, while her arms extend behind to hold the arms of a chair. Her initial gasps change into deep crying. After about three minutes when I ask what is happening, she says that she couldn't breathe, was experiencing some pain, and feeling like a baby being punished. Since she manifests no impulse to come off the stool, I push the energy-mobilization process to the saturation point be telling her to lift her pelvis on the inhalation and to drop it on the exhalation while making the sound of Ah-h-h. Persisting for thirty seconds, she suddenly yells in acute pain. She says that she is experiencing severe pain in her shoulders. I ask her to drop her arms to her side. Approaching her from behind, I place my two hands against the bundle of muscles that stand midway between the top of the shoulders and the neck. I press into the center point of intersection. After her screams subside, I ask her to lie flat out in a spread-eagle position.

After listening to Christa's description of being on the stool, I decide to continue the bioenergetic barnstorming of her peripheral armoring. I take her hands in mine while I stand behind and over her. Asking her to hold my wrists while letting her head fall back, I lift the upper half of her body off the floor and wait. She holds her breath in fearful anticipation. I yell at her to take deep breaths. After the first one, she contracts her whole body, complaining of a sharp pain in her head. The second time she tries to breath deeply, she complains of a sharp pain in her chest area between her throat and her breasts. She reveals that she has been experiencing severe pains in her upper chest for the past three days. With the third attempt, Christa is able to breathe deeply seven or eight times. At this point, I end the session by returning her upper half gently to the floor.

Such a demanding and consistently catalytic session inevitably leads to an elaborate set of delayed metabolic reactions, all of which signify an upheaval of the biological status quo. Christa came in the next day significantly dazed. She spent the first half hour describing many bizarre physical symptoms. She reported feeling more or less continuously sick. She awoke again and again during the night because of acute pains in her breasts, diaphragm, and four limbs. She kept coughing uncontrollably from time to time. Her bodily temperature kept fluctuating -- moving from burning fever to shivering cold. Christa complained of swollen glands inside her throat and groin. She experienced great stomach tension, accompanied by a nearly irrepressible urge to vomit each time she tried to eat.

I call these symptoms the 'flukey flue' -- many clients experience them at some time during their treatment. They bear a close resemblance to a real flue and are frequently perceived as such. But they vanish so suddenly that the client begins to reconsider my interpretation that they represent a massive collapse of the middle layers of the mesodermal muscular sheath. I am not certain what they signify in terms of the dearmoring process, except that their appearance means that we have reached the body's threshold for hard catalytic bodywork. Their appearance also usually means that the diaphragmatic block has been loosened. Whenever a client describes such symptoms, I either curtail bodywork altogether for the present session or administer only nurturing touch. That so many of my clients undergo them inclines me to believe that they are inevitable to the first stage dearmoring process. And the sooner a client can allow himself to experience them, the sooner the transition to second stage. Similar symptoms can also appear after very gentle bodywork sessions.

After describing her uncomfortable night, Christa begins to talk about her history of terrible dreams:

> I used to go to a psychologist when I was only eight years old because each night I was dreaming and dreaming and I was afraid to sleep. I had to make drawings of my dreams. I was always drawing people without hands. I remember being aggressive because each time I made a drawing, the psychologist said, 'The fingers, where are they?'. I had to draw them in and it was such a big, difficult decision for me. My resistance was

so great.

I ask Christa why it was so difficult to draw the fingers, given what she has learned about her own fingers. She responds :

> I cannot turn my hands like this (She extends her hands forwards with the palms up). Just with the left hand which is cramped. I am afraid to make this gesture (She extends the hands again with the palms open and upwards). To give hands to other people it would be to give my hands to do (She places both hands around her throat). ... to strangulate myself.
>
> This past night I had the impression that the only thing living in me is my right hand. I don't know why. I was holding Ilsa because I was afraid. The only thing I could do to release me was to hold her with my right hand because this hand was sensible but the rest of my body was frightened.
>
> The phantasy I had was that my right hand is like a hand that comes from out of the ground like a plant or a tree. This part is in the earth (She indicates the lower wrist upwards to the shoulder) and this part is coming out. (She indicates the wrist and hand)... I wondered last night about the sensibility of this hand and that with just this hand alone I could receive the warmth I needed.

I ask Christa to leave her clothes fully on and to lie on the mattress on her back. I lie down beside her and say: "Let's see what you do with your right hand". For the next ten minutes, Christa makes the following exploration in total silence. While keeping her eyes and head held rigidly straight, she puts her hands exploringly upon her face. After a couple of minutes, she closes her eyes. Slowly, she extends her right hand to find my left hand lying at my side. She holds it for a minute lightly and tentatively. Then she grips it as she draws my hand away from my side and rests it in her hand lying over her abdominal region. She plays with my hand a little by moving it in her fingers, at first tentatively, but with increasing spontaneity. It tickles a little, so I laugh, and then withdraw my hand.

This sequence indicates that Christa has moved towards a clearer differentiation of the extent of her distorted body image. Five days previously, she experienced her left hand as a horrible bird's claw -- essentially vulture-like. Now in a spontaneous momentary act, she recognizes that both of her hands are equally alienated from the rest of her. More significantly, she recognizes that in their state of relatively encapsulated isolation, they are just as prone to act destructively against herself as they are against someone else. In fact, they are more prone to actively manifest a destructive aggressiveness against herself. Both hands, when propelled into spontaneous action, are equally contaminated in the sense of being anti-contact-oriented both towards the inner and outer worlds of reality. Both, when confronted with the prospect of actively extending themselves outwards towards another human being, are inclined to cut all life flow moving from within outwards towards other people.

The only gesture which Christa can make which positively affirms contact between herself and another is when her right hand reaches out to pull the other to her front half, especially to her chest region. She made these affirmative movements with me in the session just described and during the previous night with her friend Ilsa. This shrunken use of her hands implies that they do not belong to her as active agents of subject-world contact. They have become relegated to limbo -- they belong to nobody. In a metaphorical sense, they have been unconsciously disinherited.

The imagery associated with Christa's right hand signals the beginning of the birth of her real, deeper self. This process includes a literal reconstruction of her own body in the immediacy of self-awareness. It takes two forms: the objective bioenergetic reconstituting of her organism and her dawning recognition of her primary dynamic feeling needs within her psychic depths. The two realms of phenomena are wholly interdependent. Hands are one of man's most unique instruments for establishing an active and humanly differentiated contact with living reality without and within. As Christa's core longitudinal energy currents are slowly awakened, her hands will be compelled from within to reach out and to actively initiate contact with other people. Both of her hands, her left more than her right, must have become charged with such powerfully conflicting impulses that she was forced to dissociate them from actively belonging to herself in order to survive with tolerable amounts of anxiety. Consciously facing these impulses alone would have been too overwhelming and catastrophic.

Christa's experience of holding my left hand in her right one gives some clues as to the traumatic origin of her symbolically cutting off her hands. After taking my hand to her upper abdomen, Christa opens her eyes and turns her head to look directly into my eyes as she plays with my fingers. And after looking into my eyes, she was even able to place my open palm against her diaphragmatic region as she cupped her hand over mine. Afterwards, she remarks :

> It was a good feeling. I looked at your eyes. I could continue to hold your hand because I didn't see any hate or pushing away. So I could touch you also.

These remarks suggest that the dissociation of her hands is linked to a failure of immediate non-threatening feeling exchange between her eyes and her mother's. Christa spoke repeatedly throughout treatment of two basic modes of interaction with her mother: her mother pushed her away or gazed at her with undisguised hatred. On innumerable occasions, her mother's hateful eyes glowered down at her when she finally came to Christa's bedside in response to her crying.

Christa probably reached out to hold her mother in these situations. Perhaps her mother would condescend to hold Christa for a short time in hopes of quieting her child. But since Christa was a very high-energy and desperately needy child, she would have responded to this small token of affection and direct contact by clinging aggressively to her mother. Christa's intense emotion and direct demand would have quickly taxed a mother so alienated from her vital feelings. Such alienation would compel such a mother to push her child away. Assuming an authoritarian stance and a cold voice and bearing, she would leave the room, once again abandoning Christa to her solitary state of chronic emotional deprivation.

III. The Vampire Mother

A pattern of interaction similar to the one between Christa and her mother includes so many mixed messages that the child remains confused and frustrated. The mother feels just enough obligation and guilt to make token gestures of meeting the child's needs for attention. But such mothers are not in touch with their unconscious hostility and contempt towards their child. Without even realizing it, they double-bind their child's emotions. They twist the child into the same ambivalence that they themselves unconsciously feel. Such mothers are unconsciously persecutory, beginning with the child's birth. They become vampire like in their progressive possessiveness as their child becomes increasingly civilized and impulse-inhibited. They breed a deep sense of distrust in the child which develops into fullscale paranoia as the child matures.

As with Christa, this paranoia often extends to the child's own body as much as to the overtures of other people. Christa developed a generalized contamination and rigidification of feeling in both body and psyche. Her body parts which came repeatedly into contact with her mother's body met with painful frustration as she was continually separated from her mother prematurely. As this process repeated itself, these parts eventually became frozen off from the inner mainsprings of vital energy flow. She was forced to armor herself against feeling her own body, especially those parts which contained the greatest concentration of double-binding negative feeling reactions. Any child who has to deflect a mother's cold and hateful eyes is forced to erect a ring of armoring around the entire peripheral surface of the body. This ring enables the child at an early age to totally repress the cruel rejecting vibrations emanating from the mother's being. Later the child similarly cuts off his hands and arms as he is continually frustrated with every active attempt to reach out for human warmth. Failure to make interpersonal contact usually initiates the armoring process. And the pain of this failure is so traumatic that the child will sacrifice his own body by bioenergetically sealing it off from the mainstream of inner life flow.

In order to reclaim her vital energy flow, Christa needed to regressively reexperience the painful conflicting feelings which flooded her with anxiety in her early relationship to her mother. This process is enabled as the peripheral sheath thaws and the core longitudinal energy currents strengthen. But even these developments are not always sufficient to bring to the surface the very early catastrophic anxieties which are sufficiently paralyzing to render a child completely helpless and hopeless. An immediate stimulus is often required. Such a stimulus emerged during our ninth session with Christa, the second session when she was accompanied by her friend, Ilsa. Christa talked about her feelings while lying in Ilsa's arms earlier that morning :

> I remembered that I had the same feeling that I had years and years ago. My phantasy was that now she takes me in her arms but this afternoon she will become aggressive towards me and it will be finished between us.
>
> The connection I make is when I was seven or eight years old my mother couldn't support me too. She was always having heart attacks since I was born and was sick. I was very bad. I was always crying and I was not a nice child. She placed me in a children's boarding school, but she didn't tell me that she would. One day she said to me that we would take a nice excursion today. I felt that something must be wrong, but I trusted her.
>
> Then we arrived at the terminal railway station and I saw my luggage there. At this moment I knew what was happening because I had been at this same boarding school before. I got out and sat down on the station platform and started crying. My mother went away, and they came from the school and said I was a bad child to be crying and that they ought to hit me. So I went to this children's home.
>
> But this feeling that she would -- never she told me that she would take me to this home when I was little. She just took me and I was there. I was so afraid that I would plead with my hands like this. (She holds out her arms clingingly). I would then have the feeling that I would have to hold her so that she wouldn't go away. (Her voice rises increasingly in intensity and pitch).

It's the last chance. The feeling is that I can only take her for a little moment and then she will go. It has nothing to do with any real hope of stopping her. It's not that I am mistrusting her as Ilsa, but what feeling comes up is absolutely unreal... It's always this fear that if I am like that bad child, they will have to give me away just like my mother did it.

I direct Christa and Ilsa to reenact the scene: Ilsa, you stand over Christa. Christa, you kneel, hold Ilsa's hands and talk the way you did as a child, while closing your eyes. After only a second, Christa begins to cry, struggling at first. But after a few seconds, she bursts into torrential sobs and poorly articulated screams of "MA MA, MA MA, MA MA." After two minutes, she grows quiet. She is grasping Ilsa's arms, just above the wrist -- she does not touch Ilsa's hands. I ask Christa to close her eyes and speak to her mother, remembering what she felt as a child, while speaking with the insight of an adult. She begins :

> I'm so afraid of myself because I know when I am bad that you will give me away, and because I am so afraid that you will give me away, I am bad. I'm crying and crying, and when I am I know that it turns against me. This anxiousness is turned against me and I cannot get out of my circle.
>
> The more you show me how you suffer on my account, the more I cry. I would cry away your suffering face... I wished that you would come to me and be strong enough to break this circle for once... and not give me away. But I knew that I had to return as a changed child or otherwise you would give me away again and again.
>
> (Sobbing in between sentences now) The home leader said it to me, 'I have to change you into a good child; and you are guilty for the sickness of your mother'. And (more haltingly now) I couldn't tell you that... but I don't know... what to do... The more you suffer like this, the more anxious I become, and the badder, and the more I cry. You did understand that I was so anxious that you would give me away, and I understood that you did give me away, and I felt so lonely.

(She is speaking more quietly now).

No doubt it was this particular set of childhood experiences which finally sealed Christa off and totally alienated her from her primary dynamic feeling needs, and, simultaneously, created the deep chronic split in her psyche. Thereafter, she had no alternative but to cultivate a cerebralized self-system which was distinguished for its submissive compliance to her mother's tyrannical will. Returning Christa to a children's home for a second time finally confirmed that she was caught in a vicious trap with no possibility of escape. Unless she could mould herself to fit her mother's image of a good child, she would again pay the terrible price of extreme deprivation and insecurity. She had no alternative but to stop fighting for her soul's inner integrity and vitality and to fashion herself into her mother's expectations.

Christa's mother was so dominated by her cerebral cortex and a perverse will-to-power centered in her upper back, that she could only relate by bullying Christa into a highly life-denying set of rigid rules of proper behavior. She was totally incapable of relating to Christa from her sympathetic feeling centers in the front half of her body except in the most insidious manner of reaching out for sympathy from her daughter. The mother's frequent heart attacks and other sicknesses were all probably psychosomatically induced. They were unscrupulous weapons for clobbering Christa's vital feeling impulses to near extinction. They were hysterically self-deceiving devices which enabled her to limit responsibility for her child. They also provided a pretext for instilling into Christa a sense of personal guilt and responsibility for her mother's physical weaknesses.

From the outset, Christa was doomed -- any behavior springing from her own vital feeling centers would be viewed as bad and wrong. In one way or another, Christa's mother was unconsciously determined to possess her daughter's soul. She was driven by a demon within, a demon which feeds on a cerebralized alienation from life and a will motivated to take revenge upon life both within and without, slowly killing any perceptible life forms. Therefore, Christa was wise to capitulate to her mother's bullying will, even though she had to repress her soul to the point of complete dependence upon her mother's values and ideals. She adjusted to a lower level of chronic anxiety and ontological insecurity that remained largely hidden from the objective consciousness of both mother and daughter, thereby maintaining a false appearance of equanimity and contact with her mother.

At eight years of age, Christa made a conscious choice to learn to adjust to her mother's petulant needs, during her second six months stint at the children's home. Thereafter, her chronic distrust of her mother became a protection against over-identification with her mother's destructiveness. Christa's response to Ilsa reveals how this deep distrust of her mother congealed into a firmly fixed attitude towards anyone else with whom she became intimately involved. Ilsa had become Christa's mediator to her fellow man, a mother substitute, older sister and guru combined. Christa had fastened herself tenaciously to Ilsa. Her ontological insecurity was so great that only now at the age of thirty-one was she able to begin to face the enormity of her distrust of other people, including Ilsa.

It was a significant achievement for Christa to allow her irrational distrust to surface spontaneously while lying in Ilsa's arms. One of the peculiarities of the paranoid position is that the individual does not begin to recognize his paranoia until the external interpersonal and social situation becomes safe. The last thing any desperately paranoid person can face is the omnipresence of the psyche's tendency to project negative fears and expectations on to one's immediate relationships. But until a person can begin to spontaneously claim the paranoid projections of his psyche, the dearmoring process cannot evolve further. The yielding of the musculature goes hand in hand with the yielding of the psyche's unconscious ego-defenses against interpersonal closeness. Christa's growing understanding of her relationship with Ilsa is an example of this indispensable element in the dissolution of character-muscular armoring: she identifies in the moment her innermost catastrophic expectations regarding Ilsa. Furthermore, she connects her present irrational perceptual distortion of reality to a very rational memory of what happened in the distant past.

Making this significant connection enables

Christa's psyche to expand its repressed boundaries of consciousness. Now she can begin to feel more fully the enormity of emotional insecurity which held her captive within her own psyche. Recognition of the degree of her bondage is poignantly revealed when Christa recognizes that her fear of abandonment by Ilsa is not grounded in the present. She also begins to crystallize how she is totally encircled in her present adult relationships because of her underlying but unacknowledged mistrust of others upon whom she depends emotionally. The perceptual recognition of her present attitude towards Ilsa represents one of Christa's first approaches to a creative experience of chaotic divergence out of consciousness into repressed unconscious material -- she confuses time and space as she incoherently lumps together what happened between her mother and herself and what is still happening between Ilsa and herself. She is on the threshold of cognitive differentiation between past emotional trauma and present perceptual distortions of reality: this is tantamount to opening up hitherto encapsulated parts of the psyche.

To return to her treatment process, Christa's words appear disoriented as she moves her limbs to reenact her half-hearted attempts to delay her mother's inevitable departure. Her voice begins to express impending catastrophe. The anxiety conveyed in its rising pitch plunges her into a chaotic divergence out of her normally focused rational consciousness. I structured physical contact between Christa and Ilsa just after Christa's psychological disorientation triggered the memory of how she used her arms to delay her mother's departure. Clasping Ilsa's wrists enables Christa to rapidly crescendo into intense infantile feelings. Her plunge into repressed feelings emanated from her primary dynamic feeling centers in her lower back regions and in her chest. Aggressive self-assertiveness from her lower back filled her partly panic-stricken, partly omnipotent screaming at her mother not to abandon her again. Most infantile screaming emanates from the lower back and represents the child's willful demand that his wishes be met immediately. But Christa's screams also contained the anguished pathos of unfulfilled longing and active reaching out for her mother's caring which emanates from the eros center in the chest.

Spontaneous surfacing of repressed emotions,

both positive and negative, inevitably unfolds when the psyche is loosened enough to permit consciousness to make connections between the uncompleted feeling past and present reality. The gates of censorship between consciousness and the repressed unconscious open. In addition, the core longitudinal energy currents have become mobilized by Christa's physical contact with Ilsa. They radiated upwards to produce Christa's externalization of affect. The direct touch between the two women catalyzed the destruction of the censor in Christa's head. In other words, the downward flowing metabolic energy current generated by the cortex was temporarily overpowered by the upward flowing core vegetative currents. This reversal allowed Christa to more fully reexperience her acute emotional impasse as her mother abandoned her when she was eight years old.

One of the signs that Christa is fully reexperiencing this event is the relative ease with which she addresses her mother immediately following her cathartic outpouring of repressed emotions. She authentically reproduces the conflicting feelings which pervaded her eight year old being with an accuracy and a depth of understanding that indicate that both her cognitive and her feeling faculties are newly alive and open to her early painful psychic reality. She was able to tolerate reexperiencing the state of acute chronic anxiety in which she lived during those earlier years. This achievement in itself has an inestimable healing impact, especially since she accurately differentiated the hopelessness of her childhood situation in relation to her mother. The more she could reexperience her childhood anxiety, the more she could confront the objective reality of her mother's tyrannical power. Christa recognizes, "You did understand that I was so anxious that you would give me away", and so begins to realize that her mother was devoid of kindness and compassion.

More attention is due to the event which triggered Christa's falling into divergent chaos: her bodily reenactment of clinging to her mother to forestall her inevitable departure. The mobilization of extreme anxiety was rapidly generated by this event -- Christa relapsed into a state of acute emotional desperation characterized by total resignation and helplessness. This state escalated when Christa was asked to hold Ilsa's arm. She became so panic-stricken that she could not take Ilsa's hands.

Reaching out for interpersonal sympathetic contact with her arms and hands produced extreme catastrophe largely because Christa was forced to sacrifice her hands and arms when she surrendered to her mother's will. All four of her limbs became split off as she unconsciously gave them over psychologically to her mother's tyrannical will. This sacrifice represents the bioenergetic price of adopting an attitude of compliance to her mother's demands. Thus Christa's adoption of a cerebralized self-system not only sealed her off from her primary dynamic Being centers, but also alienated her core regions of vital flow from her four limbs.

This double-fronted sealing off of parts of Christa's metabolism began very early. When Christa surrendered to her mother's will, she also surrendered any hope of ever satisfying her primary feeling need for unconditional positive acceptance. This primary need is affirmed when an adequately loving mother affirms the circuit of feelings which are immediately exchanged between the solar plexus of the mother and the solar plexus of the child during the holding stage of development. Christa was abandoned and rejected by her mother throughout this entire stage. Subsequently, she was continually rejected whenever she risked actively reaching out for a sympathetic response from her mother which would have signified an unconditional positive acceptance of her just as she was.

By identifying her will to behave with her mother's values and mode of being, Christa not only introjected her mother's negative image into her own psyche, but also her mother's alienation from her body into her own body. This point cannot be emphasized enough because it has been largely overlooked by orthodox psychotherapists: the psychological capacity for a prepubescent child to metamorphose his metabolic energy currents into unconscious patterns which accurately imitate the organism of the dominant parent. By introjecting her mother's psyche, Christa was forced to introject her mother's peripherally armored muscular sheath. To do this, she had not only to repress her primary dynamic feeling centers, but also to consolidate and reinforce the surface energy currents which flow down from the cortical synergist, and by way of the voluntary cerebrospinal network, spread themselves throughout the peripheral regions of the torso.

There is no doubt that Christa's mother was so constituted bioenergetically and psychodynamically. Her mother was totally blocked from expressing herself with her arms and hands from the sympathetic feeling centers in the front half of the body. Instead, she was compelled to use the bullying will to power over the other of her upper back region. This will to power induced Christa to cling to her mother in a mutuality of self-other destructiveness, thus generating and reinforcing an ongoing strangulation of both women's primary feeling centers. This is the essence of the vampire syndrome: to break the vital self-assertive center of the other's lower back to the point where the other must cling to oneself in a closed circuit of interaction that makes no contact at the freely flowing surface or at the vital core of either body.

We can now begin to grasp the real power of the Terrible Mother image when it is unconsciously introjected by an emotionally dependent daughter. The daughter adopts the same invalidating attitude towards her own life-affirmative instincts and feelings which the mother has communicated indirectly since the child's conception. The mother's basic underlying hostility becomes internalized by the daughter's prematurely awakened secondary feeling centers in the regions of the neck and pelvic-leg joints. This psychic complex becomes synchronized with the defensively organized mental circuits in the cerebral cortex to form a self-invalidating false self-system. In Christa's case, the introjection of her mother's negative image repressed her hitherto unfulfilled need for an unconditional positive acceptance by her mother, and erects in its place a viciously active intropunitive attitude towards her own unsatisfied primal needs and impulses. Adopting her mother's negative image of her, Christa actually believes that she is hopelessly bad, weak and incapable of considering the needs of others. She becomes totally possessed by a guilt-ridden and self-castigating super-ego. Such a psychological development is the quintessence of a split psyche.

More horrendous still, however, is the way in

which the incorporation of the death-dealing Terrible Mother image reconstitutes the vital metabolic forces within the victimized child. Christa's mother had undoubtedly resigned herself long before Christa was born to relationships devoid of any vestige of dynamic feeling circuits of real interchange between self and others. She had withdrawn into the citadel of her compulsively organized will. Here she remained impervious to the life-affirmative forces within and without by erecting a hard peripheral muscular wall of armoring. Christa did precisely the same thing to her own limbs by unconsciously rejecting their efforts to express feelings or need-inpulses which welled up from the mysterious inner depths of her soul. Her hands and limbs became unconsciously contaminated and perceived as grotesquely forbidden agents for satisfying her loathesome animal needs. Viewing the left hand as the claw of a bird of prey represents her psyche's perception of her body after incorporation of her mother's demonic alienation from her hands and limbs. Christa's hands and arms have become so possessed by the Terrible Mother within her that they want to strangle any vital feeling forces that still flourish deep inside her. This is revealed by their inclination to strangle her own throat -- the one important remaining outlet for spontaneous expression of her primary feeling centers.

Another example from the session under discussion illustrates the extent of Christa's introjection of her mother's values and mode of being. Christa is standing, wearing a mask which completely covers her eyes, while Katherine stands about three feet in front of her. Christa is to play herself while Katherine enacts her mother. I ask Christa to interact with her mother through direct body contact as much as possible, but I have deliberately not structured anything specific.

After breathing deeply and audibly, Christa addresses Katherine: "It is so different when you are my mother I --- OOhh". Christa has gathered in her breath with a gasp and holds it suspended. This quick, small gesture is emblematic for what shortly develops. The gesture represents an organismic tendency to withdraw in fright from the present reality. The holding of her breath allows her to desensitize her awakened senses and to numb her consciousness.

Christa has a long history of withdrawing into such states of partial paralysis -- her choked up throat and chest make breathing difficult during these times. This is a classical hysterical device for not confronting immediate reality.

After her throat valves open following an exhalation, Christa mumbles, "I am afraid... and I am not afraid". After a short silence, she says, "I am confused because I cannot see you or control how you are looking". Katherine does not move, thus forcing Christa to initiate any physical contact. Christa continues, "She took me in her arms but had a bad look at the same time, so I never knew how to be". Katherine clarifies Christa's words:

K : She held you and had a bad look at the same time ?

C : Yah. Where are you ?

K : Standing right in front of you.

Christa begins to weep quietly, her breathing erratic. Silence. Christa sighs in despair. Katherine breaks the silence :

K : I have my hand on my heart.

C : Why ?

K : Because you are so bad it hurts.

C : Yah I know... I know. I can't ask you to take me in your arms, because... you won't like me.

Christa is now speaking with tremendous sincerity and bitterness. Katherine responds :

K : Because you are so naughty, so loud.

C : I don't know what to do with you. I don't know. Give me another mama.

Christa is sniffling -- her voice is beginning to rise in pitch, while struggling to breathe in between sentences :

C : Give me another mama who is not as cold as you.

K : I could be nice to a sweet girl.

Katherine speaks matter-of-factly, successfully conveying an attitude of self-righteous aloofness. Christa bursts out loudly with considerable anger:

C : It is so easy for you to pose like this. I am such a little girl. You are the only person I have. You can do whatever you want with me. (Her voice reaches a scream) I can't touch you. I can't.

Katherine says coldly :

K : Look at you. What are you crying about.

C : I know that finally I will have to come to you because I have nothing else. I cannot stand not being touched by somebody. I know that I will have to come because you are destroying all the relationships I have. You are laughing about my neediness for tenderness. You are laughing all the time about it. I can't touch you.

K : But I do touch you.

C : It's like a dead hand you have. Heavy and dead, pushing me down. It makes me afraid... You are cold. You will eat me as cold as you are, or let me alone, one or the other.

Realizing that Christa is totally frozen and unable to reach out, Katherine places both of her extended hands against Christa's outer shoulders. She begins to push Christa in little rhythmical shoves. Immediately, Christa utters plaintively, "Mama, No, No, No, No, Mama, Mama, No, No." Her voice becomes louder and louder, sounding about fifteen years old. She bursts into deep open-throated crying which appears to relieve her growing tension as she actively resists Katherine's pushing. But after two minutes, she says, "Mama, I will be good". She can no longer resist Katherine's pressure, nor speak intelligibly. Increasingly, she cannot exhale deeply without prematurely gasping for air. Progressively swallowed by her own breathing, she becomes preoccupied with surviving through an inadequate intake of air. After struggling through this obstacle, she begins to make sounds again, but they are distinctly more regressed -- sounds from a five or six-year-old girl. But she must struggle to breathe again until she vomits some mucous. Then she continues to whine pulsatingly with each exhalation as she collapses on the mattress and finally eludes Katherine's touch.

The most important feature about this interchange is that Christa faces her still fully intact ambivalence about reaching out for sympathetic direct touch from her mother. The encouragement to use her arms and hands coupled with the physical separation between the two women polarizes an approach-avoidance chronic impasse within Christa. She could tolerate it only briefly before disintegrating into total helplessness. More fully than ever before, Christa confronted her underlying distrust and hostility towards her mother.

The mobilization of Christa's lower back center enabled her to resist her mother as enacted by Katherine. She maintained an active self-assertive stance, not relating directly to her mother's body for a commendably long time -- an eloquent testament of Christa's growing confidence and belief. Her resistance crumbles as Katherine becomes assertive and initiates bodily contact. The entire front half of Christa's torso begins to freeze in response to the growing constriction of her throat. Not only does Christa's formidable throat block become prominent, but also in keeping with the hysteric's usual pattern, her entire front half, both chest and abdomen, simultaneously freezes to strangle any core longitudinal energy currents rising expansively from her lower half. This development allows Christa no choice but to flee from outer reality.

The eventual collapse of Christa's resistance to Katherine's overtures is due to the still intact armoring in her peripheral muscular sheath. This same sheath has enabled Christa to maintain a defensive position against direct contact with her mother. It has allowed her to defend herself against her mother's hatred, her coldness, her inability to hold Christa without hostile glances, and her mother's ridicule of Christa's need for emotional warmth. It has kept her in touch with her longing for another mother. The ability to directly resist her imagined mother, however, indicates a temporary intensification of the sheath followed by a total collapse and withdrawal of interpersonal contact.

At this point in treatment, Christa is still caught in the battle between resistance and surrender. This is reflected in her response to Katherine's statement that she has behaved so badly that she is almost killing her mother's heart. Christa introjectingly accepts this assessment and succumbs: she bitterly acknowledges that her reaching out for contact is pointless, not only because her mother dislikes her, but also because she is intrinsically unlikeable. Christa has plunged into an old emotional imprisonment within her mother's double-binding stance.

Christa's continuing verbal counter-attack reveals that her mother's touch always connoted death rather than life. It also reveals the suffocating impact of her mother's vampire tendency to erect a psychological wall within Christa which made contact with anyone else virtually impossible. Her mother largely succeeded in making Christa believe that she would be inevitably disappointed if she attempted to find loving support and emotional satisfaction with anyone else but her mother. Christa clarifies this possessiveness as she acknowledges her mother's desire to eat her emotionally even as she remains overtly cold. These contradictory messages typify the demonic engulfment and absolute power of one soul over another which is chracteristic of a Terrible Mother interpersonal circuit.

Christa was reclaiming a non-distorted body image as she actively resisted her mother for a brief period of time and refused to reach out for sympathetic bodily contact. For the first time, she identified and repudiated her former identification with her mother's deadened surface energy flow. Once again we see how the healing impact of catalytic techniques involves an intensification of the body regions which are arrested by the greatest implosion of inhibition-impulse twistings of opposite tendencies. The polarization of Christa's hands and arms to actively choose either to reach out or not reach out enabled her to discover inner strengths never previously mobilized against her mother. Christa's discovery of her own creative resources is further confirmed as she resists her mother. Her deeper energy blocks inside the peripheral muscular sheath begin to prevail and push her into flight from contact only as Katherine resorts to more aggressive methods.

Chapter VI

EVOLUTION OF THE THERAPEUTIC RELATIONSHIP

The interpersonal dimension of the treatment and healing process is as complex as the client's dearmoring process throughout first and second stage. Katherine and I are wholly allied with the contemporary movement of humanistic psychology as distinct from mechanistic and behavioristic clinical approaches to working with the body of the psyche. Such approaches invariably rely upon atomistic models of human functioning which reduce and analyze man in terms of some kind of measurable machine. We believe, to the contrary, that man's inner psychobiological resources are ultimately unfathomnable, inexhaustible. When functioning in unity, they provide the wisest source of decision-making in response to all outer and inner situations of meaningful contact. Therefore, our model of full human functioning must give priority to man's uniquely self-created modes of subject-world contact.

The wise body psychotherapist, I have already suggested, always perceives and relates to the client from his own alive and intact primary dynamic feeling centers. He always allows his creative intuition to guide in the cultivation of a circuit of feeling vibrations between himself and the client which is absolutely unique in every therapeutic long-term relationship. The art of psychotherapy hinges upon the therapist's intuitive cultivation of a totally distinctive mode of interaction with each individual.

The therapist's half-conscious, half-unconscious cultivating of a therapeutic relationship thus rests upon the final flowering of his or her own primary dynamic feeling capacities in their more advanced stages of individual transformation. A therapist becomes wise precisely because his secondary intuitive centers have already been transformed into self-actualizing modes of subject-world relatedness. This achievement permits the therapist to trust his feeling centers to spontaneously cultivate a relationship which acknowledges the client's internal process, while at the same time polarizing the client's growth towards self-actualization.

The belly region of the therapist which once

functioned as an internal stabilizer and preserver of an ongoing homeostatic continuity of being develops into the Great Hara Center of the core self. The belly functions in a mature adult as the harmonizer of conflicts and the integrator of opposite tendencies. It is the seat of the mature individual's continuity of self-identity and self-esteem. From this region, a therapist is able to generate a circuit of immediate feeling vibrations which convey an unconditional positive acceptance of the client's present condition as well as for his future promise. From this region, a therapist is able to psychologically and emotionally continue to relate to the client in an other-affirmative mode which contains the fragmented psychic vibrations emanating from the client.

The chest region of the therapist which once functioned as the mediator of a totally symbiotic fusion with the mother is transformed in the mature adult into the Agape-Eros Center of the core self. From this region, a mature adult can reach out and unify himself sympathetically with the feeling vibrations and psychic space of another human being. This region mediates what Rogers calls the therapist's empathic identification with the client. This empathy never amounts to the primary-process level of intense emotional investment which occurs with total fusion between two people. Such a fusion between adults is usually reserved for passional love relationships. By contrast, the kind of sympathetic contact between therapist and client must always remain consistently secondary-process Agape-dominant, or spiritually differentiated in nature. Nevertheless, unless a therapist's primary feeling center in his chest is fully alive and integrated, he cannot generate an immediate exchange of warm and authentic feeling investment in the client's emotional pain.

The upper back region which once functioned as an instinctive tendency to distance oneself from others in order to perceive them more objectively, is transformed in the mature adult into the Logos Center of the core self. The self-actualizing adult discovers a powerful need to understand the inner and outer worlds of his experience as an intrinsic end in itself. This need transcends any acquisition of empirical knowledge gained by the inductive analytical intellect. When this logos need to understand is directed by a therapist towards a client, it manifests itself as an intuitive faculty of the creative imagination, and not as a scientific categorizer which dissects the client's being according to abstract theoretical constructs. Logos mediates Being-Cognition, not intellectually detached and operationally measurable objective knowledge. The logos faculty enables the therapist to maintain a heightened middle-in-mode subject-centered objectivity as he relates to the client's soul from moment to moment. It also enables him to verbally share with the client reflectively distilled perceptions of the client's development. A fully functioning Logos permits a therapist to practice an other-affirmative style of what Reich called ego-resistance character interpretation which never overinvades the soul of the client.

The lower back center which once functioned as a fiercely survival-motivated tendency towards self-assertiveness against outer threats is transformed in the mature adult into the Great Warrior Center of the core self. The Warrior Center permits the self-actualizing individual to create new horizons which challenge his will to competency. It is the source of man's continual striving to perfect himself with a warrior spirit of dedication. It is the medium by which a mature person establishes a long-term project whose actualization requires continual testing of resolve to complete a task reflecting unique destiny. Every long-term treatment relationship becomes an ego-transcending challenge to the therapist. His Warrior Center risks encounter so as to fecundate the client's own determination to persevere in the task of self-transformation. In the deepest sense, the lower back center functions as the spiritual will to believe and carry through to quiet satisfaction the higher purposes to which one becomes committed. Often a client is so alienated from his lower back region that he cannot even conceptualize a commitment to anything truly challenging, such as the giving up of neurotic functioning. In such cases, a therapist is intuitively obligated to affirm a belief in the client's potential for eventually standing on his own feet to maintain his ground in the face of difficult obstacles.

These four modes of interpersonal relatedness contribute to a therapeutic relationship which is fluid and process-centered rather than structure-bound. Based upon the therapist's intuitive sense of where the client is at the moment, both bioenergetically and psychodynamically, a therapist allows any one of the four modes to dominate a given transaction. Generally, any transaction involving a Logos-dominant or Warrior-dominant mode of contact is a masculine style of interaction, whereas an Agape-Eros or Hara-dominant mode is a feminine style. A therapist must be able to call with equal effectiveness upon these fundamentally different styles of interaction throughout all phases of treatment.

A structure-bound therapist is one who uses his professional position of authority and expertise to cultivate a false facade in his relationship to a client. To the extent that any therapist is not actively rooted in a spontaneously living from his own dynamic Being centers, he will adopt a structure-bound role in relating to the client. For instance, consider the structure-bound role inspired by Freud: the orthodox psychoanalyst deliberately maintains as much personal detachment as possible from any interpersonal feeling exchange with the client. The Freudians have rationalized this role largely because of their exclusive trust in reason as the only real healing power available. They only trust in the Logos authority under the domination of the analytically-oriented cerebral cortex as the therapist's exclusive medium for strengthening the client's ego to progressively conquer his id and super-ego. Therefore, a deep distrust of instinct-driven emotionality and an attitude of vigilant wariness towards the irrational id is reinforced through the medium of cerebralized analytical interpretations.

An even greater danger is presented by the therapist whose egotism blindly and falsely deceives him into believing he is more self-actualizing and other-affirmative than he in fact really is. If a therapist's vegetative longitudinal energy currents are not circulating constantly and vitally enough to permit all four of his spiritual intuitive authorities to interact with each other, he will invariably establish a relationship with a client which lacks a pre-cognitive circuit of feeling vibrations emanating between them. Only this circuit permits the client to optimally discover his own creative and self-healing resources. By contrast, such a therapist gradually cultivates a superior-inferior relationship characterized by a power over the client. This represents a subtle tyranny of one individual's will and cerebral cortex over another's. No psychotherapist is so enlightened that he knows what a client needs from moment to moment better than the client. In a generalized sense, a therapist can know what a client needs to move into and towards. And he can guide a client in that direction. However, the ultimate authority is determined by how well the therapist subjectively resonates to the unconscious wellsprings of the client's being and allows the latter to reveal what needs to be done.

Even during first stage when a therapist assumes a more directive stance, he will invariably overdominate and eventually engulf the client emotionally if his Hara and Agape-Eros faculties are not quietly flourishing within. The treatment will become therapist-centered rather than client-centered -- a fatal development for the healing process because of the excessive control and power over the client. Usually during first stage, a therapist's Logos and Warrior faculties prevail. But they must prevail lightly, always ready to be superceded at a moment's notice by the sympathetic centers. An integrated therapist never assumes a God-like authority or an intrusively bullying stance even for a moment. To the contrary, when a client's defenses have been excessively shattered and he is experiencing enormous psychic pain, a therapist should have the option to respond as a nurturing mother or as a fellow human being who gives unconditional support and containment of the client as he is.

Treatment focuses on gradually dissolving the old conditioning and rebuilding the client's soul from within the psychic orbit of the latter. This process must be wholly tolerable for the client throughout all phases. Otherwise, it becomes a mechanically grim process of pushing and pulling by outer forces and authorities to whom one entrusts oneself out of sheer desperation.

A therapist does have a great deal of specialized knowledge concerning a client's psychopathological condition. However, this knowledge comes to him from two distinct pathways: the cerebral cortex and the Logos Center. The cortex generates a clear and distinct rational inductive process, both bioenergetic and psychodynamic. By contrast, knowledge from the

Logos faculty is filtered through the primary feeling and sentient networks; it resurfaces in consciousness by way of the creative unconscious faculties. Understanding the client's psychopathology provided by the Reichian-Lowenian character types is postulated on a medical structure-bound model of observable forms and ideals of surface functioning. As such, it represents a scientific theoretical system based upon logically inductive-deductive constructs which superimpose upon the actual unique body and mind of every client a stereotyped set of abstract patterns. This classification system can be most helpful when a therapist initiates the therapeutic process and begins to gradually dismember the defended ego structure. It provides a useful shorthand for the various patterns of muscular armoring. However, exclusive focus on this model will actually obstruct the later stages of the soul-building process.

Therefore, the Reichian-Lowenian categories ought to be confined to the initial phases of first stage treatment. Thereafter, the intuitive sensibilities of the therapist's Being centers must assume dominance. Should a therapist find it difficult to stop superimposing a Reichian-Lowenian label, he has failed to establish a rich circuit of precognitive feeling vibrations between himself and the client. During first and second stage, this dynamic circuit provides the therapist with the kind of intuitive cognitive resonance which enables him to assess the degree of unconscious flowering in the client's primary feeling centers. The heart of second stage is the cultivation of the flowering of these dynamic centers through the satisfying of unsatisfied primary feeling needs. Consequently, unless a therapist is primarily guided by Logos, the client's primary feeling centers may never be fully affirmed. In fact, they may actually be extinguished in the hands of a therapist who is not really in contact with his own creative unconscious networks.

The cerebralized defense network and the accompanying rigid armoring cannot be optimally eroded without a simultaneous and progressive awakening of the client's feeling capacities for here-and-now relatedness. During first stage, most nurturing touch is intended to polarize the weak and dormant and unsatisfied feeling needs deep inside the client's organism. This is closely intertwined with the gradual awakening of the core longitudinal energy currents regulated by the vegetative nervous system. Consequently, it is difficult to separate energy-mobilization exercises generally from the more delicate fostering of the primary feeling capacities. It is difficult, that is, if the therapist is sufficiently attuned to these capacities and their importance through the medium of his own Logos and Agape-Eros faculties. Any practitioner of body techniques who does not acknowledge their existence in some conceptual-intuitive form cannot avoid using body techniques mechanically.

The same can be said for the use of consciousness-opening psychological techniques. I do not endorse the practice of character-analytic resistance analysis as taught by Reich himself. Such a practice presupposes that a therapist assumes an unnecessarily authoritarian and excessively assaultive stance. On the other hand, neither do I endorse a consistently Rogerian approach which presupposes that any attempt to confront a client with his defensive maneuvers is overly directive and therapist-centered. A consistent Rogerian attitude tends to invalidate a therapist's more masculine intuitive sensibilities -- his Logos and Warrior faculties. Without the Warrior faculty, a therapist cannot demand that a client persevere with a particular energy-mobilization or consciousness-confronting exercise until he peaks throughout his total organism. The capacity to expect the client to tolerate a limited degree of embodied physical pain is imperative for first stage catalytic bodywork, provided it is counterbalanced with nurturing, security-giving methods.

By the same token, without the self-assertive initiative arising from the Logos faculty, a therapist cannot begin to directly polarize a client's consciousness so as to become aware of his psychopathological patterns. Such an exchange involves a rudimentary polarization of the client's false self-image by the therapist's Logos capacity. A good example of this kind of interchange occurred in our seventh session with Christa. This session follows the one in which she talked about her right hand as the only part of her body which was sensible and alive. After verbalizing this discovery, Christa silently explored my left hand with her right hand. She remained in a quiet state following the session.

In fact, her interchange with us during the first half of the seventh session was low-energy enough to suggest that she had relapsed into a low-grade depression.

Perceiving Christa's sluggishness, I began to initiate catalytic bodywork, assuming a firmly self-assertive stance. For example, I start by placing her on the stool, giving her very explicit directions such as, "Make the sound of 'Ah,'" or "Move the pelvis up with every inhalation and down with every exhalation", or "Stop moving the body completely. Freeze", or "Move the head from side to side with each exhalation", or "Come off the stool and lie on the mattress". When I see that this work hardly affects her either emotionally or bioenergetically, I know that she is depressively withdrawn. This is confirmed by her self-depreciatory verbalizations which convey hopelessness and resignation. Again and again, I interrupt her remarks and direct low-key energy-mobilization exercises as she lies on her back. She responds obediently without any sign of resistance. When directed, she even immediately produces explosive sounds. Christa performs like an obedient, fearful child who would not dare to defy my instructions.

At one point, Christa begins spontaneously to explore her growing bodily and emotional responses in her lower half when making love with a man. A ring of hopefulness appears in her voice which immediately leaves as she reflects that all of her man-woman relationships have quickly terminated. Deliberately interrupting, I counter by mentioning her most recent relationship with a man which began just prior to her coming to California for treatment. I point out that he could not leave her after deep love-making until she forced him to leave because of the late hour. Christa tries to counter my countering by arguing that this man once told her that he was not able to love her even though he desired her. Her interpretation was that he could never love her because she was intrinsically unlovable. Vehemently attacking her conclusion, I postulate that he was merely being honest about his own neurotic inability to love. I also chastize her for such self-depreciatory neurotic thinking. Without giving her a chance to reply, I ask Christa to get on her feet and assume the severe starting stress position, the one in which the pelvis is extended forward while the head drops backward.

(see page 230).

Almost at once, Christa's body begins to tremor in a medium-fast, steady hum from head to toes. This indicates that her core energy currents are finally beginning to distribute themselves better and to radiate further outwards and upwards from her abdominal region. I ask her to drop her jaw and allow sound and then demand that she make louder sounds. Her sounds slowly become aggressive and uncontrolled, expressing much anger. I catalyze even further loosening of her energy flow by having Christa drop forward from her waist. After a minute, I direct her to shake her head wildly with each exhalation. As she complies, Christa mobilizes a still greater quantity of uncontrolled sound with each exhalation. But after about five explosive sounds, she suddenly stops. When I ask why, she says that she has an urge to vomit. Shoving a wastebasket in front of her feet, I respond in a half-provocative, half-serious manner, "That's what we want to get to. If you are going to vomit, vomit in this". She continues the violent headshaking as her upper half dangles in front of her lower half. Without any badgering from me, Christa heaves up mucous a couple of times. After I have directed her to lie down, Christa says, "I enjoyed this sound. I am happy because something was blocking up inside and I could feel it". When I ask her where she feels it, Christa points to her upper middle chest region below her throat on the side of her heart.

Placing one hand on the indicated spot and the other on the opposite side of her torso along her spinal column, I command her to shake her head. After a few exhalations, Christa throttles it again, explaining that she stops because of a rising impulse to vomit. As she persists in violently shaking her head, her vocal sounds assume an increasingly uncontrolled hoarseness which indicates a real collapse of the mesodermal musculature throughout her throat and chest areas. She is able to carry through to the point of physical exhaustion. Finally, to consummate the peaking of her now fully awakened energy currents, Katherine holds Christa's heels while I hold her hands. (see page 231) We lift her whole body a few inches into the air. I direct Christa to shake her head again while making sound. She manages with complete abandonment: her entire torso writhes

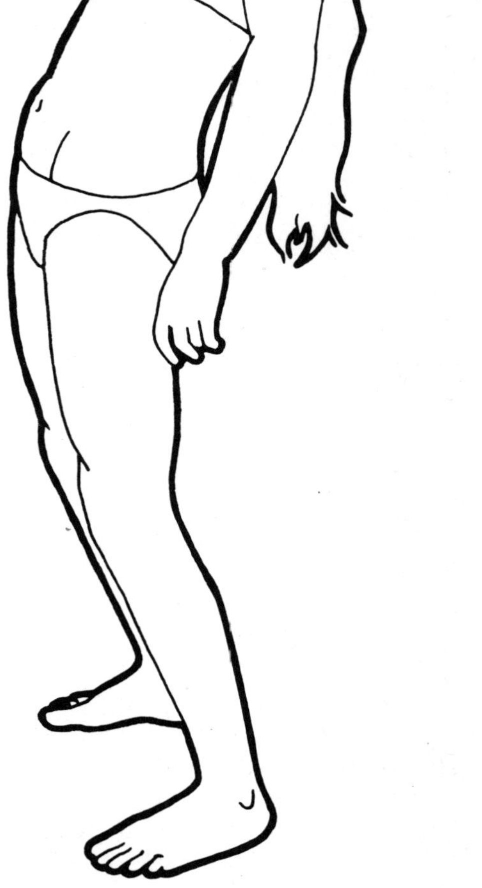

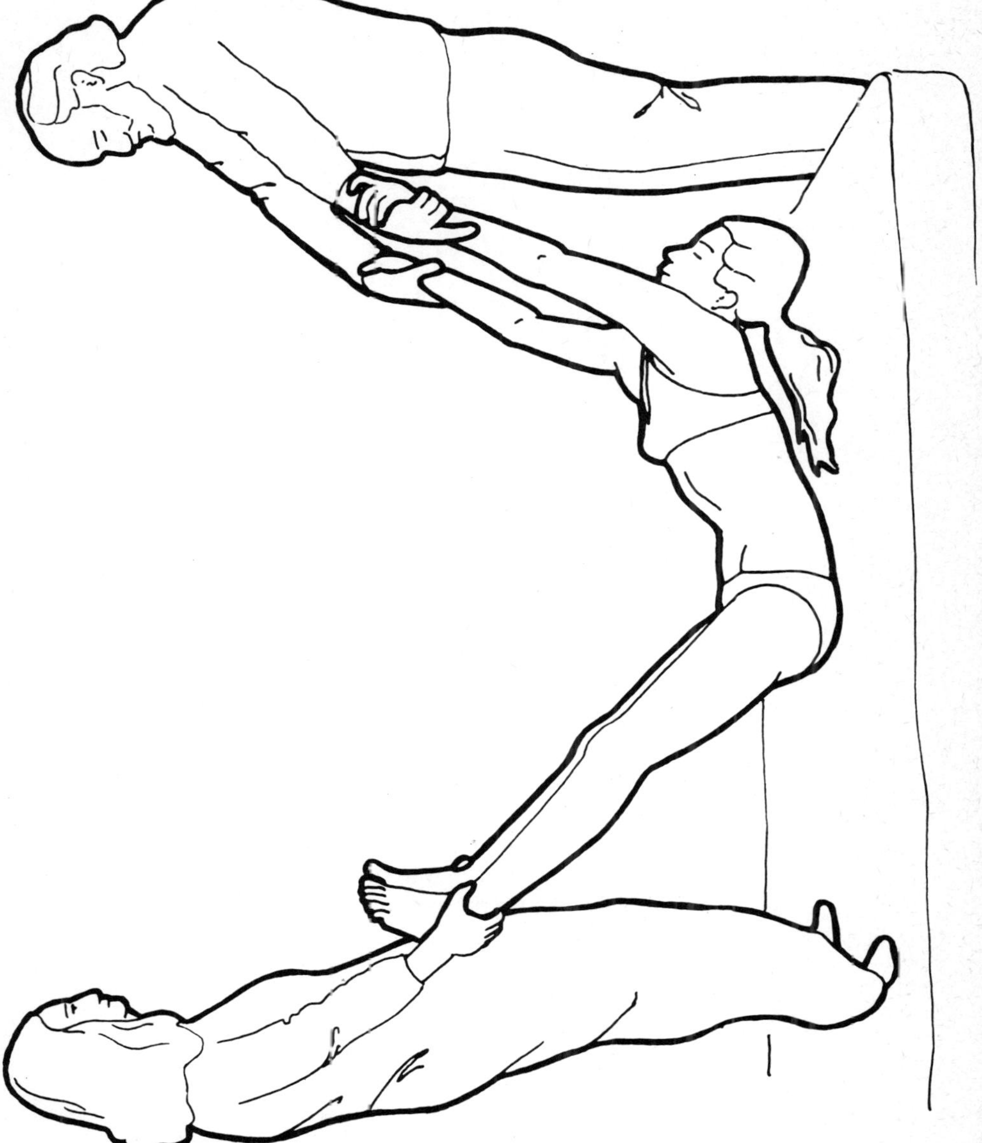

and her pelvis bounces up and down with each head shake. When these movements stop, we release our grip after letting her down. Her breathing is now deep, full, and slow, almost astonishingly so, given her recent violent movements and energy expenditure. After a brief silence, Christa speaks :

> A strange feeling I have... I'm playing a role... I can't explain. I don't realize clearly... I'm asking myself why I don't stand my ground and say this is my place and refuse to put my hands back over my head. This typifies my feeling towards men generally, that I can't do anything against them and stand my ground.

Speaking ironically, I respond, "You're passive". Katherine adds, "Helpless". And I chant, "Paralyzed and passive". Christa responds :

> Yah, and I hate it... I don't let out anything until I have so many aggressions that I'm lying on the bed and I'm crying. When I was married I would become depressed and angry and I would lie on my bed with a pillow over me and crying... So frustrated, but towards my husband so passive I was that I waited until I collapsed.
>
> There was no fight in me. He would say, 'Poor girl. She's so neurotic. We must put her in therapy as a defective'. I made myself worse than before. I never could stand up for myself... I don't believe that I have aggressions. I don't believe I do except those that I can let out in a good way. I tolerate and tolerate and tolerate the other. It should not be. I have the impression that I'm playing a role.

Me: How do you characterize that role ?

C : Passive, helpless.

Me: Child.

C : Child... It was the only power I had over my husband.

Me: Does your present boyfriend Bo see you as a passive, helpless child ?

C : Ah... no. (Uncertainly) But I know that I accepted things from him that I should not. Because I was so afraid to lose him. I should be able to take the risk to lose somebody. Otherwise I can't do anything and I'm so afraid.

With exaggerated mockery, amounting to a Cheshire-cat drollery in my total body language, I chant, "Passive... helpless... clinging... clinging... clinging." At this point I come forward to grab her two outer shoulders in my hands, trying to forcefully pull her close to my chest. Christa resists. My voice rises to a phony theatrical pitch as I say, "Clinging child." Christa yells at me good-naturedly to stop. I don't. I place both hands on one of her arms and kneel down beside her while making sounds like an angry child. I say, "Now you cling to me too". Christa flatly refuses, pushing me away. She laughs heartily and I withdraw. She says :

> Oh God. A child acting like that encourages aggressions against it... Oh, I have this new idea that when I am like that, I have my aggressions too in me, but the other who is hitting me I see to be wrong.

I remark, "You are invalidating them and playing innocent. Passive and innocent". Katherine adds, "Self-righteous". Christa responds :

> I should revolt against what you say, but I feel that you are right. I would like to change myself ... If I had legs, I could go, but I don't use them... I did the same thing with Ilsa. She told me how furious I made her when I cling to her.

Katherine says, "She's on to your game of pretending to be helpless". And when I ask, "But do you see your game ?", Christa says :

> Yes I do... I didn't see it before as clearly as now... I couldn't explain it before... It's not only my feeling of anxiety but also an unconscious need to force the other.

At this point, I abruptly terminate the psychological work of the session. We exchange social pleasantries for the few remaining minutes.

My directive, therapist-centered manner was equally guided throughout by three faculties: my scientific knowledge of Christa's character-muscular armoring, my Logos capacity for understanding her immediate response to each bodily exercise and verbal exchange, and my Warrior capacity for self-assertively persevering with the bodywork and subsequent Logos-to-false-self-image encounter. Legislated by the intuitive back centers rather than the front ones, my pervasive attitude was one of detached irony. This is obvious in my provocative confrontation of Christa's gamesmanship, but it is equally pervasive earlier as I bulldozed her through one catalytic energy-mobilization exercise after another until her sluggish energy economy lightened. All three faculties in synchrony were required to slowly polarize Christa until she could partially open herself to Katherine's and my devastating caricature of her psychological posture. This attack was only possible after she mobilized her resources through bodywork and we cultivated a partly playful, partly serious interpersonal exchange.

My bulldozer role was self-consciously imbued with the image of a provocateur. This combination indicates the extent to which my sympathetic feeling centers in my front half were resonating subjectively in response to Christa's physical discomfort and psychic pain. I maintained a certain distance and disinterest towards my own behavior while executing it. I knew that only a part of me was openly showing itself to Christa as I directed her. If I had not known this, I would have been betraying my inner sympathetic feeling centers. I was able to detach myself from myself as much as from her in order to direct this session. In some respects, it was a partial mechanization of both Christa and myself which permitted this interchange to continue, especially the bioenergetic aspects. By mechanization I mean a calculated constriction of my own and her totality of beingness. I channeled both her and me into an accentuation of a part of each of us to the point of isolating that part from each of our totalities. This process of psychological mechanization happens whenever a professional uses his specialized knowledge and authority to direct another human being into facing up to his/her defensively games-playing roles and superego injunctions. Such a Warrior-Logos-Expert stance is often necessary during the first stage of treatment.

A Warrior-Logos-Expert stance is necessary when the client's cerebralized and defended volitional centers are still dormant and need gradual polarization until they rise to the surface of both the body and mental consciousness. The session under discussion indicates a paralysis in Christa's volitional centers in the upper and lower regions of her back in response to the double-binding messages emanating from her mother and ex-husband. Her description of her general feeling reaction to men is a measure of her crippled personal will. Her personal cognition initiates this dawning self-awareness. To be sure, Katherine and I add our Logos-inspired observations to her self-exploration. We make our contribution in a deliberately caricaturing and provocative manner precisely in order to reinforce and affirm her awakening consciousness to the objective reality of her psychological condition.

We resort to the classical medium of ironic caricature to open her awareness to the truth about herself. This catalytic provocation is often extremely productive to spearhead the later opening of the primary volitional feeling centers. It is especially appropriate to first stage when the armored client is totally alienated from all four of his deeper Being centers.

I want to point out how supportive our provocation of Christa was throughout this session. I attacked her vehemently head on only once, when she attempted to invalidate the positive features of her alive relationship with her boyfriend Bo. Since her merciless super-ego was dominant at the beginning of this session, I took every opportunity to attack it. However, as we focus on her counterfeit role of the passive, helpless child, I convey nurturing support and affirmation as I over-exaggerate our ridiculing stance by attempting to embrace her as a buffoon. This exaggerated exhibitionistic self-expression indirectly conveys our empathic identification with Christa's predicament. By totally giving up our aloof detachment, we make ourselves active allies in Christa's continuing battle against her frozen passivity. My playing a child clinging to Christa enabled her to perceive more keenly how her own embodiment of this role affects the primary feeling centers of the person to whom she clings. By reversing roles, we further stimulate her consciousness to look freshly at her chronic fixation to a helpless child syndrome of interaction. By actively sharing in this process, we ease the psychic pain and humiliation of having to face the truth about herself. Our Logos-to-false-self-image circuit of contact is enriched by a certain degree of Eros-to-Eros interchange.

Three sessions later, after a long opening verbal exchange, I ask Christa to stand with a mask over her eyes and to relate to me verbally and non-verbally as if I were her ex-husband. I place myself squarely in front of her, telling her to allow her pelvis to move forwards and backwards as effortlessly as possible. I ask her to reach out with both of her hands to take my hands in hers. The fact that we are both holding our elbows in front of our torsos and our five fingers are firmly intertwined multiplies the mobilization of energy currents into our hands. This mobilization quickly escalates if one of the two parties begins to push against the other's hands. I let Christa move her pelvis for about a minute before initiating this direct hand-to-hand contact. The pelvic movements further mobilize Christa's energy currents, particularly those in her lower back region, so that when I do begin to push her hands, she shows no inclination to stifle her instinctive resistance to my aggression. In fact, she responds by pushing me with such vitality that I have some difficulty holding my own. Finally, I decide to weaken my pressing, and to yield to her growing aggressiveness so that she forces me to withdraw from the direct contact (see page 237).

The moment I disengage my hands, Christa unleashes a flood of mockeries against her ex-husband, berating him for his cowardly withdrawal during much of their four years of contactless marriage. I fuel the fire by making vocal sounds of a demonically elusive and exaggeratedly fiendish clown. I apparently succeed at reproducing the feeling quality of their actual interpersonal relationship because immediately Christa launches into a scathing attack on his elusiveness. I continue to consistently non-encounter her, playing the cowardly enfant terrible. I wildly alternate between replying with ridiculous sounds and incisive verbal remarks. Exuding contempt, they

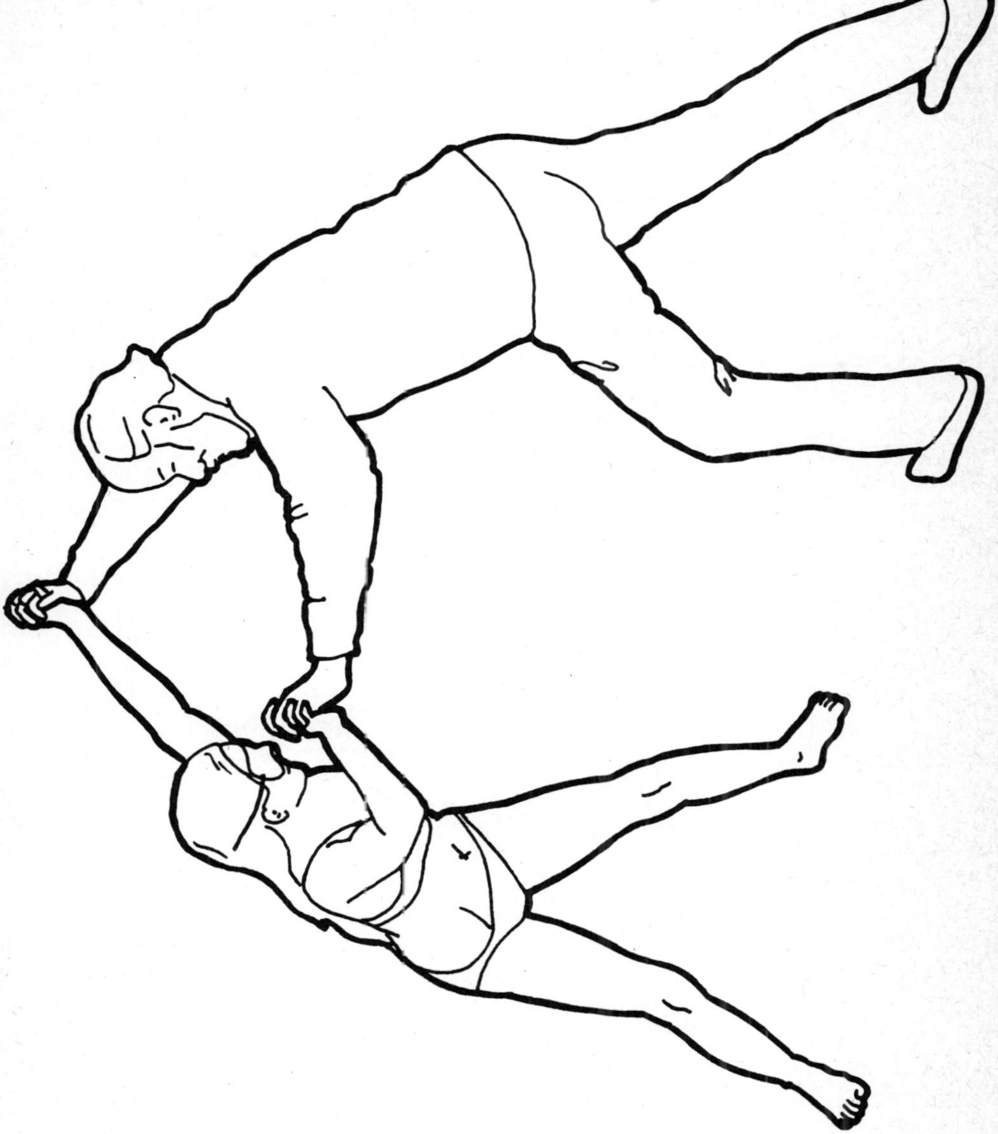

are designed to obliquely invalidate and mock her utterances. Christa responds with rather eloquent accusations against his behavior. She correctly interprets my oblique attacks and returns my sarcasm with a more blatant verbal sarcasm against him.

What is most significant about Christa's accusations is not her directly expressed lower-half defiance, but her upper-half seeing through his facade of strength. He never did engage her as his equal, but related to her as a cunning, insensitive fox which leads an innocent fawn to gradual destruction. Christa was never more paranoid than during her years with him. By refusing to engage her as well, and trying to deflect her accusations, I catalyze her perceptions to a new level of sophistication. Her Logos-inspired intuitive perception of him progressively awakens. Her observations include :

> You must learn once and for all that you cannot continue to do with people what you want. Until now you have done this. You have tyrannized everyone who came into contact with you. And with your wife you did the same because she was stupid and could not see what you were doing.
>
> I see how you are now. You can never respond to me directly. I will not be party to a monologue in your presence any more. Your replies are like dirty, devious sentences being expressed with the innocent voice of a child.
>
> You never really could praise me but always in the same sentence made me feel both elated and depressed.

If I had not so actively participated in our interchange so that Christa was consequently less reactively dependent upon my creative contributions, her behavior might have been more totally second-stage in nature. Her volitionally dominant self-expression lacked sufficient origination from within to qualify as second stage. My excessively directive part was still too first-stage in style to permit otherwise. In a sense, I was still the initiatory force behind her dawning expression of her lower and upper back primary feeling centers. Nevertheless, she did marshall all of her energetic and dynamic feeling forces and directed them outwards against me in the role of her ex-husband. This indicates an initial unfolding of a vitalization and connection of her lower and upper back centers. They are beginning to find some direct subject-world contact that is emotionally charged and rationally focused. As compared to earlier sessions, Christa's feeling capacities in her back have changed in relation to her ex-husband. There is sufficient mobilization of her core longitudinal energy currents and of her consciousness of the other to permit her to express her feelings with vitality and intuitive awareness. But she could not yet express her repressed smouldering feelings which her ex-husband had half-deliberately cultivated. However, these depths were beginning to surface. And when they surface, they inevitably have a phallic aggressiveness which is both annihilatingly powerful and subjectively self-regenerative.

The next day Christa reports that she has been thinking a lot about her past relationship to her ex-husband. She has realized that it resembled the kind of contact one establishes with a mirror: her husband played the role of a mirror in order to conceal his real feelings and thoughts. Christa says that she has been experiencing great anxiety every time she thinks about our psychodrama exchange of the previous session. I recognize the probability that her rising anxiety means that her hitherto tightly denied negative feelings of rage and frustration towards her ex-husband are pressing her psyche for more consummate self-expression. When Christa becomes stuck as she analyzes the relationship, I affirm her spontaneous showing of her fists as she reaches a moment of impasse. Encouraged to strike the mattress, she quickly skyrockets into sounds which begin to sound like an angry barking dog. Throttling them abruptly, she says :

> I have just the feeling that when I do that I prove to the other that I am crazy.

Me : Do it again.

She strikes the mattress again with both fists, making angry sounds. She continues much longer this time. After a brief silence, she says :

> You shouldn't show your feelings. You will be lost if you show them. Then they will have some-

thing concrete to take and hold against you. I know that I played this role with my husband and I used to threaten that I could leave him. I did not have to continue to stay with him and behave like a helpless child that he wanted me to be and have no communication with him even though I tried again and again and again. On the other hand, he was so brutal and cruel.

Christa begins to hit the mattress with her right fist. I encourage this instinctual gesture by saying, "Speak to him, and do that again". She responds with a voice that bellows with power and emotion :

You are so brutal. You can do whatever you want. You think that when you look sternly at other people they will fall down on their knees because they are afraid of you. You manipulate that to the utmost. You yell at anybody who does not obey your will. You play the performance of the great orator who is speaking so well and is a genius.

You are a genius, I know. But you use your genius to put down other people so that they cannot attack you. You twist the words coming from their mouths so that they cannot speak again. Afterwards, you are laughing about what you have done.. And when you were inspecting a great number of factory employees whom you were responsible for, you said to me: "That's all mine. That's all mine." (She imitates his pompous, pretentious exclamation venomously with her own voice). I was so ashamed of you. You behaved like a Nazi. I saw the hate in the eyes of the factory men. And I said nothing.

You treat others like puppets. You once said to me, "Look, we are going to go to a party, and the other men have old women, but I will show them that I have a young woman. So clean your teeth, otherwise you will have the teeth of a horse. And you must be my representative, darling".

And whenever I talked with you, it was like there was a window between us, and when I thought that I could touch you, I always hit against this window and never reached you, and you laughed about it... "Society serving me", you said. All others serving your glory. Your sadistic laughing about the anxiety you created in others and in my mother was repulsive to me.

You complimented my mother to her face, but laughed about her behind her back. She was like putty in your hands. And you learned more things about me to use against me. You twisted all that I said and she said.

When I left you and returned to being with others, I felt like a stranger, as if all other persons were far away from me. It was like I moved in this thick sticky material that stood between me and other people. I couldn't make any contact with other people for two or three days after being with you.

When I saw you again, the game between us went on again and I couldn't feel myself anymore. Then you would say, "Yes I know, you are my little light, my little light". And I felt helpless to make contact with you again.

And when we were divorced, you told everyone that I was mentally sick. You told others that you could prove that I was so emotionally dependent upon you that I phoned you each week and asked you to help me with all my academic work... You told this to all our friends. I feel you like a ghost in my back.

Christa is expressing a more spontaneous outpouring of both an object-centered perception and a great rage towards her ex-husband. She is no longer simply reacting to my provocative influence, whether bodily or psychologically. She is beginning to allow her own autonomous well-springs of feeling and intuitive cognition to guide her self-expression. She has now reached the threshold of a second stage mode of relating to her ex-husband in relation to at least two of her primary instinctual feeling centers, her upper and lower back. The longer she addresses him directly, the quieter her voice became. It is as if she needs to affirm her lower back center first, or what I call the phallic center when it functions as the medium to satisfy repressed needs for primitive aggression and active self-assertion. Then she can find the self-assurance to confront her repressed intuitive perceptions of her ex-husband.

Both Christa's phallos and logos inspired faculties have begun to flower. Now she can express what she has felt and perceived and even believe her expressions. This is a significant achievement for Christa who throughout her marriage was unable to clearly acknowledge or believe in her perceptions of her husband. She began increasingly to doubt their objective validity because he remained totally impervious to her tentative overtures for real encounter. In order to rout out Christa's deeper intuitive cognitions, it was necessary to awaken her more primitive aggressive instincts and to allow them to unite with and give support to her expression of long-buried and half-believed perceptions.

This polarization of the two back half feeling centers is the real objective of all our catalytic techniques during first stage. When the core longitudinal energy currents are alive enough to harness themselves supportively to the differentiated expression of hitherto dormant feelings, the buried emotional-instinctual needs of the psyche begin to emerge and manifest themselves with increasing urgency. Second stage is distinguished by the emergence of a hierarchy of unsatisfied instinctual needs associated with a previous alienation from the primary feeling centers. This emergence quickly becomes converted into a capacity to allow these needs to function as the essential initiators of self-expression. Their satisfaction becomes the foundation of a new identity. During first stage, the prime mover is ultimately the therapist working catalytically to penetrate the chronic rigidities from within. During second stage, these chronic rigidities have loosened enough to enable the deeper psychological needs of the repressed soul to surface as the deepest needs of the individual.

Second stage is the appropriate time to meet the unsatisfied needs from the uncompleted emotional past. These needs are of four kinds: 1) the need to take an independent stand and to express one's independence self-assertively in direct interaction with the alien other; 2) the need to separate and distance oneself from others to the point where they can be perceived and understood in an object-centered manner; 3) the need to unite with and at the same time empathically flow with the core being of another person in a circuit of exchange characterized by reciprocity and mutual caring; 4) the need to submerge oneself totally from time to time in one's own being-for-oneself to find a sense of harmony and self-completion so tangible as to engender a genuine acceptance, respect, and liking for oneself just as one is. The first need corresponds to the phallic or Warrior principle, whose nucleus is the lower back region. The second need corresponds to the Logos principle, whose nucleus is the region between the upperback, the primitive brainstem, and the cerebral cortex. The third need corresponds to the Agape-Eros principle, whose nucleus is the thoracic cavity region. The fourth need corresponds to the Hara principle, whose nucleus is the abdominal region.

These four basic needs are not the same as those described earlier as characteristic of an infant's healthy instinctual tendencies for contact with his mother -- these are primary-process and totally primordial in nature. The needs under discussion represent a distinctively matured differentiation of the former. They are more secondary-process in the sense that they presuppose an integration between conscious and unconscious, cortical and subcortical levels of functioning. The recognition and satisfaction of these four needs transforms the undifferentiated child within into a growth-motivated adult. Perhaps the best way to describe this metamorphosis is to say that the progressive emergence and satisfaction of these needs during the second stage of treatment represents the refined humanization and maturation of the four primary feeling capacities. In the last analysis, these capacities are too primitively subject-centered, too instinctually impulsive and too resistant to an integrated hierarchical organization of the total personality structure to function as the enduring boundaries of a mature adult's sense of self-identity. They must be superceded by higher-level capacities for synthesis, organization, and the concentration of cognitive consciousness in order to qualify as integrated expressions of an adult personality structure.

Usually, the two fundamental needs mediated by the upper and lower back feeling centers emerge into the foreground of consciousness first. The two fundamental human needs of the sympathetic feeling centers in the front half break through after the back half. This sequence has many causes. For a person who has not been able to stand on his own feet or to trust his own intuitive feelings and perceptions of others, it is less psychologically painful to open himself to the here-and-now experience of these personal deficiencies. This is particularly true of most neurotic syndromes in which a powerfully unconscious will-to-struggle-through-and-survive has prevailed. This will is mediated by the cortico-cerebrospinal circuits moving downwards and outwards from the head. They stand in chronic opposition to the more fluid and vital impulses of the viscera.

A reversal of this priority of flow to a flow from the lower half upwards usually initiates the satisfying of the most demanding need of the neurotic position during the first stage of treatment -- the need to penetrate the tyrannical reign of the false self-system localized around the overloaded cerebral cortex. Not until this reign of absolute supremacy is undermined from within and below can the fundamental needs associated with the primary feeling centers begin to appear even briefly in the foreground of consciousness. Most successful first-stage catalytic work awakens the core longitudinal energy currents. But their simple mobilization is not sufficient for healing. They must radiate and impact the reign of the cortico-cerebrospinal network. The more a client can move out of his head into the repressed feelings and unsatisfied needs of the uncompleted past, the sooner a gradual disintegration of the false self-system can begin. It is much more tolerable for a neurotic to fall out of his head into a full experiencing of his unsatisfied volitional needs for confrontive feeling contact with and separation from others than it is to resonate in beatific pleasure and fullness of investment with others or to withdraw totally into oneself and there sympathetically resonate with one's own creative depths and richness of Being.

Empathic tenderness towards self or others is far more frightening to the typical neurotic because it involves a greater divergence from the chronically convergent and ego-defended functioning which characterizes an intact false self-system. As compared to breaking into logos or phallos needs, a divergent breakthrough into the sympathetic feeling needs mediated through the chest and belly always entails a greater distance of psychological movement towards vulnerably regressive states of being. This is partly because the sympathetic feeling needs were always more potent at an earlier stage of development than the volitional ones.

When compared to the aggressive needs of the back, it is far more frightening for most neurotics to open themselves to the love needs of the front half. The subject-world polarization of the front half presupposes a much finer, slower, and longer lasting charging of the psychoorganismic totality. This polarization also presupposes a greater expansion of the boundaries of contact between subject and world because they are less harnessed constitutionally to the cortical-cerebrospinal circuits of cognition which superimpose a convergent ego-defended rational order upon the objective world. Agape-Eros and Hara are far less governable by reason, even in a relatively unarmored individual. They are the watering grounds for the creation of irrationally plastic and subtly refined sensory-motor-affective circuits of contact and resonance with outer and inner realities. They are the primary agents for the more fleeting and delicate predispositions of the mature adult -- roughly, they mediate the more feminine and artistic traits and abilities. Their crystallization as achieved individual virtues is therefore the consummation of the higher self-actualization process. Their consummation yields the most exquisite pleasures as well as the most aesthetically and religiously meaningful experiences available to mankind in contrast to the more solidly structured virtues and abilities mediated by the two back centers. In summary, most neurotics are usually not able to fall out of their heads into a here-and-now experiencing of their unsatisfied love needs until after their deeper volitional centers in the back have strengthened notably. The id-regulated sympathetic needs of the front half are intrinsically more frightening when first satisfied than the ego-integrative needs of the back half. There is nothing more frightening in the world to a neurotic than actualized true love, whether for others or for oneself.

Chapter VII

THE EMERGENCE OF THE FRONT HALF

The second stage of treatment challenges a therapist more than first because a client now begins to fall out of his head into the newly discovered feeling needs of his soul in the process of becoming. It is a time of becoming more than being -- the basic trend is towards a differentiated opening of consciousness to the feeling depths within. Since these feeling depths are composed of opposite inclinations naturally polarized to counterbalance each other, and since the emergence of each one is usually a piecemeal affair, second stage can be justly depicted as the period of productive or nonproductive chaos. The more differentiated becomes the emergence of one of these fundamental needs, the more this stimulates the emergence of the totally opposite need. The ensuing psychic process is characterized by broad oscillations from one extreme feeling constellation to its absolute opposite.

Because the newly discovered feeling needs fluctuate between opposite constellations, a client needs the greatest empathic identification and unconditional positive regard from his therapist during this period. The therapist must both contain the growing fragmentation and disorganization of the client's ego and facilitate the further opening of consciousness to the unexplored, unowned, and uncompleted feeling depths within.

The opening of the phallos center in the lower back and the accompanying capacity for increasing perceptual objectification of past and present interpersonal relationships eventually triggers the emergence of the opposite need -- the need to love and to be loved by others. Because this need can only emerge very slowly and hesitantly, second stage usually is the longest of the three stages, perhaps two to three times as long as first stage.

The delicate emergence of the need to love and to be loved is tied to the greater delicacy of opening the primary feeling centers in the front half. Some psychodynamic reasons for the slowness of this process have already been suggested. These reasons are supported by bioenergetic structural and functional patterns. The front half of the human body is regulated by the finest interpenetration of fluid and neural pathways of communication, whereas the back half is regulated by a less delicate coordination between the cerebrospinal voluntary nervous system and the larger muscle groupings. Consequently, the hormonal, cardiovascular and involuntary vegetative networks play a more predominant role in the metabolic regulation of energy currents coursing through the front half of the body as compared to those in the back half.

For these reasons, nurturing styles of direct touch are far more productive during second stage than first. Once the barrier to energetic and fluid flow between the central and peripheral regions of the armored body have been loosened, nurturing direct touch will mobilize a much greater polarization of the longitudinal energy currents to move into the front half of the body. Second stage is the time for optimal use of both nurturing and catalytic touch, since the front half usually shows the greatest movement towards softening during this period. The front half of an armored organism is especially impervious to softening as long as the peripheral muscular sheath remains intact. This is not because the armoring is any greater in the front half than in the rear, but because of the psychological reality that the front half contains the sympathetic feeling centers.

The remainder of this chapter will focus on Christa's discovery of her heart's need to love and to be loved and her belly's need to love herself as a woman. In her case, this process could not happen until she confronted more fully the severe deprivation and frustration of both of these needs in her relationship to her strong-willed mother.

The tenth session began and ended with a sustained period of softly nurturing direct body contact between Christa and Katherine. The initial contact sprang from Christa's description of her growing awareness that she had been unable to sustain any positive feelings for herself since her dramatic previous session. Christa's recognition of her pathological inclination to invalidate her newly emerging positive feelings indicated a need for more direct affirmation of those parts of her organism which cultivate positive subject-world contact -- the sympathetic feeling centers in the front half.

Furthermore, her slower alternation between positive and negative feelings indicated that she was perhaps ripe to experience our direct healing touch applied to her front half without the need to defend against the touch. Apparently, she could now permit her sympathetic feelings to have a limited but real period of subject-world dominance, free from the ruthless criticism of her cerebral cortex. I knew that the pleasure-pain threshold must be lowering because she was able to sustain a positive resonance with herself and her environment at least long enough to recognize her pathological need to destroy this resonance.

I ask Christa to lie on the mattress with a mask covering her eyes and to hold her arms gently in the air ready to engage anything they find waiting to receive them. I ask Katherine to softly hold Christa's hands. Christa becomes filled with sadness and warmth all through her body as she sheds silent tears. After ten full minutes, both women withdraw their hands. Christa expresses her enjoyment of the exercise and talks about how easy it was to make direct body contact with Katherine as compared to her real mother.

Shortly thereafter, I encounter Christa as her ex-husband as described in the previous chapter. This encounter is followed by some good work on the stool. I make some Logos inspired remarks about how she is beginning to allow her hands to reach out and enjoy direct physical contact with somebody else. Then I structure the first total body holding exercise of her treatment. Both women lie on their sides facing one another. I ask Christa to reach out and draw Katherine to her unclothed chest and belly regions and to hold her as if she were her own mother. Christa does not hesitate and the two women tightly embrace for nearly ten minutes. Katherine initiates the disengagement. They both fully collapse, lying silently side by side. Christa's response indicates that her armored pleasure-pain threshold is definitely lowering -- she maintained contact with Katherine's soft but very alive torso without any inclination to escape. Her silence following the separation shows that she has been able to use the total body holding to her best advantage and to relax yieldingly to the touch.

I wait in silence to see if Christa will speak. She continues to lie immobile with her eyes closed. After about three minutes, I ask Christa to allow herself to be held in Katherine's arms as if Katherine were an ideal mother figure. This is a more threatening exercise than the preceding one because it exposes a client more fully to the repressed feeling needs of his front half. Katherine sits upright with her back resting securely against a pillow that rests against the wall of the consulting room. She guides Christa into a position where her back lies across Katherine's lap. In order for the two women to embrace chest-to-chest, Christa must turn her torso towards Katherine, allowing Katherine's arms to fully encircle her upper half as Christa rests her face against Katherine's front shoulder and breast.

For Christa to relax into this mother-child embrace represents a new landmark. It means that her entire peripheral muscular sheath is losing its brittle rigidity, allowing invasion from the melting forces radiating from Katherine's front half. For Christa to tolerate this thawing of her sheath while in Katherine's arms for at least ten to twenty minutes would significantly impact her unconscious distorted body-image.

Christa slowly lets go of her self-conquering controls and begins to progressively relax in Katherine's arms. The two women continue in this position for twenty minutes, while I silently watched. After Katherine moved away, the two women were so at ease with their newly established circuit of vibrations that they chatted lightly and gayly for the last five minutes of the session without enlisting my participation. (see page 251).

Christa begins the next session by describing her experience of happiness following her contact with Katherine :

> Yesterday after the session I felt very happy. The last time when you held me in your arms (She looks at Katherine directly). I think it is the first time that I didn't feel any pain. I wasn't sad. Not any mixup of being happy and at the same time feeling sad. I enjoyed this feeling of happiness and warmth. I never felt it before.

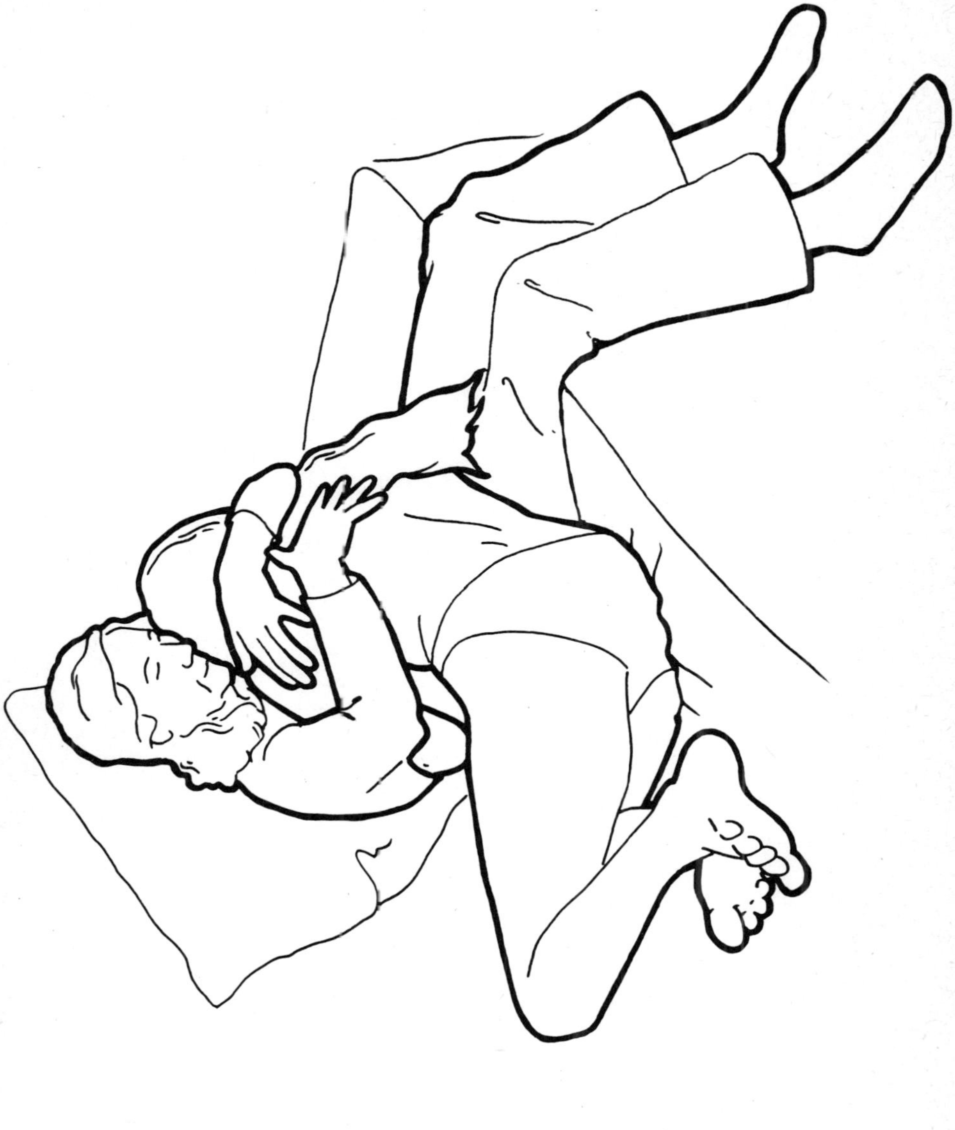

Before the more I was happy the more I felt this pain was like a fire. The intensity of the happiness was like a fire which gave pain... I think this sadness is a kind of anxiety, but I can't explain why.

Also when we were on the mattress before I was always afraid to first touch somebody else. I would wait for the other to come to me because I was always afraid that it could be disagreeable to the other... Yesterday I saw that it was easier to go to somebody with touch than before.

I have always had the phantasy that when I give my hands like that (She extends her hands outwards) the other person would slap them down. I am afraid that the other could think that I am being too aggressive with them.

With men when I was a young girl it was the same. I was afraid that the man could see that I was interested in him, because I thought that never could he be interested in me. And it was not only with men, but with every human being except the young people I am working with. And yesterday I was happy to see that it was easier than I thought.

The encounter work between Christa and me in the role of her ex-husband was valuable but totally overshadowed by the outwardly non-dramatic but tender body contact between Katherine and Christa. The essential difference between the two kinds of transactions can be characterized by the fact that actions speak louder than words, but silent actions speak still louder than actions accompanied by words. Another equally relevant explanation is that Christa's unconscious hierarchy of unsatisfied needs are changing -- her need for aggressive self-assertion is becoming surpassed by the opposite need for human warmth and tenderness.

The significant impact of Katherine's soft, warm, and tender touch upon Christa's subjective feelings suggests an internal shift within Christa's psyche towards an opening of consciousness to the needs of her front half. This does not mean that her volitional needs of her back half have been fully satisfied or strengthened, but simply that their greater satisfaction automatically triggers the progressive conscious emergence of the next most potently unsatisfied feeling needs. Abraham Maslow's formulation of a hierarchy of prepotent needs helps us to understand the long and complicated second stage of treatment. This process also conforms to the law of alternation already discussed: the human psyche naturally swings from one feeling-cognition complex to its extreme opposite to the extent that each complex represents a partial expression of the totality. For Christa to rant and rave and verbally attack her ex-husband or her mother in the safe context of our consulting room is an extremely onesided mode of self-expression.

Regardless of the techniques used, the psychic pendulum swings between extreme opposites. A skilled therapist can direct this inevitable swing in a positive direction if he directly polarizes not the pathological opposite, but the life-affirmative instinctual opposite set of responses to those of phallic aggression. In Christa's case, the pathological opposite set of responses came from her intropunitive superego. Her cortical-cerebrospinal circuits of ego control could have filled her with self-recriminations following her inordinate and unrealistic expression of anger towards her former husband and mother if Katherine's tender holding had not deliberately awakened life-affirmative feeling resources. If a week had elapsed between these two sessions, Christa would probably have retrogressed into her pathological cortical defenses, both regarding Katherine's tender holding and Christa's aggressive self-assertiveness towards her ex-husband.

Christa's description of her former response to happiness is an incisive psychological statement. Happiness was like fire -- a burning pain accompanied such feelings. This penetrates the very heart of the armored neurotic's fear of the softer positive feelings generated by the primary sympathetic feeling centers. Such positive sympathetic feelings are too good to be true in their sheer blessed beneficence. As such, they are too threatening to the defended ego's need to suffer and struggle. Furthermore, they are too physically painful to endure for more than a brief period of minutes because they presuppose a subtler, deeper and more fluid circulation of energy flow throughout the total torso. Usually the pattern of this endodermal enhanced flow is more vertical than horizontal, and the latter circulates from back to front or from front to back around the body at both ends of the torso.

Such longitudinal rotations of energy flow are especially prevalent during the second stage of treatment when the deeper thawing of the energy blocks between the front and the back halves of the body are most in dominance. Their appearance signifies a breaking down of the old compartmentalized energy currents operating in the front half and between the front and rear halves of the torso. The rushing of an enhanced energy flow in the form of longitudinal currents stands behind the subject's progressive disidentification with his cortical-cerebrospinal circuits and an increasingly focused conscious perception of being flooded with intensely burning kinaesthetic and proprioceptive sensations rising from below.

Christa's core longitudinal currents are now strong enough to sustain a circulation of flow rising upwards from the abdominal cavity and extending between the back and front halves of her body without evoking a neuromuscular tension reaction which burns like fire. The earlier psychological opening of her lower back region and her capacity to actively face her former tormentors is due to the expansion of her core longitudinal currents to the region of her lower back. These same currents subsequently expand further to embrace her entire torso.

Once this four-directional circulation of core energy currents awakens, a client is ripe for the opening of consciousness to repressed needs for love, both from and for others and for self. It is a biological reality that the internal awakening of the front half with a greater circulation of energy flow facilitates the secondary emergence of all four primary instinctual feeling needs, both in terms of past uncompleted personal relationships and unrealized present relationships.

This link between psychic and bioenergetic events is demonstrated by Christa's experience following her eleventh session as described in the last chapter. During her twelfth session, she moved into a more consummatory and cognitively object-centered expression of rage and frustration. Christa received no direct nurturing touch during this session. Christa's first words during the session were unintelligible except for the single phrase, "This need for warmth from the other". She is so introspectively embroiled with this phenomenon that she mumbles. She describes her preoccupation with this unsatisfied need during the three days intervening since the last session. The need literally swamped her consciousness: 'I felt like a cripple with this need for warmth. It made me feel anxious all week-end." This need was so dominant that it almost intruded excessively in all her immediate interpersonal transactions. She realizes for the first time that she has always expressed all of her feelings with a manic compulsive intensity which left her feeling completely empty afterwards. She experiences this emptiness as a big hole in her middle.

This accurate self-revelation was made possible by a change in Christa's internal chemistry. It has slowed down to a steadiness of ongoing excitation which enables her to perceive the discrepancy between her presently felt need for interpersonal warmth and her former manic defenses against acknowledging the need. Her perception of her former inability to open herself so as to receive sympathetic warmth and tenderness from others implies that she is now opening up to her underlying need in all her present relationships. This can be explained bioenergetically as a psychological concomitant to the establishment of a four-directional circulation of fluid energy flow between her front and back metabolic regions, above and below the diaphragm. This circulation slows to a rhythm of excitation and equalization which permits the subject to feel in the immediate moment the primary feeling needs emanating from the front half of the torso.

Christa's dawning recognition documents this development :

> I take nothing for myself. I have a very unbalanced life. I never stay with myself, but all is happening between me and the other. I take all from the other and give all to the other. It's like a current going through me, but not staying in me.

I cannot wait for something growing up within me. I have to give it out instantaneously. In my work I am always running after my ideas.

This has to be the origin of all my intensity. Until now I felt this intensity to be a good thing. I have always had a good feeling when I'm giving out rapidly to another person. Yesterday I realized that this rapid giving out is neurotic too, so it made me feel kind of hopeless again.

Her words are still confused, but Christa is moving toward the discovery that she has never before allowed herself to surrender to and to enjoy a more receptive intake of the sympathetic positive feelings from others. She is, in essence, discovering within herself her natural need for relationships which permit her to relate in a self-surrendering mode as much as a giving and taking self-assertive mode. To open oneself to receive positive sympathetic vibrations from others amounts to a surrender of the coping egoic will and the affirmation of the sympathetic feeling vibrations emanating from the heart. It is very difficult for the armored neurotic to abandon his will and to allow his sympathetic feeling impulses arising from his heart center to mediate the subtle inclinations towards meeting the I - thou aspects of the other. The neurotic fears surrender to primitive sentimentality and a virtual betrayal of his egoic pride and absolute self-sufficiency.

The self-surrendering feeling needs are far more intrinsically frightening to the neurotic ego-defenses than the self-assertive feeling needs. They involve a greater opening out and exposure of oneself to the uncertain here-and-now immediate response of the other. They presuppose a greater willingness for vulnerable self-exposure to the immediate feeling reactions of the other. They require greater courage and a greater willingness to risk the unknown world of other people than the volitional needs of the spinal column region.

Christa is beginning to recognize her personal truth: she possesses no sense of inner continuity of self-identity, no essential sense of 'meness' or reliable beingness-for-oneself. She has known this intellectually for a long time, but never before has she been able to feel it in terms of her immediate interpersonal relationships. She newly experiences her intensity of givingness as an effort to fill up from outside her own inner emptiness. Although not fully formulated, she is beginning to feel at the level of the primary feeling needs the absence of a sense of self-love as mediated by a fully flowing belly center. The discovery that she is totally incapable of containing her inner life and allowing it to quietly unfold and provide her with internal resources for self-enjoyment and reflective contemplation is behind her awareness that her compulsively driven externalization of her inner life represents a defensive flight from the inner self. This penetrating self-revelation was enabled by the opening of Christa's delicate front half and its progressive emergence in consciousness.

Although all the previous sessions contributed to the initial unfolding of Christa's front half, the decisive catalyst was Katherine's direct touch during session ten. This is confirmed by Christa's two dreams preceding session twelve. In the first one, she dreams about Giovanni, a European medical doctor whom she has known for some time and who is also in Berkely for individual treatment with us -- Christa enjoyed a new depth of contact with him the day before the dream :

> I dreamt last night that Giovanni and I were lying on our beds and we each had to die. We had some pills for dying. Some person, I don't know who, gave more of them to me than to him, but still I couldn't sleep or die. Then Giovanni said to me: "That's your neurotic structure that prevents you from dying and keeps you alive. You are thinking all the time, and feelings are coming up in you and because you are so neurotic you cannot die". This made me extremely anxious in the dream to hear from him, and then I realized that I would have ahead of me to undergo great pain in my loneliness and awakeness and that Giovanni would have the good fortune to die but I could not.

Christa's second dream occurred after she went back to sleep after awaking from the first dream :

> I was coming home -- I don't know where 'home'

was -- but as I entered I saw that there was a little child, a baby, lying there. I instantly recognized that it was my baby, my little tiny child. I thought to myself in the dream: 'How could I forget that I have a baby. I have been falsely telling others that I have no baby.' I took this baby from its bed up in my arms and held it close to me and I was so sublimely happy. Just deliriously happy. And when I woke up I was very disappointed to find out that it was not true, that I do not really have a baby of my own.

Christa's actual conversation with Giovanni the day before stimulated her new discoveries which are articulated in both dreams. The pills for dying refer to our treatment sessions -- the dying relates to the gradual dearmoring process. The psychodynamic essence of this process is the eventual extinguishing of the false self-system which functions in relative isolation in the cerebral cortex and upper back regions. Giovanni made several observations to Christa about their mutual neurotic condition which indicated that until both of them got out of their heads and into their bodies, they could not give up their neurotic split. This observation is echoed by Giovanni's statement in the dream, "You are thinking all the time, and feelings are coming up in you and because you are so neurotic you cannot die." This ties in with Christa's realization that she is compulsively driven to externalize all of her ideas with others without allowing herself to reflect upon them first in terms of their feeling impact upon her own inner psyche. What she does not yet realize is that she is describing how her false self-system has been compelling her to discharge her internal tensions and total alienation from core feelings through a manic ventilation of an overstuffed and chronically agitated intellect.

It is the death of this isolated and overcharged intellect which Christa's creative unconscious is newly translating into the essence-like, symbolic language of dream. At present, she is unable to understand what the dying refers to. This indicates that she is not yet dearmored enough to tolerate a massive loss of ego control and flooding of her heavily intellectualized consciousness. But she is becoming aware of the contactless way in which she has been relating to others in the past.

Initially, Christa found the second dream equally as perplexing as the first one. Like the first, the second dream arose from her deepest psychic depths. Too many psychic and bioenergetic defense layers prevented it from entering Christa's rational consciousness with any immediacy of feeling or intuitive significance. Christa still has a long road to follow before her core intuitive faculties are directly accessible to rational consciousness. She could not perceive that the tiny baby symbolizes her own buried deeper self free from the tyrannical control of her overcharged cortex. The dream is primarily prophetic -- it points to future developments with an uncanny perceptiveness. It is stating that when Christa learns how to assume a basically sympathetic and positive mothering role towards her own buried feeling depths, she will discover her deeper self within. It is also saying that she will do this one day with the same ease with which in the dream she spontaneously picks up the lying child and holds it to her breast. It is also saying that to the extent that her front half thaws, she will discover the lost child within waiting to be born through acknowledgment and nourishment.

Christa responds with silent tears as I ask her to return to the dreams at the end of the twelfth session. After a minute of silence, she says, "The important thing was that I could be a mother who could give out this warmth to the baby." She acknowledges how hard she has been with herself all her life. Suddenly, she speaks with great but controlled pathos :

> I never could contain myself. Never. I hated myself too much for that. I can't imagine how to be good to myself. I hated myself all the time. Sometimes I had the phantasy I was killing myself. Sticking a sharp long knife into myself and cutting my body to pieces.
>
> Whenever I behaved badly with someone else, I would have this phantasy. Always afterwards some kind of suicide phantasy. I was very cruel to myself in these phantasies. I would take a razor blade and slash my wrists. This has been going on since I had problems with my husband. I used

to hit my head when I was alone. Phantasies of throwing myself under a train down to the last detail.

After having the phantasies I always felt emotionally released and could sleep better. But how I would punish myself and others in revenge in my phantasies. But I just realized that I have not had one since being in California. Instead I am having phantasies of how I will remodel my apartment when I return home.

Christa is moving one small step closer to experiencing the split between her false self-system in her head and her primary feeling centers in her torso. For her to acknowledge on a feeling level her chronic self-hatred and its uncontrollable manifestations presupposes enough opening of her front half to sense her total absence of tenderness towards self.

Increasingly during the last three sessions, Christa is becoming aware of the more subtle imbalances in her personal experience. This opening arises from her front half which is becoming charged with energy rising from the abdominal wellsprings of her endodermal vegetative currents. This development is not merely a mechanical opening of the feeling centers themselves and an enhanced capacity for sensory-motor-affective responsiveness from moment to moment. Rather, it is the enhanced flow of internal interaction between cognitive consciousness and the kinaesthetic sensations issuing from the frontal metabolic regions themselves. These changes involve nothing less than a total reconstitution of the neural pathways and the comparatively greater interaction between the central nervous system, the cerebral cortex, and the vegetative nervous system in synchrony with the core longitudinal currents. The basic trend of this total biological reconstitution process is towards a progressive weakening of the cortical-cerebrospinal alliance of forces and a simultaneous strengthening and vitalization of the visceral-vegetative alliance.

The stronger the visceral-vegetative alliance becomes, the greater internal emotional security and self-reliance Christa will experience on an immediate feeling level. This is because the belly center is the seat of the deeper self's sense of ongoing continuity and stability. Once the visceral effector organ network deep inside the abdominal cavity is awakened and allowed to circulate its slow-moving currents of blood-synergized energy flow, a person can face any amount of painful psychological material and tolerate the anxiety of confronting it in consciousness. This is because after the encounter, the visceral-vegetative currents will be able to spontaneously surpass the cortical-cerebrospinal emergency-oriented forces and absorb them through the process of equalization into its nurturing-restoring radius of influence. The belly is the great equilibrium-making center of the human organism. To the extent that an individual becomes truly dearmored, the belly center heals all excessive tensions created by the cortex -- it equalizes and integrates them into harmony.

Christa makes another move in this direction during her thirteenth session. She experiences a direct sensory awareness that she has to repress her inhalation because her mother is sitting on her chest and throat regions. This connection occurred after I touched her on her center chest and middle abdomen nurturingly for over ten minutes while she lay on her belly on the mattress. Her spontaneous connection was incited by the fact that for several minutes as she lay motionless while my hands touched her, she began to cough compulsively shortly before the acme of each breath. The cough had a peculiarly hoarse and hollow sound which generally correlates to the initial loosening of a chest block. Although Christa experienced no pain in her chest or belly regions while being touched, she found the slight pressure of my hand on her chest "irritating" because it reminded her of her mother's pressure on her. She pointed to her upper chest just below her throat, an area which my hand was not touching directly.

Christa's connection between these three phenomena heralds the beginning dissolution of her firmly armored chest region, between the middle and upper central thoracic area. This interpretation is borne out by what happened about fifty minutes later. While phallicly addressing her mother, Christa spontaneously recalls how she felt an impending attack of nausea everytime her mother touched her. In order to quell the nausea, she suddenly held her breath and swallowed so that her mother could not see what was happening. Christa does this reflexively at the moment of consciously recognizing the process. I immediately ask her to repeat the quick intake of breath, holding, and covert swallowing several times in rapid succession. After about eighteen times, Christa has become so choked up that she is forced to cough explosively.

Christa struggles to recover her normal breathing cycle, coughing and gasping like someone possessed, an echo of her response during our initial sessions. Now she cannot restabilize her breathing cycle until she vomits mucous from her chest area. Even then, it takes another minute before she can speak to her mother :

> You have never given me any self-affirmation with your touches. You were possessing my body in any way you could find. You came into my bathroom and watched me until I would throw you out. I was so terrified by it.
>
> You were putting these medicines in my vagina. I couldn't do anything. I would push you away again and again. You would come saying, "I am your mother. You cannot be ashamed about your mother seeing your vagina."
>
> I feel now this nausea and I could vomit. I have the impression now that you were coming and you would like to suffocate me. I had to be what you wished I should be. I had to be the other part of yourself. You were looking at me in a way that I feel ashamed when I see your staring eyes like that. I felt like an exhibitionist when you looked at me. My first impulse was to hide myself down there. (She points to her genital area.) You have to tell all to your mother.
>
> It was not a sexual coitus, but it was like a coitus of the soul. You have to tell all to your mother. You swallowed up all of my problems, all that was coming out of me, and at the same time you were hating me because I was not the reflected image of you. I would not be it. I was just your alter ego.

Here is another link to Christa's distorted body image which caused her to erect a peripheral muscular sheath in order to preserve whatever integrity and freedom of choice possible. The most striking feature about Christa's outpouring is her recognition that her mother tried to fully possess her very soul, a kind of spiritual incest. This recognition was catalyzed by delicate polarization of Christa's energy blocks below the peripheral muscular sheath in her chest area. Apparently, her mother's attempts to possess her daughter emotionally were always contradicted by contactless approaches to direct body contact with Christa. Christa was never so completely alienated from her feelings that she could not dimly sense, however nebulously, the counterfeit, double-binding intent of her mother's touch. Christa's front half was never so completely desensitivized that she could not register at the immediate sensorymotoric level that something was askew. Christa literally froze her feelings altogether in response to her mother's approaches, in order to keep her inner feelings to herself.

Recalling the spiritual incest manifested in Ronald's case as presented in the earlier chapters, we remember that it is the sympathetic center of the upper half -- the heart region -- which experiences the most exacerbating contradictory messages emanating from the double-binding, love-needy parent. On the one hand, the parent articulates lofty ideals of love and devotion to her dear child and cultivates a kind of spiritualized love relationship more suitable to adult lovers than to parent and child. But such verbalized expressions of love are sharply contradicted by the actual behavior and circuit of unconscious feeling vibrations emanating from the parent's body, because the love is the largely willed expression of the parent's cerebralized self-system.

Victimized by her mother's spiritual incest, Christa had no choice but to freeze her heart center in order to retain her emotional thread of integration. It was a matter of life-and-death emotional survival that she harden her entire front half against her mother's vampire approaches. The effect of this hardening was to kill her own dynamic feeling centers in her front half and steel her back centers in chronic resistance against her mother's counterfeit sympathetic investment in Christa's personal welfare. The coughing, nausea, and vomiting are incipient vegetative release reactions which begin the long and tortuous process of melting Christa's protective armoring until she can fully acknowledge her heart, and later, her Hara.

Christa's outpouring had an enormous impact upon her psyche. A tiny crack in her hardened chest began to allow seepage of stagnant, muddied waters. After the session, Christa continued to process memories of long-buried feelings of revulsion and disgust which had clogged her gastrointestinal tract for years. The damming up of her chest and natural breathing cycle resulted in part from continually swallowing the nausea and disgust generated by her mother's innumerable physical approaches. In our session, Christa was able to finally experience these feelings to the point of intolerable discomfort. Since Christa's phallic center had already begun to thaw, she did not react passively to this discomfort. Instead, she brought her rich imaginative resources as well as her primitive self-assertive instincts to confront her many negative feelings and painful memories.

The capacity to autonomously process hitherto chronically repressed psychic material is peculiar to the second stage of dearmoring. It signifies that at least one primary feeling center in the back half and one in the front half are making contact due to the functioning of the core longitudinal energy currents. A self-regulative balance of movement between opposite modes is now possible without the therapist's presence. Christa's heart center is beginning to open in response to the significant opening of her phallic center.

Christa begins the fourteenth session by describing how she has processed alone many painful memories :

> When I felt this morning how my mother had carved me into becoming her image of me I became so furious that I lay on the mattress and started pounding it. Afterwards I had this phantasy -- it was from a movie I once saw.
>
> It was about this man who had snails in this room and he forgot that he had left them there. He entered the room and slipped and fell because of the slime of the snails covering the floor. They covered the walls, the lamps, everything

in the room. The snails then came over him more and more. He cried out, but they kept coming and even went inside of him. They came from every part of the room and encompassed him.

This was the same feeling I had this morning in relation to my mother. I have to push these things away from me, but like the slime of the snails it is so sticky and not easy to push away.

Since the last session I have been feeling this nausea that I would have every time my mother came close to me. (She gasps and holds her breath audibly.) When she was touching me, it was like a coming and a going away at the same time. She couldn't really touch me in a good way. It felt so strange. It was not real....

It was a touch which neither soothed me or made me feel warm, but always made me feel tense. From the age of twelve I can remember her coming to me in my bed to give me a kiss. I had the feeling to become suffocated because it was not that she had come to really give me something, but she was waiting for me to give her something -- to show her my child-like feelings of love for her.

She stood there stiff and waiting, watching and controlling. It was so different with my father who I would wait to come home and would run to and leap into his arms and collapse in them. But I see my mother standing and watching me. Sometimes I forgot to kiss her. She would say: "You don't give a kiss to your mother ?"

I felt a power coming from her as she waited for my kiss. No spontaneous gestures she was making, but waiting. Waiting. I felt this tension in the atmosphere that she would eat me up... After last session, I felt like this (She gasps and sucks in air as if she cannot breathe) and I could hardly breathe.

Christa is moving into a new dimension of subjective feeling reactions which are more delicate and more subtle than the grosser emotions associated with the back half of the body -- rage and aggressive anger. Neither are they in the same category as the fear emotions of anxiety, panic and apprehension -- emotions which manifest a shrinking away from the immediate outer world and a withdrawal inwards as far away from the sensory outer environment as possible. Christa's new feelings refer clearly to a subject-world context whose ambiguity was one of its outstanding characteristics. Her feeling ambiguity contained a sinister and perverse quality because it hid more than it revealed of her mother's chronically ambivalent and underlying possessive feelings towards Christa.

Christa is now beginning to face the enormity and the subtlety of her mother's vampire engulfment of her feelings. Vampires suck blood, and they also deprive their victim of any capacity for sympathetic feelings towards others. Both of these processes filtered through Christa's being every time her mother hovered over her before the goodnight kiss, waiting for Christa to take the initiative. It is fascinating how Christa could remember the feeling constellation of those moments: tension arose from her mother's menacing presence; irritation erupted at the mother who "would eat me up". Until now, the feeling was mercifully repressed from Christa's consciousness -- such a cannibalistic feeling constellation would have been too acutely painful to bear. The connection between her mother's physical approaches and snail slime suggest an enormously perverse set of vibrations radiating unconsciously from her mother. And the fact that they were not acknowledged by her mother multiplies the perversity of the vibrations. Just such a perverse set of contradictory vibrations induces paranoia.

As the primary feeling centers of the front half begin to thaw, a client usually becomes vulnerable to regressive states of paralysis. These states may take the form of depressive stupors or floating states of relative mindlessness. To the extent that these divergent collapses are related to the gradual unwinding of the chronic energy blocks in the front half, they are partial spontaneous returns to original pathological states of total paralysis. As such, they are to be encouraged by the therapist -- the sooner they appear in the client's daily living, the sooner the long period of second stage can run its chaotic course.

Christa, for example, had to struggle against collapse into a state of partial regressive paralysis following her thirteenth session, largely because of the opening of her chest center. Describing this struggle at the beginning of the fourteenth session, she felt proud not to have succumbed to a fullscale depression. She was able to stay consciously in touch with her uncomfortable psychic feelings and her mother's ghostly presence. Although she phantasized about doing so, she did not collapse into an anxiety-stricken infantile helplessness which would have compelled her to run to Ilsa for emotional containment and physical contact.

Paradoxically, if she had been more fully into second stage, she would have been less able to control her need-tendency to collapse into a divergent regressive state. Although she would have been less likely to turn to Ilsa for help, she would have been unable to prevent herself from falling into a formless stupor. Her intact armoring enabled her to arrest this need to collapse into a mindless state of chaotic, anxiety-giving formlessness dominated by repressed feelings from the unfinished past. Since Christa had to terminate treatment with us before she arrived in the more advanced phases of second stage, our description of her is prototypical of the first half rather than the second half of second stage. The essential difference between these two parts of second stage is a greater loss of ego-cortical control during the later period which is accompanied by the appearance of menacing archetypal imagery and other bizarre and forbidden manifestations of the collective unconscious. These latter phenomena will be discussed in a later chapter.

Since Christa's partial feeling paralysis progressively revealed itself as she talked, I asked her to go on the Lowen stool. Placing her on the stool would awaken her dynamic volitional centers in her back and hopefully mobilize her newly discovered phallic forces. She welcomed my suggestion, saying that she was aware that she could not access her more primitively self-assertive powers. Hearing this, I decide to use an especially potent energy-mobilization technique. As she lies with her upper back on the stool, I ask her to put her arms down by her side. I take her hands in mine, bring her arms backwards over her head and hold them. The direct body contact in this position on the stool polarizes energy flow more quickly than when a client grips the inanimate arms of a chair. This technique is not to be used with clients who have not begun to thaw in at least two of their feeling centers. If used prematurely, it will overwhelm the metabolism, arousing the emergency-oriented secretion of large amounts of adrenalin. (see page 269)

As expected, Christa was not bioenergetically overwhelmed by this exercise. It penetrated her energy stasis in the region of her chest and throat, but in a tolerable way. This position exerts such pressure on the upper chest that it literally blasts open from within the dominant short-circuiting pockets of stagnant energy flow. In Christa's case, the greatest arrestment was in her throat area. At first she talked calmly about her different reactions as a child to her father as compared to her mother. When I asked her to hold my hands as tightly as she could, she became silent and began to hold her breath for the first time since getting on the stool. After making barely audible sounds, she mutters, "I feel suffocated. The old thing." And then the barely audible sounds resume. Since they do not grow louder or more frenetic, I realize that her organism is adjusting to the stepped up energy polarization. Instead of splitting, her endodermal energy currents are gradually unifying to produce an encounter. While remaining on the stool, she says in a vital, assertive manner :

> I didn't know who I was. She was always destroying my own image of myself as a woman. She always told me how impossible I was, so that I would remain a child for her I now think. I couldn't see when a man was nice to me because I couldn't believe it.
>
> She said, "All people are not true to you. Only your mother is true to you." (Christa's sounds signify psychic rather than physical pain).
>
> I will not be broken down. I have had enough. (More sounds of pain with each exhalation, but nothing intense). I'm just sad when I see her. Her whole life she could not do otherwise, but it was not good for me what she did. (Shifting, she says directly to her mother).....I will not tell you.

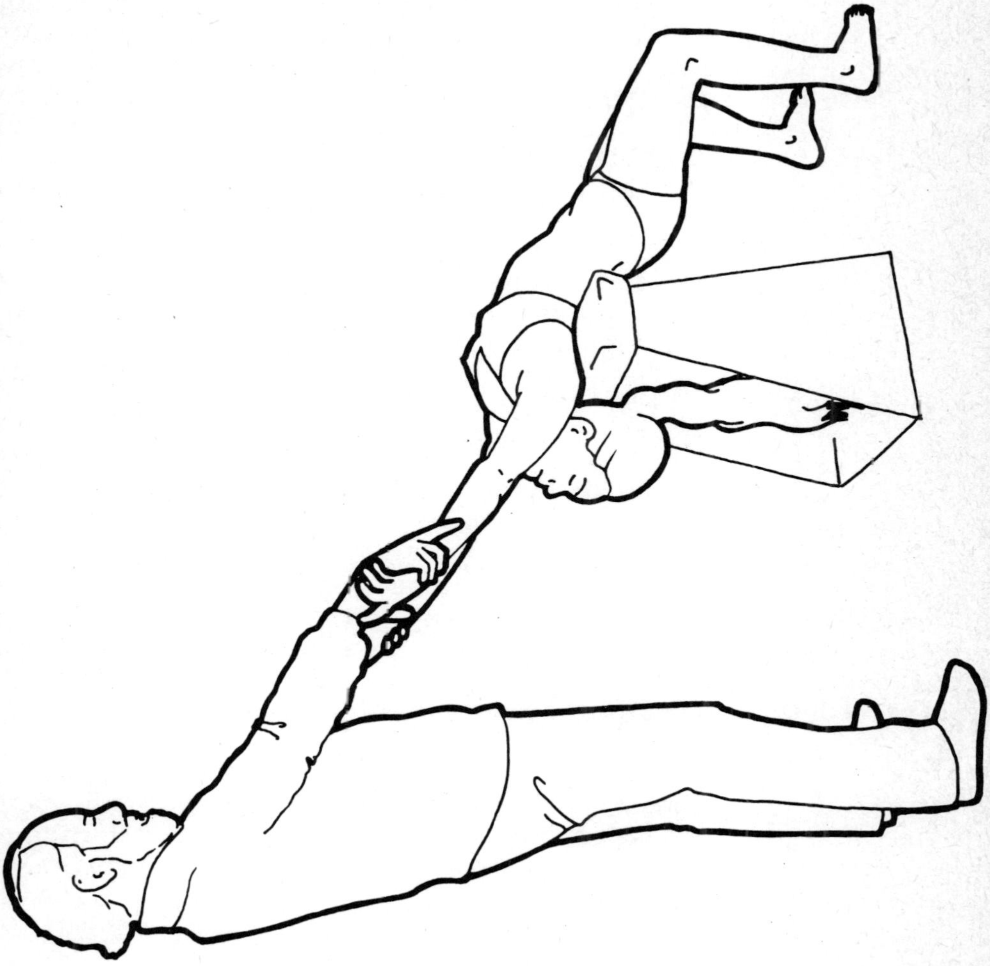

Such an encounter presupposes a pattern of energy flow which encompasses the entire neural and metabolic totality and forms a figure-background excitation gestalt. For the first time, Christa recognizes that her own false self-system resulted from introjecting and identifying with her mother's image of her. Until now, Christa could not perceive this fundamental truth. This significant breakthrough in the Logos capacity could only come after her feeling capacities in her lower back and upper front half had softened. Only now can Christa begin to see that she has actively colluded with this insidious formation of a self-invalidating self-image by openly sharing much of herself with her mother during her formative years. Having connected with at least three of her core feeling centers, she can see her complete and pathetic ensnarement in her mother's destructive lies about herself. The opening of her Logos capacity is tantamount to reversing her negative image of herself: it enables her to trace it to past identifications with other people's negative judgments about herself and to her naive trust and belief in their distorted verbalizations.

Christa must have sensed her need to pursue such a conscious confrontation because she had no inclination to come off the stool. After twenty minutes, she said, "I'm staying on this stool in order to get the feeling out." She needed her back centers polarized as much as possible to be able to carry through her confrontation. She continues :

> You were always stopping me, always stopping me all the time. "You have to be good. You have to be good. You have to be good. Your husband is so good, your mother is so good." (Christa's voice expresses considerable intensity, but it never reaches an hysterical pitch.)
>
> And they are not so good. It is not true... She was always distorting the truth in order to manipulate me into doing or not doing something, either to hinder me or to push me. Never was she telling the truth. She was always telling something coming from her hidden motives. I think she doesn't know what it is, the truth. She doesn't know her truth too. (Christa makes a loud sound of disgust and then speaks with a moaning lamentation.)

I can understand how bad she felt. I can understand. I know how bad she is feeling in her neurosis. I know it, but I cannot help her. I cannot. I will be myself. I will not be depressed and a child all my life. I would be happy. I would find a man who is not like my mother is. (She cries openly in halting sobs that gradually free themselves).

I can't anymore. I can't anymore... I saw everything through my mother's eyes and not through mine. I was not myself -- never. Just in my work was I myself. (Christa begins to express a reflex to vomit, repeating it three times without actually vomiting. Almost gagging, she yells instead to erase the need to vomit).

I feel this coughing in my body and this vomiting is just my mother's hand on me. Go away! Go away! No! No! Go away! Go away! (With each exclamation, Christa lifts the entire lower half of her body, pounding the floor with both feet simultaneously. This achievement requires an enormous mobilization in the pelvic girdle. Her exclamations are loud but focused. There is no break in her confrontation with her mother as she continues.)

You have not lived your life, I know. But I will live my life. I cannot die because you could not have yours. I cannot. And don't kill my father together with you. But that is his problem that he has married you. I cannot help my father either. (Her voice has assumed an angry tone that is equally defiant in its strident harshness.)

I will find my eyes, and my hands, and my feet, and not be your image. And I can breathe. It's hard but I can. And it is not true that I am so impossible as you said. That I let myself be taken by men like a thing, not a human being, but like an object, a thing.

I ask, "What's that? What did she say?"

She said: "Your neck is so thick, your legs are so bad, your walking is like a soldier, your hair is terrible, your behavior is terrible." And because I believed her, I let myself be taken by men like a thing, like a, a...

I add, "Like a possession. She said those things to you before you were married?"

Maybe it began when I was twelve or thirteen years old. She compared me all the time with my cousins who were so beautiful. I am not so beautiful, I know. But I can't be. It's not my mistake. I am myself. I can make something of myself. I am not looking like a model. I know it. (Actually, on occasion, Christa would be regarded as a strikingly beautiful woman.)

You punished me for not remaining a child. You wanted me to remain a child because when I became a woman you would lose me. You would not let me grow up. I was not allowed to go out. I had to stay at home with you. You gave me not much love because if I had enough I would be able to go away and become free. You kept me dependent upon you. You said that I am bad looking, that I am not a woman, that I will never be a woman, that I will never have a man, that nobody will ever like me, and that only you will ever understand me.

After remaining on the stool for forty-five minutes, Christa decides to lie down on her belly. Immediately, she begins to cry freely and robustly. Without encouragement or direction, she continues to address her mother, her face looking down into the mattress :

You hated me because I liked other people more than you. Even when I was a little child it was the same. I liked to be with my cousins, and I would cry whenever they would leave after visiting us. You would then scold me after they left for crying, saying, "You are an impossible child. I am so ashamed of you." All the time it was the same after they left.

I was so afraid to be alone with her. I would not be alone with you. You could do with me whatever you liked. I had nobody. The others would never believe me because a mother is right and never the child. You knew this. You were playing with my feelings. Playing all the time. You were playing. Playing... Playing.

(Christa's voice has grown progressively louder and more intense. By the time she says, "playing," it has reached an hysterical level of intensity as she begins to shriek briefly. Then she cries openly and continues her heart-felt confrontation with her mother.)

I did not know that you could not tell the truth. I believed you. I believed you. I could not like you. All the time I could not. You made a cripple out of me. When I was looking at myself in the mirror, I was hating myself. I was crying when I was seeing myself in the mirror when I was seventeen and eighteen years old. I saw myself through your eyes.

And, when I ask what she saw in the mirror, Christa says :

I saw just the picture that my mother had made of me. I saw my neck as long, my hairs hanging down, my face was not laughing nor charming, and not attractive. I was so tall. I saw my legs as thick and clumsy. Just as she had told me.

A neurotic split client must face his false self-system both objectively and subjectively. That is, not until he can both cognitively perceive and immediately feel it can he rid himself of his false self-system and complete the dearmoring process. Furthermore, he must perceive it objectively in terms of its introjection from others, while at the same time feeling its presence within his own past and present perceptions of self before he can finally extricate the distorted body image.

The capacity to perceive objectively the neurotically split essence of one's childhood tormentor and its subjective effects upon one's feelings, a capacity which Christa illustrates here, is mediated by the intuitive Logos faculty. The center of this faculty is the primitive brain stem, unimpeded by the bullying tactics of the cerebral cortex. The primary foundation of this center is the self-other confrontation facilities of the upper back. Christa's phallos center and Logos center interpenetrate as she convergently focuses upon her mother's being while feeling the anguish of previously introjecting her mother's being. Having experienced this functionally integrated synthesis, Christa has reached a point in the dearmoring process which is probably irreversible.

Christa's intuitive and convergent focus upon her mother's being begins the final phase of extrication from the perceptual system superimposed by her mother with which she has identified. Unlike the primitive externalization of first stage treatment, this is a highly complex process of object-centered, cortical-subcortical synthesis. Her intuitive faculties now penetrate to the essence of many past situations which were formerly completely misinterpreted. Her perceptual rendering of those same situations is becoming totally reorganized. Such a revolution in cognitive awareness presupposes an enormous internal convergence of biological and psychic forces. In all probability, Christa had many similar insights about her mother's being prior to treatment. However, these insights had not acquired enough substance to produce the complete interior reorganization and object-centered focus of prior cognitive moulds.

The four-directional fluid circulation of Christa's core longitudinal energy currents is the key which allows her to imbue her perceptions of her mother and past situations with such personality-changing substantiality. However, the movement of these currents alone cannot permit her to cognitively reconstruct and recreate the past in a novel and liberating manner. Simultaneous with the penetration of objective reality, Christa's primary dynamic feeling centers and the basic human needs which they mediate must also be brought to pleasurable satisfaction. The emergence of Christa's long deprived and frustrated need for authentic love and caring from her mother stands behind her driving determination to finally come to terms with her mother's heartless being. She is motivated by an instinctual inclination to feel her own unsatisfied need for reciprocal love and respect. The unconscious objective of Christa's newly awakened heart center is the final purging of her own false self-system, one of whose hidden premises is that she is intrinsically unlovable except by her mother. Her chest region instinctually and humanly compels her to confront the painful reality of her mother's total alienation from her own sympathetic feeling centers.

Another psychic breakthrough in Christa's gradual shedding of a core-alienated self-image occurs in the wake of her instinctual propulsion towards extrication from other people's beliefs. The latter is a more elemental reconstituting process -- at the bioenergetic level there emerges a rebalancing of ongoing self-regulative powers between the two antagonistic energy currents, the mind-brain and the visceral effector organ network. The more Christa can consciously face how she introjected not only her mother's values and ideals, but her very same patterns of energy flow and mode of embodied interaction with others, the more she can extricate herself from an identification with her mother's dominantly self-and-other-destructive cortico-cerebrospinal alliance against her own primary dynamic feeling centers. This process is vividly revealed as Christa blurts out: "I saw everything through my mother's eyes and not through mine." And also, shortly thereafter, when she says, "I will find my eyes, and my hands, and my feet, and not be your image. And I can breathe. It's hard but I can."

As Christa removes the veils from her eyes and sees from her intuitive Logos-guided frame of reference, she begins to shed the cortico-cerebrospinal circuit of subject-world cognition which has previously entrapped her. Her former mode of being has been imprinted upon her cortical synergist from without -- what the gestalt school calls 'confluenting'. She has been enclosed in a cortical conditioning which amounts to a total brainwashing by her mother. The elimination of this brainwashing can be measured by the extent to which Christa replaces her old conditioning with the four intuitive faculties of her creative unconscious. This process, which culminates during the third stage of treatment, is capable of infinite stages of transformation. Christa's distorted body-image emanates from identification of her own vision of herself with her mother's other-destructive visual perception of Christa's body. The nucleus of Christa's blindness regarding her own body and its natural needs and impulses is the introjection of her mother's eyes. This blindness has even extended to her perception of her visible outer shape and beauty.

In the last analysis, what the orthodox Reichians call an energy block in the eyes is reducible to an introjection-imprinting process which is more than passively reactive to the negative feelings stemming from the eyes of the tormentor. The additional component is an unconscious identification with the eyes of the dominant tormentor. Until this psychic identification is unmasked in conscious awareness, fully focused upon, and subsequently extinguished by the creative intuitive faculties themselves, no amount of energy-mobilization work with the eyes as such can dearmor their energy stasis. These observations critique those body methods which primarily emphasize a direct approach to loosening specific muscles and nerve groupings around the eyes of a client with an eye block. In contrast, I have found that the energy stasis in the eyes will disappear only when the intuitive core faculties begin to invade the false self-image complex itself under the guidance of Logos.

Chapter VIII

CHRISTA'S COLLAPSE

I. The Collapse As Experienced

Christa's marshalling of such a rich assortment of forces while confronting her mother with her vehement eloquence took a heavy toll upon her economy. A relapse was almost inevitable. The swing from one psychic state to its extreme opposite is especially characteristic of the long second stage. The emergence one by one of the dynamic feeling capacities is usually demanding enough to mobilize the opposite set of forces. These opposing forces are direct expressions of the still intact armoring. In Christa's case, the opening of her Logos, Eros, and phallic capacities in synchrony against her mother is eventually short-circuited by her belly region -- the other primary region of her torso still encased behind layers of repressed conflict.

So far, we have not systematically touched Christa's lower half. She has been too cut off from her upper front half to be able to yield with any depth to any direct touching of her abdominal or pelvic areas. We have learned through working with many paranoid hysterics that it is particularly hazardous to touch the lower half before the upper front half has begun to yield and the false self-system to significantly unwind. Otherwise, the client's response is usually dissociatively erotic. They experience a whirlwind of genital sensations around the rim of the peripheral muscular sheath which threatens to overwhelm their ego controls, thus causing a panic dissociation. This reaction results from the client's chronically overcharged genital area, centered on the clitoris. When any part of the belly or pelvis, either back or front, is touched, the overcharged libido generates a massive pseudo-erotic response in defense against any deeper penetration of the severely armored pelvis. We knew that Christa's sexuality was relatively undeveloped. Suspecting that her pelvis was severely armored, we did not touch her lower half until the fifteenth session.

Christa spent the first hour of this session talking with vitality and penetration about her mother and her newly discovered good feelings about men. I ask her to lie on her belly after removing her outer garments. I prepare her for being touched :

"Before we touch you, I want you to allow yourself to stay open to your creative imagination in terms of the past as well as the present. I want you to phantasize now in advance what it will feel like when we touch your pelvic area."

Kneeling on both sides of Christa, Katherine and I wait half a minute before placing one of our hands between her body and the mattress over the central muscle grouping located in the middle of the upper front leg where the leg joint meets the abdominal wall. We place our other hand on the back half side of this point over the gluteus maximus muscles towards the outer sides of the buttocks.

Christa does not move nor speak for a long time. After about five minutes, I ask what is happening. I sense a progressive constriction of her breathing cycle. Her silence is ominous, suggesting that she is withholding. Christa replies somewhat cautiously and enigmatically, saying only that she is not enjoying the touch. Our touch is slightly catalytic -- we are rotating our four fingers in a circle. We began this after discovering that the pelvic muscles both front and back are extremely taut. We rotate the hands which are touching the pelvic-leg joint in the front of her body while keeping our hands touching her buttocks completely immobile. When moving one hand, we usually stabilize the other in order to balance the catalytic and nurturing effect. (see page 279).

We persist with our direct touch after Christa says that her discomfort arises from sexual phantasies. When I ask about the phantasies, Christa denies having them. She suggests that our touch resembles her mother's -- it is not tender and resembles an animal approaching her with ambiguous intentions. I suggest that we are evoking her sexual paranoia which is concentrated in the pelvic-genital area. Christa asks for elucidation. After offering a brief example, we say nothing more. Sensing that she is not conscious of her sexual paranoia, I do not force the idea. It is always unwise to implant ideas that clients have not already arrived at in the form of embodied immediate experience or direct intuitive reference.

Christa begins to cry for about three minutes

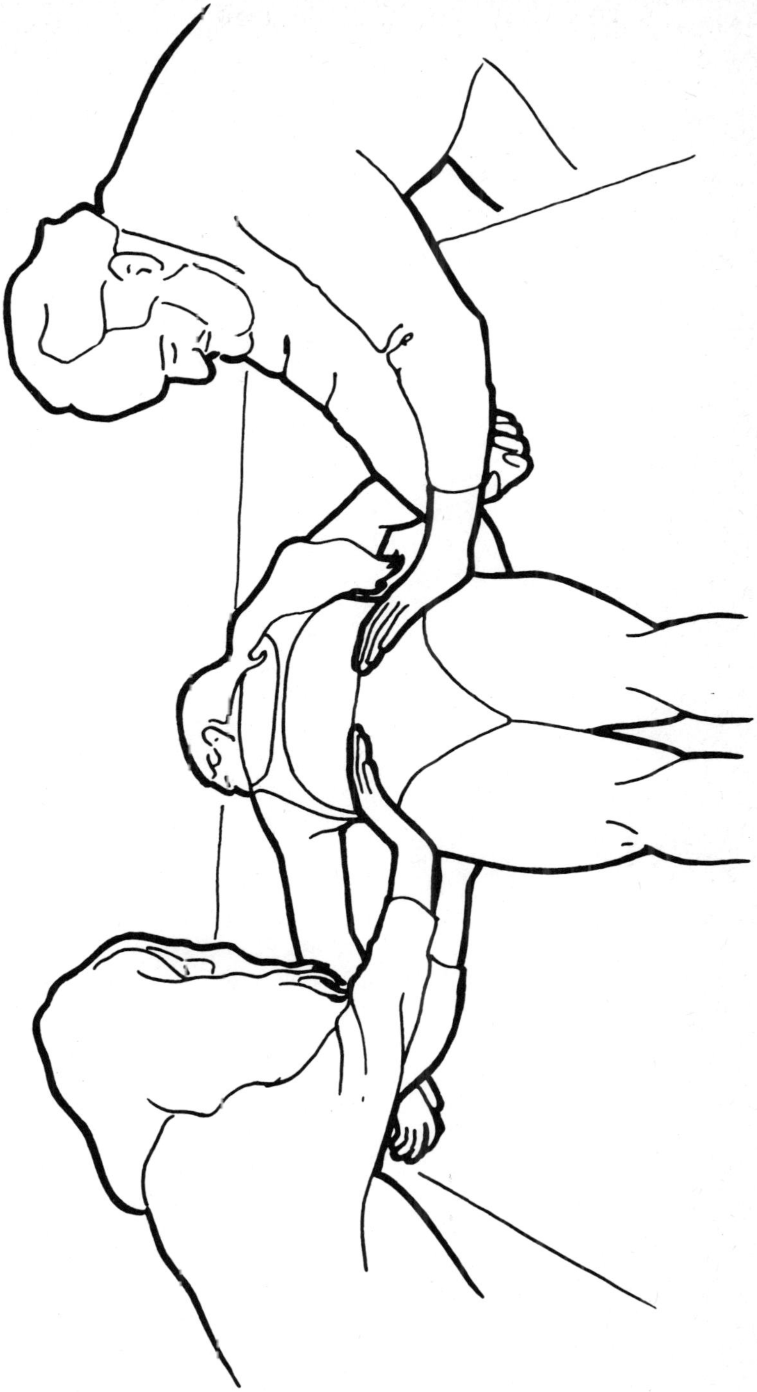

as we continue to touch her lower half. When I ask what's happening, Christa whispers, "I can't describe it. I don't think I can trust myself. I feel paralyzed." Katherine and I respond by moving to the other side of the room. After remaining motionless and silent for another two minutes, Christa says, "I have a feeling that I can never go out." This remark suggests that not only has Christa become paralyzed from anxiety, but also that she has begun to regress to childhood experiences of fear and anxiety. Although no longer touched, Christa remains fixated in this scattered, semi-helpless feeling state. I finally ask her to turn on her back -- this is twenty-five minutes after having first touched her.

Another ten minutes pass while we touch Christa's belly and pelvic-leg joint areas as she lies on her back. Again, she moves out of contact. After prompting, she says that she feels far away and disembodied. Her relative disembodiment is accompanied, as it usually is, by irrational and fragmentary phantasies and images. For example, she imagines, "My mother and husband coming to me together and taking me with them because I am like them." Dejectedly, she speculates that she has been incapable of perceiving any boundaries of personal separateness between herself and her mother and between herself and her ex-husband. This objective observation is reality-centered. Like paranoia syndromes generally, paranoid hysterics are especially prone to eradicate any semblance of separation between themselves and others on an unconscious feeling level. Simultaneously, they entertain fleetingly in consciousness very negative projections and distorted perceptions about the other person. There is a general absence of firmly structured boundaries between themselves and their primary love relationships.

Instead of transforming her valuable insight into a feeling conviction, Christa uses it to flagellate herself, maintaining that she is too hopelessly paranoid to ever discover her own boundaries. She questions whether she has ever touched her male lovers in a way that differs from the uncertain, ambivalent manner in which both her mother and her ex-husband used to touch her. She even questions her growth-enhancing movement during the past two weeks, worrying that she is as deeply paranoid as her mother and her ex-husband believe. In summary, Christa becomes entangled in a self-defeatist state of fragmentation and negativity typical of an ego-disintegrative depressive-paranoid stupor. Her sudden tailspin can be attributed outwardly to the fact that Katherine and I have touched her for the first time in her pelvic region with maximum impact. We have evoked a reaffirmation of much of her remaining armor.

The extent of Christa's rearmoring throughout her organism becomes clear forty minutes later as she does some straightforward energy-mobilization exercises on her feet. After over ten minutes, her contricted breathing eases only slightly. Realizing that she needs something more dynamic to release her depressive-paranoid stupor, I stand in front of her and have her place the open palms of both her hands in mine, interlacing her fingers in mine. As I start to push her towards the wall, she shouts, "No" several times as she resists with greater and greater vehemence. However, this work is not sufficient to get her out of her head into her body. Christa spends the remainder of the session ruminating about her fears of becoming psychotic and how both her mother and ex-husband actively fed this fear.

Three days later, Christa instantly reveals that she has remained psychologically fixated in an ego-disintegrative state. After sitting silently for several minutes, she cries and then says in a subdued voice :

> The first thing to happen to me was that I woke up in the night after the last session because I couldn't stay still in the same position for longer than two or three seconds.
>
> I was afraid to wake Ilsa and so I got out of bed and went on the floor. There I rolled around constantly, going from one position to another. I couldn't stay in my body. It was as if somebody was piercing me and holding me down in the same position, and I couldn't stand it so I had to move. I would cry out. Maybe for an hour it went like this until finally I did breathing and stress exercises for half an hour.
>
> It was then better, and when Ilsa woke up I asked her to give me a little massage and she did. There were tensions -- deep ones -- coming up here

(She points to her diaphragmatic muscle in the front) and moving down here. (She points to her genital region.) I felt better after the massage and could go back to sleep.

Christa's psychophysical reaction is a delayed response to our direct touching of her pelvic-abdominal area during the prior session. This is a good example of what we earlier called a vegetative release reaction. This kind of reaction represents an initial discharge response of the endodermal vegetative flow to a group of muscles which are beginning to dearmor for the first time. After being touched, the chronic hypertonicity contained in armored muscles often does not begin to release until several hours afterwards. Severe tonicity usually lessens in the form of a secretion of toxic wastage into the blood-vascular network from the muscles themselves. In turn, this sets off a counter hormonal reaction which is responsible for Christa's extreme physical restlessness and her sensations of being pierced and held. Her experience proves conclusively that her pelvic-abdominal regions were indeed severely armored.

Since last session, Christa has been feeling emotionally confused, scattered and suicidal. Reviewing her sexual history from a self-defeatist perspective, she realizes that she is like her mother, a basically non-sexual person. She describes how her mother convinced her that any kind of direct touch between herself and another woman, including her teen-age girlfriends, was clearly homosexual. She describes her excruciating guilt whenever she touched one of her girlfriends. Her suicidal desires arose after she impetuously clung to Ilsa again as if she had no inner resources to restore her sense of separate self-identity. On several occasions, Ilsa responded with fury to Christa's possessively clinging behavior. And when Ilsa spoke of hoping to find a boyfriend, Christa had a major hysterical attack. Christa viewed such a development catastrophically -- she could not believe that Ilsa would continue as a close friend after finding a boyfriend.

Responding to Christa's confusion and desperation, Katherine and I touch her upper half as she lies on her belly. Christa reacts with spontaneous coughing, leg-kicking, and arm-pounding, coupled with a little gasping. However, for the most part, she continues to whine and beat herself with critical comments indicative of severe isolation in her cerebral cortex. The session ends with Christa tenaciously clinging to her self-defeatist attitude despite our efforts to guide her towards a more positive outlook about her future relationship with Ilsa.

II. Four Stages of Divergent Functioning

Christa's chaotic collapse during the four days under discussion is basically a divergent experience -- it represents a collapse of her usual egoic self-identity. The disintegration of her usual controls was as constructively disorganizing in many ways as it was emotionally painful. To give up a false self-system and its accompanying set of ego-defenses, a client must periodically collapse out of his normally cortex-dominated mode of convergent functioning into increasingly chaotic, but nevertheless, creatively productive divergent modes of functioning.

There is much confusion in contemporary circles of psychotherapists about the positive value of divergent or essentially id-like irrational modes of functioning. The orthodox Freudian distinction between ego-integrative and id-disintegrative modes of functioning has negatively branded all instances of id-like irrational modes of being and becoming as pathological. Freud believed that any one acting without rational control is indulging in instinctual impulses which are dangerously infantile and destructive. Such experiences he regarded as symptomatic of neurotic functioning, or functioning in which the rational ego is too weak to maintain adequate control over the childish and unscrupulous id. I have arrived at precisely opposite conclusions. I contend that until the neurotic can permit himself slowly but progressively to let go of all ego and super-ego controls, he will never discover his deeper creative resources. Orthodox practitioners must eventually realize that their understanding of psychopathology is topsy-turvy. They will continue to flounder in mediocre clinical results until they recognize squarely that the tyrannical cerebral cortex, in league with the anti-libidinal super-ego, are the agents and the maintainers of psychopathological functioning.

Liberation from psychopathology cannot begin until a client can risk falling out of the Apollonian heaven of logical certainties and incandescent ideas into the dark, nebulous, unknown Dionysian world of embodied feelings below the diaphragm and in the front half of the torso. The fall from the clear light of the rational mind into the darkness of the unconscious depths is a divergent mode of functioning. In order to heal his split, a neurotic must fall into the depths of hell and the chaos of the lower and front halves when sexualized. He must descend into the amorphous realms of instinctual sensuality in the belly and pelvic regions. Here, there are no clear and distinct forms, but watery vagueness and sluggish undertones of feeling and sensations. Anxiety always accompanies such divergent falls into limbo. For example, Christa could not shake it off -- no matter how hard she or we tried to mobilize her volitional centers, no matter the degree of her Logos-inspired insights, no matter the extent of Ilsa's warm responsiveness.

Ultimately, divergent modes of functioning consist of a fall out of the convergently organized upper back half into the swirling chaos of the repressed id located in the front and lower halves. But the id, unlike Freud's depiction of it, provides its own mysterious ground of order and stability. This order and stability is totally disjunctive, if not irreconcilable, with the rational order generated by the mind-brain. The human psyche is fundamentally dual. Half spirit and half animal, man must live in perpetual tension between two kinds of order and stability which are generated in an integrated being. At peace in both realms, an enlightened adult fully acknowledges these two levels of functioning and self-regulation. This is the art of remaining rational while at the same time authentically remaining centered in one's core regions of being with Hara as the nucleus.

Jung called these two realms consciousness and unconsciousness. I prefer to regard them as the convergently focused and divergently irrational networks, or the Apollonian and Dionysian realms of the creative unconscious. In order to balance these two ultimately irreconcilable levels of functioning, man must allow each to dominate alternatingly. Without divergent modes of functioning, man cannot actualize all of his creative potentialities. There are two kinds of experience as one falls into his creative depths below the head: the passional-divergent-primordial unconscious below the diaphragm and the spiritual-convergent-creative unconscious above the diaphragm. Only the person who explores both realms will find the alchemist's <u>lapis philosophorum</u>, the philosopher's stone of inner wholeness.

Tension is an inextricable part of human nature, no matter the degree of personal individuation. The transition between the two realms of Dionysian-regulated and Apollonian-regulated functioning inevitably contains life-long conflicts for the truly creative soul. Future study of these transitional experiences in either direction across the diaphragm is essential to an eventual understanding of the human psyche. The process becomes increasingly less excruciating the more integrated a person becomes. As the neurotic split heals, the journey loses much of its terror. Nonetheless, a cleavage always remains between the spiritual and passional dimensions of human existence. Escape from the tension inherent in this duality of being is possible only by totally denying power to one or the other side. Such an achievement pays the exorbitant price of diminishing human creative potential.

Stabilization of the self-actualizing process only comes when an individual can tolerate a process of alternation between convergent and divergent modes of being and becoming. This is especially true during the long second stage of treatment when the false egoic self-image is slowly supplanted by a deeper, soul-centered self. The latter is strengthened and crystallized by the humanization of the primary feeling centers. This process is accompanied by a reconstitution of the cortical capacities -- they form a new and more integrated kind of convergent functioning. This type of convergent functioning is not grounded in the head, but in the four intuitive faculties of the deeper self. When functioning in polarized interaction with the differentiating capacities of the cerebral cortex, the domain of these faculties includes both unconscious and conscious psychic realms.

The process of dearmoring, or creative disintegration, is four-fold. During the first stage, the defensively organized ego loosens in the form of abortive tailspins of divergence into the chaotic swirl which is the character-muscular armoring at an unconscious, primary-process level. Such momentary tailspins are described in detail in the next section. Designated as 'primals', they are usually characteristic of the earlier phases of treatment, but not always. During the second stage, a client begins to fall far more substantially out of the ego network into the chaotic depths. These divergent modes always involve making secondary-process contact with one or more of the four primary feeling needs. This contact is never simple or clear, continuous or substantial. For example, during her four-day collapse into a regressive paranoid-depressive impasse, Christa sometimes identified with the intropunitive super-ego forces of her old false self-system and sometimes more nebulously identified with her alienation from her need for self-esteem and self-acceptance. Such experiences are bathed in chronic high anxiety. They involve a wild swing between conscious and unconscious perceptual frameworks and between a convergent-equalization and a charge-discharge-driven energy patterning. The feeling constellations and intuitive cognitions are too fleeting and too fragmentary to provide terminal subjective satisfaction. They are a mixture of primary-process and secondary-process psychic phenomena.

During the third and fourth stages of creative disintegration, the deeper self has expanded although it has not yet stabilized, and remains, at best, erratically dominant. However, convergent modes of functioning are no longer maintained at the expense of the psyche's need for divergent functioning. Tension still exists between the two experiential modes: the sharp boundaries of the outer environment contrasts with the limitless, more universally interconnected contours of the inner world. However, this conflict can now be tolerated with some pain and anxiety, even in spite of the spontaneous emergence of numinous-like instinctual forces that are transfigured as archetypal images of an unknown and frightening nature. They enter consciousness after a tremendous implosion of contrary psychic tendencies explodes the psyche into fragments, producing dissociative-like states of altered consciousness. During the third and fourth stages of dearmoring, the emergence of these instinct-driven archetypal forces can be most disruptive and anxiety-arousing. Therefore, a therapist must know what he is doing and what is happening internally to a client. Otherwise, both will collude in an effort to intellectualize and paper over the underlying productive crisis which is occurring between the depths and the surface of the psyche.

Self actualization comes only after a client has experienced all four distinct kinds of divergent modes of functioning. Each kind usually but not invariably unfolds in a progressive continuum. The first kind can be classified by the popular term, 'primaling'. The second, which occurs throughout the second stage of treatment, relates to the opening of consciousness to the repressed primary feeling needs below the head. The third kind, which consists of confronting the negative or shadow faces of the collective unconscious, occurs in the latter half of second stage. The fourth kind, which consists of confronting both negative and positive faces of the collective unconscious during sexual lovemaking, occurs towards the end of the second stage of treatment and sometimes during the third stage. Bioenergetically, this development occurs as the core longitudinal energy currents penetrate the diencephalon region of the primitive brain stem and unite the cerebral cortex with the lower and middle brain capacities.

After a client has assimilated these four distinct kinds of divergent functioning, he is free to function alternatingly between convergent and divergent modes, moving from one to the other without great turmoil. He knows how to accept being Apollonian-rational much of the time and irrationally Dionysian for briefer periods. He prizes equally his convergent-spiritual-creative dimensions and divergent-Dionysian-creative dimensions. Acknowledging their dual and ultimately disjunctive co-existence, he does not try to consistently balance the two different sets of dimensions. Although at times the two realms unite to permit peak experiences of a higher internal and external synergy of beingness, they must always drift back into their autonomous spheres. There can be no permanent union between the pure-white unicorn of the upper half and the dark-savage lion of the lower half. Consequently, any permanent structuring of one's identity as harmoniously unified is illusory. At best, a dialectical balancing in the long run between intrinsic ontological opposites is attainable.

III. The Difference between First and Second Stage Divergent Modes

First stage divergent states are autocentric, whereas second stage ones are more allocentric. Autocentricity means a primitively feeling-dominated mode of experience in which the subjective frame of reference occupies both the foreground and background of awareness. This primary-process mode of subject-object relationship is distinguished for its absence of any clearly differentiated objective reality. For example, Christa's experiences during the first stage of her intensive are feeling-dominated and autocentrically subject-centered. By contrast, allocentricity is a more rationally structured form-dominated mode of experience in which the objective frame of reference occupies the foreground of awareness while the subjective frame of reference occupies the background of awareness. This secondary-process mode of subject-object relationship is distinguished for its focus of a differentiated cognition upon some objectified reality. The objective reality can be either inner or outer world. If inner, the medium of objectification involves the use of images, symbols, feeling memories, perceptual constructs, or localizable sensory sensations. If outer, environmental realities directly present themselves in the form of perceptual gestalts as received by the senses and cortex.

When Christa was uncovering her distorted body-image but still unable to objectively perceive it as such, she was functioning in a chronically autocentric mode in relation to her body-image. She was never able to cognitively grasp the distortions themselves. All she could do was to experience their crippling impact upon her feeling totality. The rapid succession of coughing, gasping and crying generated by her energy-mobilization work was primitively feeling-dominant. Therefore, its meaning was centered in a gross discharge of bound-up energy.

This mobilization, or 'primaling', is essentially the polarization of a counter energy arousal. The purpose is always to obliterate the stimulus of arousal and to produce a primitive, partial, and very short-lived equalization of the mobilized energy throughout the totality. Expression of qualitative feeling does not distinguish this catharsis so much as the underlying discharge of the abnormally high tension overload of the cortico-cerebrospinal circuit.

An example from Christa's second session illustrates this psychobiological process of charge-discharge mobilization of the body's intact armoring. For the first thirty minutes, Christa talked about her extremely labile fear that Ilsa would leave because she could no longer tolerate Christa's clinging emotional dependency. Christa had slept very little the night before because of her fear of impending abandonment. I tried to make Christa focus on her subjective feelings of anxiety regarding this catastrophic expectation. Simply by talking about these feelings, Christa's body began to tremble. Her overt body expressiveness prompts me to say, "Are you trying to stop shaking? Don't. Don't stop it." After asking her to remove her outer garments, I give the following instructions :

> Lie on your back please, and we will sit on either side of the mattress and we will watch you. Bring your knees up and put your feet together. That's right. Now maybe you remember the exercise we call the jellyfish... Yes, that's right. Let's see you do the jellyfish... Allow that tremoring to continue.

During the following two minutes of silence, Christa continues with the exercise. Her extreme silence tells me how rigidly intact her peripheral muscular sheath remains -- it prevents her from relaxing even enough to allow a natural breath sound. For this reason, I ask her to allow the sound of Ahh with each exhalation. She complies immediately, and is able to sustain about ten exhalations accompanied by the sound of Ahh, but with extreme breath control, a control revealed by her automatic, drill-like perfect timing of the inhalation and exhalation. Asked to allow a longer sound, she manages to sustain a slightly longer sound and exhalation for about seven breaths before she begins involuntarily to choke up completely in her throat, so much so that she is forced to start coughing and to break the exercise. After she recovers from the coughing, I ask her what she has been aware of. She responds :

> I had the impression -- (she suddenly gasps in mid sentence) that I cannot breathe.

I extend my hand, asking her to hold it. After a minute's silence, Christa says :

C : Sometimes I would not breathe anymore. I would just stop it.

Me: When ?

C : When I'm thinking that the other will go away because I am so bad. (She gasps with sound). When I'm thinking that he would not stay with me, I see myself with a great open mouth and I can't scream or say anything.

Me: Hold my hand. When did this last happen to you?

C : Last night. When I cry, first I can't breathe. It gives me a good feeling not to be able to breathe anymore. But then I become afraid that I can't breathe even though I enjoy not breathing ... I feel so great a tension that I don't know what to do with my hands and legs and body. Sometimes I begin to hit myself with my hands.

Asked to resume the jellyfish while making the sound of Ahh, Christa emits two exhalations. On the third, she begins to cough hoarsely and uncontrollably. She struggles to recover her composure so that she can continue the jellyfish, but she never succeeds. Instead, her coughing grows louder and deeper as her body progressively convulses. After three and a half minutes, she suddenly manages to stop the coughing. Again, I ask Christa to resume the jellyfish. After two 'Ahhs', she starts to cough again. Seeing that her legs are beginning involuntarily to draw up into her torso into a foetal position, I encourage her to continue to draw them up. And when they are up, I ask her to make the sound of Ahh with each exhalation. I repeat my instruction, and each time her Ahh becomes louder. I raise my voice in order to make it louder than hers, shouting vigorously, "Louder... Louder... Louder", three times, once after each of her exhalations. Her 'Ahhs' become interspersed with coughing and crying. After about half a minute, her crying assumes a distinctly infantile sound and rhythm which resembles a tiny infant who is both screaming in rage and simultaneously gasping for breath. This continues for another full minute when Christa suddenly becomes silent. The silence lasts for thirty seconds. And then, Christa begins to weep quietly. Katherine says softly, "Say it". Immediately, Christa begins to sob and cry "Mama --Mama--Mama--Mama--Mama". Between each "Mama", she cries hysterically, the sound moving rapidly up and down the vocal register. After a minute, Christa becomes silent, and then says with complete logical coherency, but with the voice of a young girl :

> I have a strange phantasy... that my mother would kill me. I don't know why. She never did... But I couldn't live... (She gasps in horror) unless I fought. I had to fight against death. I don't know why. Oh I'm so afraid... Don't go away..... (Silence of two minutes).
>
> No matter how much or hard I cry, she doesn't come. No... No... (Silence of three to four minutes until Katherine asks what she is experiencing).
>
> I'm in a dark room. There is nobody. I have no hands except the fingers of an animal. They can hold nothing... I would like to fight against something, but there's nothing there to fight. Nothing... Or to get out. There's nothing to get out of, nothing to do...."

Most 'primaling' is a massive contraction of the intact armoring against the possibility of a greater opening of consciousness to overwhelmingly painful psychological realities, past and present. One of two occurrences enable this massive contraction: either the high chronic vigilance level of the metabolism relaxes, or else, a dynamic mobilization of the energy flow loosens the armored mesodermal muscle layers. Both phenomena occur from the moment Christa begins the deep breathing exercise. Her compulsive coughing and gasping signify that the armored sheath is softening. Nevertheless, these are nothing more than incipient vegetative release reactions as compared to the tailspin regressive dedifferentiation of functioning into which Christa plunges precisely at the moment when she reaches a psychodynamic breaking point. She is forced to move out of a defensive convergence into a divergent mode. Her wails for 'Mama' represent a bioenergetic discharge and retreat from a massive mobilization of chronically impacted psychological and energetic forces. Like cathartic release generally, 'primaling' always arises as a flight from conscious confrontation of instinctual and psychological forces frozen within the organism. It is a natural safety valve.

The uncontrollable screams and body thrashing of primals are surface manifestations of an externalization of and release from massive contractions of the armor. They facilitate the healing process by loosening the still intact peripheral muscular sheath or deeper network of rigid energy blocks. Particularly with severe armoring, they are a necessary form of productive divergent functioning. For example, charging up Christa's already overloaded cortical-cerebrospinal ganglionic circuits precipitated her regressive struggle to breathe. Her reflexive coughing and gasping escalated her energy economy to the point of plunging it into massive collisions of energy flow deep inside her metabolism. This in turn triggered a massive surface discharge of a portion of these jammed energy currents. This discharge took the form of infantile cries which resembled those of a tiny baby less than a year old.

Christa's infantile expressions can best be understood in terms of a definite pattern of her energy economy in relation to her intact character-muscular armoring. The expressive behavior cannot provide us with any coherent or profound understanding of the broader process of personality transformation which is involved. This is particularly true during the first stage of the dearmoring process when all change-producing bioenergetic and psychological movement remains embedded in a primary-process matrix. To be sure, Christa's infantile cries represent a reliving of early trauma and expresses partial relief from the tension mobilized. But both the charging and the discharging of the tension mobilized is what is significant -- not the mental contents of the release.

Primaling makes possible a non-differentiated and hence non-objectified subjective experience in the here-and-now of one's underlying helplessness and inability to feel anything except in the most desperately divided fashion. Primaling amounts to a primary-process convulsing of one's unacknowledged inner emotional rigidities. It cannot be more convergently crystallized than as a tailspin of the psyche into feeling the anguish of one's chronic emotional and bioenergetic impasse.

Hence, it is not surprising that Christa totally lost contact with her rational faculties when she was possessed by the primitive reflex reactions of coughing and gasping. Her regression to an infantile expressive discharge had no psychological significance except as it permitted release of a large amount of chronically bound energy from within her peripheral muscular sheath. This release is expressive of a massive clonic convulsion of the entire peripheral sheath. A clonic convulsion presupposes a massive contraction and charging up of the metabolism, followed by a massive discharge of some of the freshly mobilized encapsulated energy stasis. Such a discharge also represents a dedifferentiated excitation and expansion from the center to the periphery of the organism. The dedifferentiated excitation gestalt allows two benefits: deepening of the organismic trend to maintain an ongoing homeostatic distribution of energy charge throughout the organism, and a temporary reduction in the high chronic tension level in the cortical-cerebrospinal ganglionic circuits.

Goldstein's postulation of three distinct stages of dynamic energy patterning provides a scientific basis for the differences between autocentric and allocentric, or primary-process and secondary-process modes of divergent functioning. Autocentric divergent functioning is paralleled by a charge-discharge-driven energy pattern, whereas allocentric divergent functioning is paralleled more by a convergent-equalization energy pattern. One of the unique characteristics of first stage divergent functioning is the total absence of any kind of subject-object-structuring. No convergent differentiation arose from Christa's regressive fits of coughing, gasping, and crying. In fact, Christa moved directly into a dedifferentiated equalization of the tension generated by her expressive behavior. In other words, she moved directly from first to third stage of a creative encounter as postulated by Goldstein, entirely leaving out the second stage formation of a differentiated figure-background excitation gestalt.

As long as a charge-discharge-driven energy pattern is present, an individual is for the most part incapable of generating any kind of creative differentiated encounter with some immediate objective inner reality. Severe armoring prevents awareness from focusing upon some inner objectified reality long enough to yield a stable sensorimotoric object. An armored neurotic is so fixated to the uncompleted and non-identified feeling past that he can tolerate only the briefest exposure of his focal consciousness to immediate embodied feelings and sensations. He is too chronically restless and self-consciously preoccupied in a narcissistic, autocentric mode. Therefore, he is unable to simply receive the objective inner world with sufficient cognition to focus his attention long enough to even receive his feelings and sensations of the moment with any kind of clear recognition. He remains mentally idea-fixated and cerebrally structure-bound, or else lost in chaotic swings from one disconnected feeling to the next.

Goldstein provides a solid physiological foundation for a neurotically defended species of convergent functioning. He attributes it to a functional dedifferentiation of the entire neural substratum which arises from the relative isolation of the cortical ganglia from the remainder of the organism. The relative isolation initiates a series of two types of mentalized responses to impinging stimuli: responses that are stimulus-bound, and responses that alternate labilely between opposite reactions. Both of these defective responses are a cerebralized mental substitute for the unfolding of a second stage process of figure-background subject-object differentiation in which immediate interior feeling needs and sensations define the object of focus. In other words, the high degree of chronic tension which already overloads the cortical-cerebrospinal ganglionic circuits of the armored neurotic precludes any stabilizing figure-background excitation process that extends organically throughout the entire neural substratum and has the capacity to focus upon subcortical embodied processes. Instead, chaotically dedifferentiated and alternating mentalized responses are elicited by each new stimulus. Such responses deprive the subject from establishing any sensorimotor contact with subcortical interior realities in and for themselves.

For example, this complex set of responses occurs as Christa becomes fixated to a repetitive archaic pattern in which she cannot breathe every time she phantasizes that someone is about to abandon her. Her not wanting to breathe, scream or talk represents a massive hysterical paralysis of vital instinctual resources. A stimulus-bound response to the catastrophic fear of abandonment causes her to divergently regress to a state of emotional helplessness and passivity. Yet within this helpless state, she is further fragmented because of absolutely opposite feeling reactions to the same subjective state: she simultaneously fears it yet deliberately cultivates it by holding her breath. These diametrically opposed reactions fluctuate so rapidly that she cannot consciously identify with either one. She becomes enveloped by a chaos of opposite reactions, precisely as Goldstein describes it, because of the total encapsulation of her infantile trauma from the rest of her psychic structure. Therefore, when faced with such opposite extremes, she understandably obliterates the immediate psychic impasse by plunging into a massive functional dedifferentiation of secondary-process psychic contact.

But Christa can only briefly sustain the discharge of her chronic excess energy level. After about half a minute, she swings into the opposite response to the same stimulus -- turning away from her emotions, she suddenly stops screaming to focus on her phantasy that her mother tried to kill her. Her reflective consciousness is surprised by the fresh revelation. Goldstein's explanation for this phenomenon of simultaneous stimulus-boundedness and a proclivity for rapid alternation between extreme opposites is a brilliant one. However, a full explanation of the phenomenological and bioenergetic dimensions of the situation requires exploration of the blood flow, a subject to which we turn in the next chapter.

Chapter IX

CREATIVE REGRESSION AND THE EMERGENCE OF THE BLOOD FLOW

I. The Crucial Importance of Deceleration

The primary agent of communication of the endodermal functioning is the blood-vascular network when synchronized with the glandular-hormonal and autonomic networks. Reich, while appreciating the significance of the endodermal processes in terms of their autonomic components, tended to dismiss the instinctual power of the fluid blood flow. Otherwise, he would not have postulated a sui generis libidinal energy known as orgone.

When Christa plunged into a regressive primal, she discharged the build-up in her peripheral muscular sheath. But something else must have allowed her subsequent stark phantasy which penetrated her unconscious depths -- the idea that her mother tried to kill her. The phantasy points to some traumatic event which happened during her first six months or perhaps even during the intrauterine period. I believe that her frozen fluid blood flow was directly polarized. It rose from deep within the visceral effector organ network to release the massive collision of psychological forces which operate in the ectodermal and mesodermal cortical-cerebrospinal circuits.

The greater the quantity of blood flow mobilized, especially when it is newly released into the mainstream of motile longitudinal energy currents, the slower becomes the entire process of adaptation and responsiveness. This deceleration critically impacts the texture of subjective psychic experience. It provides the endodermal foundation for Goldstein's formulation of the basic biological law of equalization. As an individual sheds his armoring, his entire biological pattern of energy deployment shifts from cerebrospinal-ganglia dominance to blood-vascular dominance. The regulative system of the blood flow is a much slower and a much more constancy-oriented network than that of the cerebrospinal ganglia. It is a much wiser basis of self-regulation. It is the only regulative bioenergetic system that ensures an ongoing continuity of embodied identity and fulfillment.

A corollary of these basic postulations is that the less the armoring, the longer lasting and more complexly creative become the psychic reactions to a divergent psychological collapse. The two examples already presented of a first stage and a second stage divergent tailspin will elucidate this general principle.

One of the most striking features of Christa's first-stage primal is the relative disjointedness and rapidity of sequential psychic movement that characterized the whole experience. Several partial developments unfolded in rapid succession, abounding in erratic leaps from one set of psychic contents to the next without rhythm or meaning. The initial tremoring of her whole body remained unconnected for her experientially with her succeeding fit of violent coughing and massive contraction in her throat. The most prominent aspect of her body's behavior to enter her awareness was her great difficulty in breathing. She experienced no connection between her hand grasping my hand and her realization that she often experiences not wanting to breathe. There was no experiential continuity between her self-image of a gigantic open mouth incapable of screaming and her subsequent regressive infantile screams.

The disjointedness is so extreme and rapid that Christa cannot register any cognitive meaning or feeling during the session about her ambivalence towards her impulse to stop breathing. By the same token, she cannot look at her self-defeating introjection that any human noises are bad. Likewise, she cannot evaluate her abrupt and involuntary shifts from convulsive coughing to a quiet foetal position which is followed suddenly by her outpouring of infantile rage. Most pertinent of all, she cannot connect my escalating, "Louder. Louder. Louder", to her subsequent total loss of control and movement out of convergent functioning. Finally, she made no sense out of suddenly stopping her screaming and her subsequent phantasy of fighting for her life against her mother's will. She could not even begin to explore the murder phantasy throughout the remainder of the session. This is especially noteworthy since it was much later during the same session that Christa's hand made involuntary movements which she experienced as the primitive thrusts of a terrible bird of prey.

In all probability, both the claw-like movement of Christa's left hand and her image of herself as an inhuman creature with animal claws lying in a dark room arose from an actual traumatic event which occurred shortly after her emergence from the womb. But her chronic cerebrospinal ganglion tension level had to diminish considerably before she could allow her creative unconscicus to spontaneously focus upon these two distorted body-images -- a development never reached during Christa's intensive.

In contrast to Christa's first stage primaling, her second stage divergent collapse differs in its sequential pace. Only after Katherine and I had touched Christa's pelvic area for twenty minutes did she express emotion. The expression when it did come was nothing more dramatic than quiet weeping punctuated by occasional coughs. And it took twenty more minutes of the same touch before Christa could definitely identify her subjective feeling state as paralyzing fear.

Ten minutes after we began touching Christa's pelvis, she clarified her sensations :

> It's like my mother this kind of touch. It's not coming clearly.

Her voice is extremely calm, as if she were utterly detached, looking down upon the touch from her head. I respond :

<u>Me:</u> You mean that it's ambiguous and unclear what the intention is ?

<u>C :</u> Yah. It's like an animal is coming, and I don't know what it wculd do.

I quietly reflect :

<u>Me:</u> That's paranoia... Your whole body has had to realistically armor itself against the intentionality of your mother's touch -- against its unclearness and the mixed motives that you have sensed in your mother's touch. Do you understand me ?

<u>C :</u> Yes, but I don't understand how my paranoia is showing itself now.

<u>Me:</u> She has cultivated a paranoia in you that you are

realistically justified in having.

Katherine adds :

> But it generalizes to other people -- all other people.

C : Yah, I agree. It does generalize to all other people.

This interchange shows how fundamentally impassive and imperturbed Christa remained in response to our direct touch. She evidenced no outward signs of either resistance or yielding. And only after another five minutes did her breathing cycle begin to indicate a bioenergetic response of withdrawal from the here-and-now. And it required another ten minutes of relative silence before Christa could respond to my inquiry about the nature of her paralysis :

> It's like a feeling that I can never go out... I don't know what's happening.

It does not matter whether Christa is referring to psychic imprisonment during early childhood or in the here-and-now. The important point is the subsequent chain of psychological processes.

After turning over on her back at my suggestion, Christa began to cry deeply, the sound coming from her lower half and containing great vegetative release. For several minutes, she allowed the vital and sustained weeping which was entirely free of manic-hysterical overtones. Then she described her experience :

> I felt myself far away from everybody. I have such difficulty to even describe it. It is like my mother and ex-husband would come and take me away because I am like them...
>
> Oh I know, I always had the great difficulty when living with him to know whether my perceptions were my phantasies or a response to the objective reality. Now I have the impression that I will never find the truth because I am sick too.
>
> I know my husband's paranoia because I have it my-

self. I don't find myself anymore. I cannot trust myself. I don't know if I touch others like my mother or not. Probably I am like her. Probably the other does not like my touch because it is like my mother's...

Maybe I always find men who have great difficulties to accept the relationship because my paranoia is hindering them. I never found out. To me it was always the most terrible thing never to find out what is objectively true. I never discovered the reality in my relationship to my mother or to my husband.

I feel that all that I did was unreal and just an extension of my imagination. I didn't know when I was married or with my mother what the objective boundaries were. I never knew where she was or where I was separately from her.

A total blurring of boundaries between the subject and his or her object-relationships characterizes most forms of paranoia. This disintegration of boundaries in Christa's case is so great that she cannot trust her own intuitive or cognitive perceptions of the relationship. She cannot accurately sense who is doing what to whom. Christa continues to explore her paranoia for another five minutes when she remembers with a sudden rush of fear how she has been wondering for years if she is really crazy. Her inability to trust her own perceptions was reinforced by both her mother and her husband who never lost an opportunity to indicate that she belonged in a mental hospital.

There were so many such incidents that it took Christa another fifty minutes to recall the more emotionally incisive ones. They all contributed to her growing uncertainty. The longer she lived with her husband, the more she could not and did not trust her own feelings. This uncertainty was enhanced whenever she tried to share her feelings with either her husband or her mother. For instance, they consistently invalidated her feelings that her marital sexual relations were in any way unsatisfying. Her husband's games-playing and double-binding assertions reached a pitch of mystification that convinced Christa on several occasions that she was going psychotic. Her fear and confusion finally compelled

Christa to leave her husband.

As Christa explores her fear of going crazy, Katherine and I touch her upper and lower abdominal regions in a nurturing manner. When Christa finishes her verbal exploration, I direct energy-mobilization exercises on her feet which are designed to reground her in her lower half. The exercises are only moderately effective. They do succeed in strengthening her phallic self-assertive capacities in her upper back. However, they do not have the power to disentangle her from the underlying depression which has been gradually building up from deep within.

Christa's paralyzing depression continued to linger and evolve over the next three days until the next session. She even entertained thoughts of suicide several times during the week-end. The thoughts were never so consuming as to propel action. They revolved around the return of her former pattern of wanting to possess and emotionally cling to Ilsa. However, the interesting feature was that she did not disintegrate to such desperate fragmentation that she could convince herself or Ilsa that she had no freedom of choice regarding her behavior. After a partial regressive return to her clinging syndrome, another part of her found her behavior so intolerable that she was able to stop acting out. She even achieved enough distance to see how she was pulling Ilsa into her own self-created impasse. Her Logos faculty, supported by her newly discovered phallic power, unconsciously guided her to move into her own psyche. There, she could perceive with figure-background object-centeredness that she was projecting her own internal chaos and panic onto Ilsa. So, instead of throwing herself at Ilsa's feet, she went to Ilsa for quiet nurturing contact and spiritual understanding. Her anxiety level lowered enough to allow deep sleep, her first in several days.

Christa's experience represents one kind of creative regression during second stage divergent functioning. A creatively regressive experience differs from a non-creative one by the extent to which it includes some kind of novel differentiation of subject-world contact between the client and his inner world. In this case, Christa's differentiation successfully modified both her outer manner of relating to Ilsa and her inner self-perception of her tendency to project and distort her own uncompleted emotional past onto her friend. All creative regression is stamped by a novel emergence of contact with interior objectified reality. It fluctuates between allocentrically organized and autocentrically primary-process modes of cognition and being-in-the-world.

In the same vein, all first-stage primals are characterized by a basic tendency to eliminate the presenting reality and to non-creatively regress to an autocentrically dedifferentiated state of pure feeling-dominated infantilism. This is true of emotional catharsis regulated by the underlying psycho-organismic need to discharge and obliterate an excessive chronic neural tension that has been freshly mobilized by a novel stimulus. The need to equalize the bioenergetic differences in excitation between the armored and isolated parts that have been stimulated and the remainder of the organismic totality is so prepotent that it must be satisfied before less biologically survival-oriented needs can assume regulative dominance.

Christa's use of her low-grade paralyzing anxiety triggered by our touching her pelvic region during the fifteenth session was indeed most productive. She did not contract her peripheral muscular sheath so as to obliterate from consciousness her disintegrated feeling state of imprisonment. Instead, she was able to consciously focus on this familiar feeling state. The focus enabled her to subsequently explore its implications in terms of her adult intimate relations. Rather than collapsing into a preverbal state of helplessness, Christa opened her adult secondary-process consciousness to her immediate feeling state, and allowed herself to identify in her phantasy with her husband and mother as being as paranoid as they.

This required courage and creative imagination. She allowed her Logos and phallos needs to unconsciously maintain sufficient dominance to enable her to confront the full anguish of her marriage as her mother hovered in the background. The need to understand and the need to confront painful emotional realities could now begin to guide Christa because her intact armoring was never aroused to the level of threat which would have caused her visceral effector organ network to assume total consciousness-negating command. Instead, the core longitudinal energy currents held firm against the paralysis Christa was entering. They managed to keep the fluid blood flow circulating rhythmically throughout her cardiovascular system.

At the same time, however, her partial feeling paralysis somewhat constricted her cardiovascular system. This paralysis reawakened her cortical synergist to partially excite the cortical currents to reinforce her characterological tendency to intellectualize her own feelings into distorted phantoms -- especially her inner actuality. She became inundated with negative feelings towards her present divergent disintegration largely because the merciless critic in her head was fighting against any further object-centered focal attention upon her mother and former husband. The intropunitive super-ego is the last bastion of the neurotic self-system to crumble before the rising healing power of the fluid blood flow of the lower half. In an instant, it seizes upon any weakness in the dawning core self and attempts to squelch the new self. In this instance, it defended against penetration of the formidable pocket of encapsulated energy in Christa's uterus. Her paralysis was just sufficient to enable her bioenergetic economy to seal off any immediate opening in this pocket. However, this did not refreeze the dynamic energy circuits of her back and their corresponding unsatisfied primary needs.

Nor did Christa freeze her chest region from me and Katherine. She could have easily done so by asking us to stop touching her pelvic area. She allowed us to polarize her lower front half for over one and one half hours. This was a significant achievement, given the degree of defendedness in her abdominal-pelvic region. Her achievement was made possible by the solid and continuous sympathetic rapport, or positive transference, between the three of us. Christa accepted my interpretation of her response as evidence of her paranoia. Never resisting, distorting, or denying my interpretation, she allowed it to sink deeply into her psyche. For the first time, she scrutinized her paranoia.

The most important circuit was our empathic identification with Christa's body's very real confusion and trauma regarding its inability to determine the intentionality of touch, particularly in her belly and pelvic areas. Our support during Christa's confusion enabled her to slowly and clearly recognize that our touch did not excite her sexually. However, she was never certain whether our touch was really tender and non-possessive. She was left dangling with the suspicion that no matter who touched her pelvic area, she might interpret it as aggressive or erotic. This suspicion led her to the decisive discovery that her mother's brainwashing had convinced her that all direct touch was forbiddingly dirty. She also connected her mother's touch to a cold, alien reptile. But she could not fully process these insights. She could not yet recognize that her encapsulated abdominal energy predisposed her to distort and defend against yielding to any form of tender, nurturing touch. She had no choice but to see all touch to this part of her body as ambiguous and threatening.

Another instance of creative regression happened the evening following Christa's fifteenth session. She awoke in the middle of the night to discover that her body was so agitated that she could not stay still. This incident was discussed in the previous chapter to illustrate a delayed vegetative release reaction. The intensity of the reaction was so extreme as to indicate a breakthrough of her abdominal energy vortex deep inside the endodermal layers. It was a distinctly second-stage bioenergetic breakthrough because it went deeper into her body than the peripheral muscular sheath. She could have easily become so paralyzed with anxiety that she would not have trusted her blood flow to guide her to the right breathing exercises to bring about relative equalization of the massive energy discharge. Without trusting the blood flow, she could not have resolved the stabbing pains in her abdomen. But her crowning creative act was to realize that she was still too tense after the exercise to return to sleep and that she needed the healing power of direct touch to quell her internal turmoil. She also sensed that she needed to be touched specifically in the pelvic and abdominal regions after discharging the severer tensions in those areas and that it was important enough to risk asking Ilsa to do this. Once the deep pocket had released, she not only tolerated the direct touch, but unambiguously enjoyed it for the first time in her life.

Having identified three distinct examples of creative regression in a divergent mode, we need to analyze what each has in common. Each involves a long and multi-dimensional second stage of differentiation of a creative encounter with interior objectified reality. This contrasts to noncreative regressive experience which is devoid of any meaningful stage of focused differentiation.

The second common trait is the conscious alternation between both sides of the still prevailing psychological split. Usually a split psyche refers to some continuing arrestment of flow between cortex-controlled inhibitions and fluid blood-flow-regulated instinctual inclinations. Bioenergetically, all psychic splits during the second stage of dearmoring refer to some kind of intact chronic collision of energetic currents moving from the head downwards and from the visceral effector organ network upwards. However, neither of these two characteristics accounts fully for the objective complexity. A third characteristic is the struggle for supremacy between the cerebralized self-system and the growing demands of the primary being centers for satisfaction of the needs for core-to-core relatedness. This polarity is the fundamental psychodynamic process at work during the transition from neurotic to healthy functioning.

The unconscious realms are far more inexhaustible in their richness and disjunctive complexity than the linear-like, single-track, computer-programmed rational cortex. The instinctual need-tendencies provide man with his capacity for feeling-charged subject-world investment and relatedness -- never the rational cortex. The fundamental guarantee against the resurgence of neurosis is the rediscovery of these primary capacities for a here-and-now richly complex and changing constellation of feeling circuits between oneself and others. This rediscovery represents a freshly created synthesis between primary-process feeling capacities and secondary-process thinking capacities. A dialectical tension must ensue before the optimal balance between them can be permanently stablized.

Two basic developments emerge as one travels this road of rediscovery. The first is the gradual stripping away of the cortical structures to allow the progressive descent of consciousness into the body's primary capacities for feeling relatedness. Direct polarization of the chest, the belly, the lower back, and the neck, head and upper back regions awakens the unsatisfied, inborn need-tendencies for relatedness. These awakened tendencies become the primary motivating force to propel the ego-disintegrating movement towards creative regression. The need to disintegrate and regress is an instinctual endowment to the extent that man has become alienated from his natural primary needs for feeling relatedness. As such, it represents the very antithesis of a weak ego or a sick psyche.

The second development emerges simultaneously at a less conscious level -- the building of emotional security within the client through interaction with the therapist. After penetration of his isolated cortical-cerebrospinal circuit, a client needs safety for further dissolution of the false self-system. Unless the therapist can authentically accept, respect and affirm the client, a client cannot give up his cortical controls to the point to enable a creative, id-affirmative, regressive exploration of past relationships.

This need for emotional support and intuitive understanding is illustrated in Christa's fifteenth and sixteenth sessions. Without it, Christa could not have confronted the painful realizations about her past fears and suspicions of others. She needed our intuitive understanding that her body's response to our touching her lower half was paranoid. Just as much she needed our continuing emotional support of her relative feeling paralysis and acute psychological confusion. We conveyed this support at two levels: through our direct touch, and through our sympathetic identification with her psyche's progressive disintegration. We freely allowed her to live out both sides of the split between her cerebralized self-system and her already awakened capacities for relatedness. We did not stop her in any way, whether through detached comments or a diversion of her mental torturing of herself into body-centered activities.

We did not stop her painful recognition that her extreme emotional fragmentation caused her to distrust her own feeling perceptions of her ex-husband again and again, thereby augmenting her confusion and paranoia. However, towards the end of the fifteenth session, I did make a rather emphatic little speech to the effect that she was not now in the midst of finally going psychotic. I was responding to her verbalized fear that she was deteriorating into absolute paralyzing helplessness. I did not try to talk her out of continuing to move into this helpless state, just her belief that to enter this state meant that she was finally going psychotic.

And throughout much of the sixteenth session, we allowed Christa to beat herself mercilessly this way and that, particularly regarding her possessive emotional dependency upon Ilsa. Christa was convinced that she would lose Ilsa's friendship if Ilsa formed a relationship with a man. Christa's ensuing wholescale anxiety attack was so disorienting in its whirlwind ferocity that she was willing to do anything to prevent Ilsa from involving herself in a primary love relationship with another person. Christa found it difficult to be physically separated from Ilsa for even half an hour. She entertained phantasies of suicide after realizing how she utterly depended upon Ilsa's love for any continuity and security of self-identity. She had never perceived the extent of this absolute dependency with such clarity. Perceiving it now enabled Christa to take some distance from herself at the critical stage and stop herself from her infantile clinging to Ilsa.

Christa could disengage from her self-defeating, compulsively desperate symbiosis with Ilsa once she lived it out fully to uninhibited emotional extremes. Her divergent functioning removed the normal fetters of egoic self-control. She became engulfed within repressed fragmented impulses and need-tendencies that had unconsciously determined her behavior towards others since childhood. Ilsa had become her substitute positive mother more than Christa could have previously acknowledged. By falling into the chaos of feeling-centered impulses and needs in the relationship with Ilsa, Christa was finally beginning to experience the internal chronic conflict that has characterized her psyche since the earliest years. The creative quality in this regression is that it facilitated opening her own consciousness to the collision between her false self-system and her primary needs for feeling relatedness with Ilsa. Her deeply hidden feelings of absolute dependency were now at last actualized in her interpersonal exchange with Ilsa. Two conditions enabled Christa to tolerate this extremely painful situation. The first is that her usual psychic equilibrium was acutely upset while her fluid blood flow was coming alive. The second was Katherine's and my emotional support and understanding throughout Christa's progressive disintegration.

A client cannot disengage his emotional fixation to the nonexperienced feeling past until he can perceive every past relationship from at least two points of view: the prevailing viewpoint when the defensively cerebralized self-system was dominant, and the viewpoint which emerges as he becomes able to divergently regress into his dynamic feeling centers. The chaos and pathos characteristic of the long second stage of treatment arises from the oscillation between these two very different perceptions of the same objective reality. Christa is caught in a whirlpool of contradictory feelings and distorted perceptions as she focuses with increasingly greater subject-centered feeling resonance, and paradoxically, at the same time, with greater allocentric objectivity upon her relationship to Ilsa, to her mother, and to her ex-husband.

To complicate matters, Christa cannot even experience these relationships with any enduring stability of feeling. Her feelings constantly shift from one mode of relating to its opposite. As each of her four primary feeling circuits is awakened, she must undergo a new set of feeling-centered dominances which invariably distort both the subjective and objective poles of her experience. This can madden the logically oriented intellect. At the very least, it predisposes the client to bouts of depression, partial feeling paralysis, and episodic breakdowns of adequate day-to-day functioning. Yet it is absolutely indispensable to heal a neurotically split psyche.

Stable guardian of continuity, the belly center is the foundation for a deep liking and respect of self which can thrive independently of other people's feelings and reactions. Christa has been totally bereft of any high regard for self since birth. Our polarization of her severely armored abdominal region begins a major assault upon her still intact characterological rigidities. She has no choice but to retreat into her intropunitive super-ego, the citadel of this intact rigidity. This last-ditch stand is another indispensable development which the neurotic client must endure :

> All the old relationships I have been having I have destroyed because I can't grow up as I should. I can't believe in myself because of my anxiety. I am full of phantasies about society's opinion. (Her whines are interspersed with little sobs).
>
> I don't know what I can do with a relationship to a man. I am afraid that the same thing will happen that has happened until now. There will be only sexual release and no real contact. (Sobs). I would like to have just the tenderness from Ilsa. Oh, but I can't give her enough to keep her. (The crying intensifies).
>
> She won't stay with me, I feel it. I hurt her so much these past few years. But I could not do otherwise... Never in my life could I really enjoy a relationship, never from my feelings because I would be filled with these paranoid phantasies.
>
> If I had a close boyfriend, I am always afraid that Ilsa will turn her back on me. I am also afraid that a boyfriend would leave me if I had a good relationship to Ilsa. I am so confused about this. (She cries openly again).
>
> I would not like myself if I were Ilsa and had to live with me. I would not like this hysterical-paranoid woman that I am -- so possessive. I am just waiting after each session after she has been with you for her to go away, for her coming to me and saying that she finally sees how I really am...
>
> I'm just gone away from my body now. You can do what you want with it. I'm no more there. (Sobs). I don't know where I am. I would destroy this body. I hate it.

Christa cries hysterically for a few seconds, and then relapses into silence.

Polarizing Christa's abdomen has exacerbated her neediness for some kind of ontological feeling security, throwing her into a whirlwind of irrational and archaic phantasies about losing Ilsa's friendship and love. Since Katherine and I have been working intensively with Ilsa as well, we know that Ilsa wisely perceives Christa's situation. The last thing Ilsa would do would be to abandon Christa. Ilsa felt increasingly the burden of Christa's pathological emotional dependency, and wanted to see this dependency diminish.

II. Confronting the Armor in Focal Consciousness Furthers its Elimination

Another distinguishing feature of divergent creative regression is its facilitation of immediately contacting the armoring itself. This direct contact can occur either at the psychological level of facing one's past and present characterological rigidities, or at the physiological level of feeling one's chronic muscular rigidities. Either way, focus shifts to the chronic tension and accompanying subject-world avoidance-oriented maneuvers of the false self-system. This process seldom occurs until the bulk of the armoring has loosened to the point that ego controls totally crumble during periods of divergent functioning -- usually not before the middle and advanced phases of the second stage of treatment.

The client must become able to actively feel the chronic collisions and short-circuiting vortexes at the bodily level. Furthermore, the client must perceive in the here-and-now in the form of objectified cognitive structures and images the accompanying psychic impasses. These two developments must occur before the armoring can be irreversibly eliminated. There are no exceptions to this psychodynamic principle. A client's intuitive Logos capacities must awaken to the armoring itself prior to its elimination.

During her sixteenth through eighteenth sessions, Christa progressively confronted her distorted body image. The most important aspect pertains to the loosening of the deep chronic tension in her abdominal-pelvic regions. Christa talked about her experience following our sixteenth session :

> Yesterday something strange happened. After the session I went back to the hotel and lay on my bed. I felt more and more depressed and was afraid that I couldn't extricate myself from it. Then I realized that I was waiting for the great

Malcolm Brown to rescue me and take me out of my depression.

I then thought that I cannot wait for another person to help me out. I asked myself what I could do to help myself, so I began to do exercises. I found myself holding my legs upwards in the air and they started to tremor wildly. Then I was lying on my back with my pelvis back and my feet into the mattress. (She has arched her whole back with her pelvis being held off the mattress high in the air).

My legs began to shake again unexpectedly. It happened so suddenly that I was terrified -- terrified at first. There was intense red in the eyes when this shaking was going on. Greater and greater became the shaking. I went from the floor to the bed because the shaking was so great and the floor was too hard.

My hands did the same and began to shake too. Then I stood up and did the exercises you showed me. For more than two hours it went on, and I stood up and lay down, stood up and lay down.

I had the impression that I had to do all this movement in order to shake something permanently out of mee -- the tensions in me. Much of the time I was laughing and crying and... finally when I put my head back resting the top on the mattress I asked Ilsa to touch my lower back and buttocks and I didn't feel any tension there as I had felt before shaking for the two hours.

Christa is beginning to increasingly trust her fluid blood flow as an inner guide. She is blossoming like a delicate flower in the midst of discovering her inner resources for opening to the objective world. The extreme arching of her spinal column permitted the opposed energy currents in her abdomen and lower back to burst through their encapsulation and to release themselves into the mainstream of energy flow moving longitudinally up and down the front and rear of her torso. The short-circuited energy gradually made contact with the main core river of flow. (see page 313)

Seeing intense red before the eyes always indi-

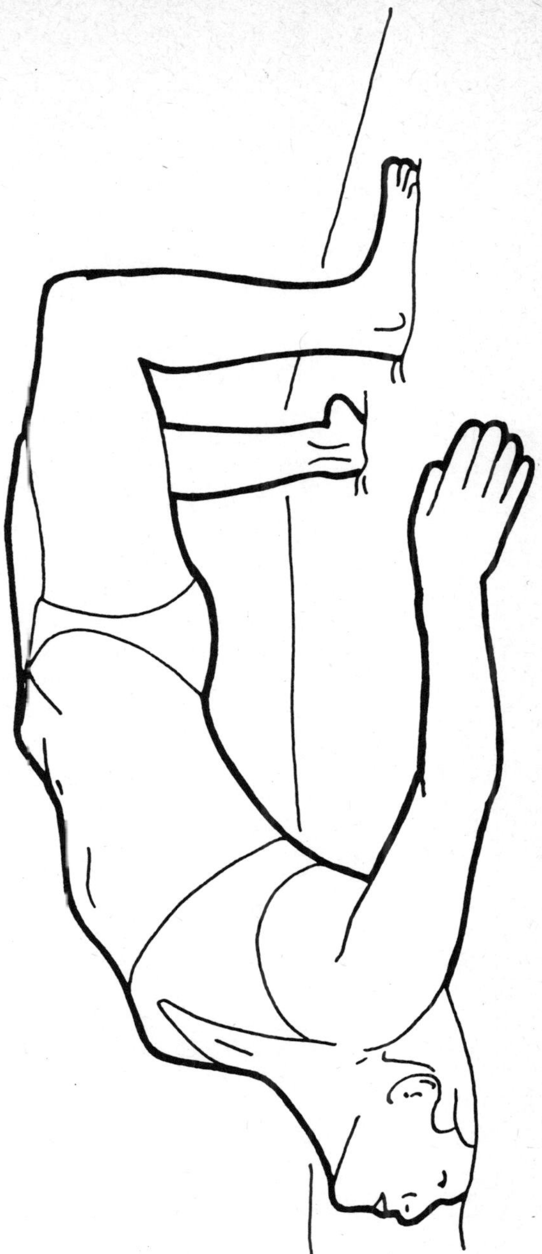

cates a tremendous energy transformation. This is the sensory after-effect of a noteworthy increase in quantity and modification of quality of enhanced blood flow infiltrating the head region. The blood-vascular network is coming to life as a harmonious whole, an experience which sharply contrasts to a willed effort to bring oneself alive. Christa's initial reaction of terror when the tremoring began was replaced by joy and abandonment as she began to laugh and cry interchangeably.

It is one thing to pump an increased supply of blood into the head through willed physical performance. It is quite another matter to see red before one's eyes while undergoing undiluted involuntary tremors throughout one's total organism. Persisting effortlessly and ecstatically for two hours, Christa reaches a point of deliriousness which can be characterized as an altered state of consciousness in which the pulsatory coursing of the blood unites every part of the body and the soul in a peak experience. Peak experiences mark authentic liberation from one's armoring. They usually occur during the middle and advanced phases of the second stage of treatment. During third stage, they become less intensely climactic and organismically dramatic. Psychologically, they cleanse internal impurities.

Christa's perception that she was shaking something out of her system is quite accurate. She spoke more of her experience :

> It was like I was imagining my mother's face when I first became terrified. When I first lay down I actually saw her face before me. It was like shaking out her -- expecially her touch.
>
> It was a feeling I never knew before. It was very strange for my body to be going on without any control from my head. I allowed it to happen by itself. I never knew before that my body has its own laws which you can trust and allow to happen...
>
> Something like in my sexual life, but this was more completely a going on of my body by itself. It was two things for me, a shaking out of my mother and all of this tension I get into when I have a conflict about some other relationship.

I didn't know anymore where I was with all that, but just listening to my body as if it were an entity in itself.

Christa's former depressive state has reversed strikingly into an almost ecstatic peak experience of unification. The differentiated psychological content is still secondary and somewhat vague, but unimportant compared with her dramatic reversal of attitude. The day before, Christa felt her alienation from her body with such venom that she hated it and wanted to destroy it. And now, twenty-four hours later, she felt an unconditional acceptance of the autonomous healing powers of her body independent of her cerebral will.

The most significant feature of this happening is Christa's contact with the unique physiological patterning of her armoring. This feature makes the whole experience a divergently creative one -- it involves a discriminating consciousness rather than an act of mindlessly primitive cathartic release. She knew her involuntary tremors were releasing her abdominal-pelvic region. This is why she subsequently asked Ilsa to touch her lower back and pelvic regions.

After acknowledging how enjoyable her whole experience had been and hearing our clinical judgment that she was in the midst of dissolving her pelvic block, Christa shyly revealed the following :

Something else I have to tell you (She giggles like an adolescent girl). My vagina part was more open after the shaking. But at first when I felt it there was great pain during the shaking. Then later I felt the whole space inside for the first time in my life. The tension was gone. It felt so good. (She titters again).

Me :
Open... That's a new sensation for you ?

C :
Yah. The first time I ever made love I didn't feel anything in the vagina part... Sensations only came much later. I have had difficulties until now to have an orgasm in the vagina part rather than in the clitoris. I have to be careful because the orgasm in the clitoris was coming

so quick that I had to stop it or it would be over with before the man had climaxed. (She laughs with embarrassment). Especially when I had not made love for a long time, once I had a clitoral orgasm I could not afterwards have an orgasm in the vagina.

<u>Me:</u> Afterwards ?

<u>C :</u> When I had an orgasm in the clitoral region, my orgasming was finished. So I felt bad about it... And I think that probably until now I have been chronically cramped and tight in my vaginal area. I realized this yesterday after the two hours of shaking.

<u>Me:</u> Yup. You did realize that yesterday? Good. That goes with having a pelvic block.

This new development reflects several fundamental bioenergetic principles. It is rarely productive to work on the so-called Reichian seven rings of armoring in a linear fashion, starting with the ocular block and systematically working down to the seventh and final segment, the pelvic block. The human organism, even when severely armored, does not function according to these seven laterally horizontal segments. Instead, it functions according to a set of cylindrical layers of energy flow which move longitudinally up and down the entire body. Reich only paid partial attention to the cylindrical structure of the human organism, whether armored or not. In the armored organism, the peripheral muscular sheath forms the same cylindrical shape that is present deeper inside the central regions of the metabolism -- the alimentary canal beginning at the mouth and ending at the anus or what Gerde Boyesen calls the id canal.

Our direct polarization of Christa's abdominal area focused upon the voluntary muscles innervating the abdominal region, front and back. It facilitated massive compression of the encapsulated pocket of vortexing energy deep inside her abdominal cavity, which eventuated in the inner release of her pelvic block. Both the peripheral voluntary musculature and the innermost tubular endodermic layer in the abdomen triggered Christa's later spontaneous mobilization of core longitudinal currents which opened her pelvis area for the first time. It rarely works to attack the muscular armoring directly. It is more efficacious to polarize the region that contains the greatest concentration of armoring from both sides, above and below. The endodermal cylindrical layer below Christa's diaphragm should be worked on directly, not her genital skeletal muscles. Polarization of this diaphragmatic region permitted Christa to loosen her vaginal cavity while cultivating the massive shaking of her lower half.

Christa's armored peripheral muscular sheath caused her reflexive predisposition to exclusively clitoral orgasms. It is coupled with a predisposition to exaggerated cutaneous sensations throughout the body's skin surface in response to direct touch. The armored sheath situated in the middle of these two cylindrical layers functions like an impenetrable wall between the center and the periphery of the organism. The result is to flood the cutaneous ectodermal layer with quickly spreading volcanic sensations of blood flow and eroticized excitation, simply because the mesodermal wall prevents any novel stimulus from passing directly into the core depths of the metabolism. Once again, we see that armoring accelerates the pace of the body's performance in response to novel stimuli, thereby diminishing the depth, richness, and complexity of creative subject-world encounter.

Christa's awareness of her own interior psyche expanded in response to her shaking experience:

> During the shaking exercises yesterday I was aware of this possessive part of myself. I had difficulties to face it during the exercises. But even before last session I had already begun to realize how possessive and how fixated on one person I was. I was always rejecting the knowing of it.
>
> The other thing was that while doing the exercises I was very aware of my paranoia... I have always been obsessed with the idea that other people are watching me whenever Ilsa and I touch each other, and that other people will think that it is a homosexual kind of touching and kissing.
>
> And that is precisely what my mother thought about any direct skin contact between two women.

And at yesterday's session when I was talking I fell into the same emotional state which I was in when I was sixteen and seventeen years old. Then I never knew if I was homosexual or not, if I will finally be able to live with a man, if a man could ever accept me.

All this confusion yesterday I couldn't understand or explain. And I felt exactly the same way for the first time at Friday's session (the fifteenth session) when you both touched me here. (She points to her lower half) Ouuuuuuuuuew! It was so terrible that feeling to have to go through all over again... All the confusion, isolation, and anxiety that I went through whenever I should touch a woman or a man at this age when all touch was forbidden. The strong need I had to feel somebody, but not being allowed to find anybody because all body contact was blocked by my mother because I believed her.

I comment :

Me :
She set up a barricade of distorted beliefs around you.

C :
Yah. It reminds me of the dream I used to have repetitively as a child. I am running around the dining room table and my mother is chasing me from behind. Then her face becomes elongated and her whole body grows taller and taller until she enclosed me completely on all four sides just as if she were a high tower.

Me :
When did you have that dream ?

C :
When I was about seven or eight it first happened. It was a black tower, and this was a dream that I had often for about four to five years. I would wake up in terror each time I had it.

Christa is beginning a higher feeling-cognitive synthesis between many parts of her present psychological makeup and her past history. She is reexperiencing the low-grade depressive-paranoid impasse catalyzed by our first touching of her lower half during the fifteenth session. But what a difference between the earlier confusion and interpenetration of opposite feeling-tendencies and her present perspective ! Christa's differentiations are now rising directly out of her here-and-now wellsprings of feeling. She is beginning to make historical connections to the formative past -- especially her incorporation of her mother's belief system, and her subsequent and still intact image of herself as unworthy of anybody else's embodied love for her, whether sexual or spiritual. To make these connections while tremoring ecstatically throughout her organism means that all four of her core intuitive-feeling being centers -- those peculiar to the endodermal cylindrical layer -- are beginning to instantaneously catalyze each other in a fertile and largely unconscious way. Christa's Hara being center is beginning to slightly awaken and to give greater substance to her already awakening Eros, Logos, and Warrior circuits of intuitive-feeling awareness.

Christa is following the usual sequence of personality change: the initial felt change occurring in the body's pattern of rigidities as a consequence of the discharge of chronic tensions is succeeded by a partial return to the psychological impasse which up until now could not be confronted fully in consciousness with feeling. Christa could face the immense confusion of feelings and false self-image belief systems which were resurrected all at once by our touching her lower half only after partial cleansing of chronic tension in her abdominal nerves and muscles. Her inability to test her paranoid phantasies by fully engaging others is directly linked to the condition of chronic energy arrestment that had been actively but unconsciously preserved in the no-man's-land of her abdominal region. Alienated from her Hara being center and consequently lacking any real belief in herself and her autonomous capacity to enjoy and love herself, Christa really was nothing more than an extension of her mother's and others' belief systems. She had absolutely no sense of herself as being-for-herself because she had no core feeling center from which she could nurture herself alone.

Christa's next two sessions are outstanding for her advances towards full functioning. They bear splendid testimony to the healing power of touch. Subsequent to Christa's two-hour shaking experience, she makes further penetrations into her false self-image. From the ashes of temporary collapse, Christa emerges to carry through the positive gains made prior to the divergent retrogression. Such is the nature of the long second stage of treatment -- partial, brief collapses of the psyche into total confusion and chaos are followed by an unfathomnable Phoenix rebirth and return to a positive merging of hitherto unconnected forces. Their progessive integration heralds the final fall of the neurotic super-structure.

Following her naive rendering of seeing in dreams her mother transformed into an engulfing black tower, Christa did vigorous bodywork for the remainder of the session. I had her stand on her feet and rock her pelvis forwards and backwards until she could make improvisational movements stemming directly from her body's needs. Spontaneous improvisational movement is far more effective in mobilizing the blood flow in the viscera than rationally premeditated exercises. The latter remain constantly in surveillance by the watching cortex, and reinforced by the super-ego's critical scrutiny. There is the real hazard that the client will mistake his movements as body-centered, when,in fact, they are subtly controlled by the cortex.

From her initial starting exercise, Christa moves gradually into improvisational movement: she bends forward from the waist on the inhalation, and on the exhalation throws her upper half and head upwards and backwards while simultaneously bringing her pelvis forward. (see page 321) This movement presupposes a high degree of energy excitation throughout the organism before it can become a dynamic but effortless pleasure-giving exercise. Christa was able to move progressively towards it in a matter of a few minutes. Her surrender of cortical-cerebrospinal controls to the body's immediate needs as mediated by the visceral blood flow indicated that she was finally ready to risk a do-it-yourself exercise designed to make her blood flow spin so fast that she would become dizzy to the point of losing her sense of balance. I asked her to improvise a way of rotating her entire body in a circle while her arms extended straight upwards into the air. She managed to pivot with great velocity to the extent that her blood flow overtook her neural gangli, causing dizziness and slight nausea. This represents a distinct personal

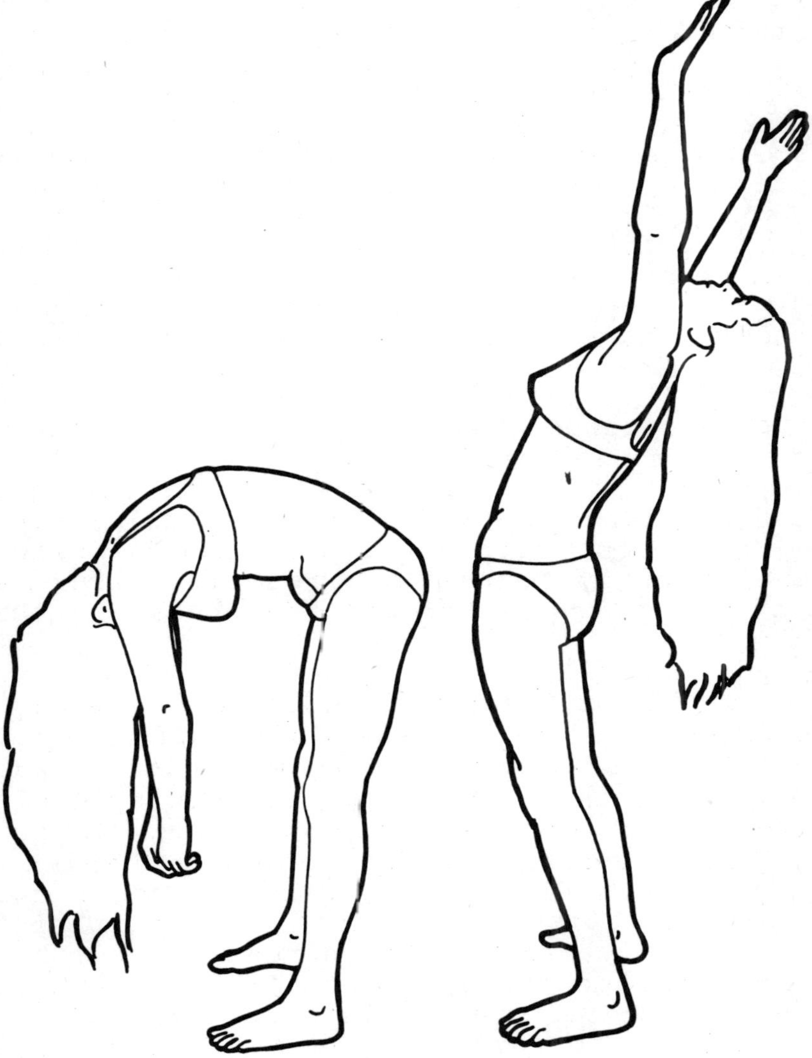

achievement. Hysterics are especially fearful of any kind of excitation of their blood flow throughout their entire body. Unconsciously propelled by their fear, they quickly become overcharged and skyrocket the energy release to an explosive level of intensity that hardly diminishes their underlying chronic tension.

Instead of skyrocketing her energy charge, Christa slowly mobilized her core longitudinal currents. This indicates a striking dissolution of any barriers between the central and peripheral regions of her metabolism. This development was further confirmed by the blithe manner in which Christa lay on the stool for forty minutes. The loosening in her armor was even more evident as she later lay on the mattress as we touched her pelvic area in a nurturing manner. She began to pound her pelvis with such vigor that she vomited several times effortlessly. Christa's vomiting indicates a clearing out and fresh relaxation of energy blockages in the region of her chest inside the endodermal layering of the alimentary canal. It is almost inevitable for every compulsively rigid characterological type to have to go through a period of spontaneous vomiting before the alimentary canal is free from chronic tensions which block the longitudinal energy currents from traveling with optimal motility upwards through the chest and throat regions.

The vomiting triggered a notable worsening of Christa's headache that she had been suffering from since her two-hour shaking episode. Her headache is accompanied by shivering, coughing, and pulsating. When we touch her head, Christa complains of sensations of heat rushing through her head which are intense like fever. Finally, she experiences a muscular spasming in her throat that is so painful that she shrieks. We discontinue the direct touch. Christa rapidly recovers her energetic equilibrium, launching without any directive from us into some magnificently vital slow-moving improvised movements of her total body, including her limbs. The session ends.

During the first part of the eighteenth session Christa talks about how well she has been feeling for the last twenty-four hours. She did some more exercises and vomited twice while doing them. She also was able to localize kinaesthetically definite sensations of a barrier in her diaphragmatic region. Try as she might through further exercise, she was unable to break through the barrier to relaxation. It was her first time to definitely desire to make the energy flow inside find a passage through a certain part of her body. This indicates a noteworthy opening of consciousness directly to her inner energy collisions.

Partly because Christa has been trying so hard to work on her chronic front half tensions, I ask her to take off her clothes and allow Katherine alone to touch her softly. I believe that Christa was trying to bulldoze something to happen to her energy economy that could not be accomplished through further do-it-yourself exercises. She needed to be touched softly in her front half, furthermore, by Katherine rather than by me, in view of Katherine's softer nurturing touch. Shortly after Katherine administered a very soft style of touch, Christa began to cough eruptively in a hoarsely loud and uninhibited manner. This is a frequent response from a front half which has become totally desensitivized at the endodermal layer and is in the midst of becoming awakened.

I ask Katherine to take Christa's legs in her hands while standing upright at one end of the mattress as Christa continues to lie on her back. Katherine holds her feet and legs firmly so that they cannot move. Christa begins to struggle to free her legs. I am holding Christa's two hands and arms behind her head, anchoring them firmly to the mattress (see page 324) -- she does not struggle against me. Christa rages about her feet and legs being held. She starts to kick, pound and yell with great zeal, breaking into an extremely phallic berating of her mother for forbidding aggression. Her tirade is both solidly focused upon objective reality and dynamically powerful. She sounds and behaves like a ferocious female cougar who has been chained to the ground. With little difficulty, she manages to tear herself loose from Katherine's grip several times.

Recovering quickly from this exercise, Christa says in an uncharacteristic cavalier tone that she feels like having a temper tantrum. I leap to my feet, grab the tennis racket in the corner, quat on my haunches, holding the racket back over my head. Suddenly, I leap into the air as I bring the racket

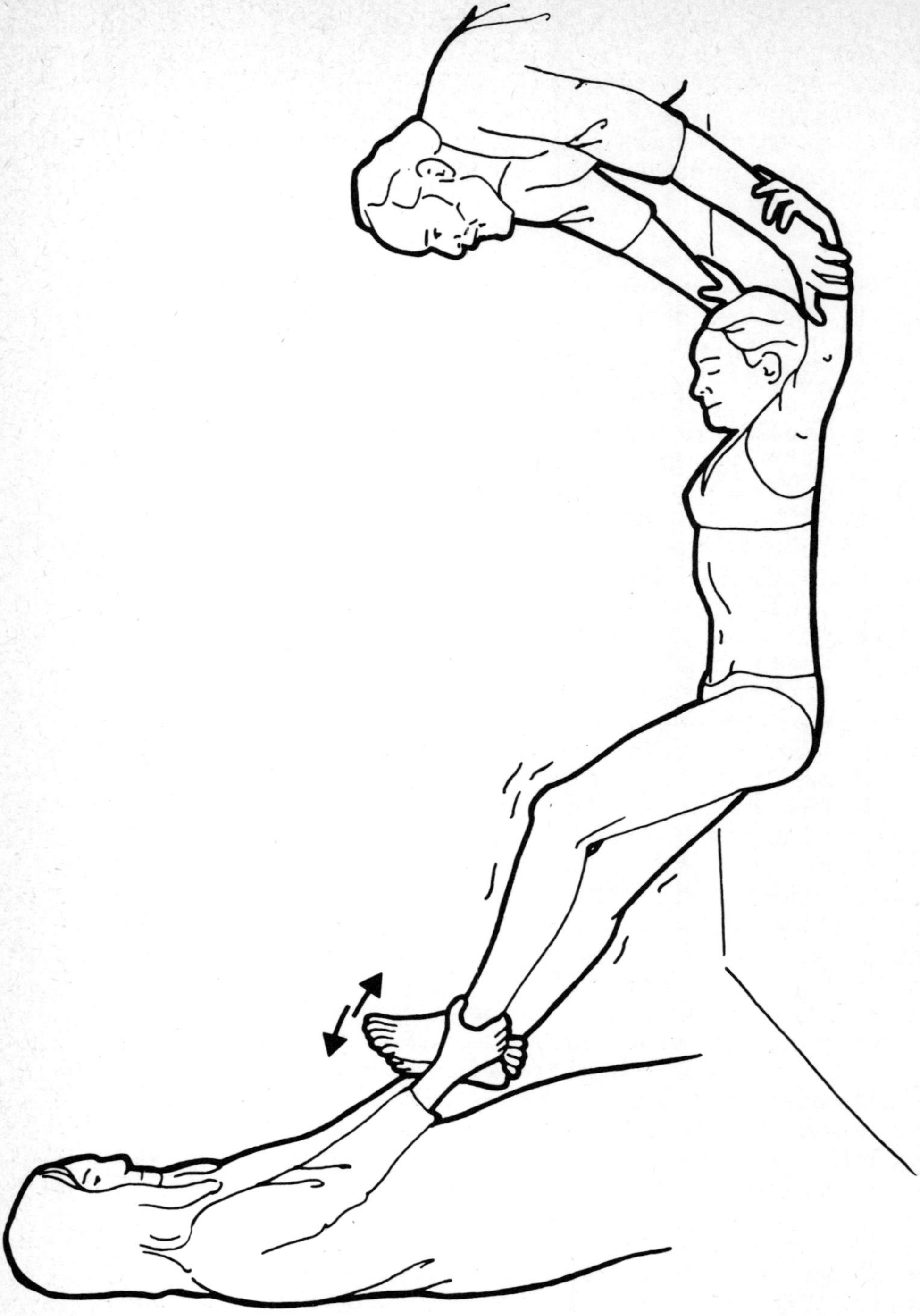

forward as assertively as I can so that it strikes the mattress in front of me with maximum impact. I yell at the instant the racket engages the mattress. I tell Christa to do as I have done. She really gets into it with a wild, barbarian rage which is manifested on her face and throughout her body. Finally stopping from exhaustion, she lies on her back. After a minute's silence, I ask her to talk to her mother. We do not touch her or come close.

> You didn't like the bad child in me. Never you did. You wanted to turn me into a good, good good child. I couldn't be aggressive against you. Whenever I was assertive with you, you broke it by making me feel guilty. Never was I allowed to be BAD. (She screams the word). Never I could.
>
> This is the first time that I have enjoyed being BAD against you. I can see your face -- terrified by my aggressiveness. Next you will have a heart attack. That's your game, not mine. You were always free to go out of the house. Why didn't you go out? You were afraid to leave the house alone. You couldn't let me go out alone either.
>
> But you were watching me and you came and were nice to me until I stopped yelling. Then you were gone. Never could I enjoy just moving and being myself as I felt. It was always stop and stop and STOP and STOP and STOP. (She beats the mattress with her clenched fists, yelling in synchrony).
>
> And when I was too loud, but enjoying myself, then you were telling me not to be so loud because there were other people around who would hear me... You could not understand that being a bad child was not only against her majesty, my mother, but that it was simply a child enjoying herself. You turned it into a tragic drama, my so-called badness, and you were the suffering model of a mother who was being tormented by her bad child.
>
> You broke up my natural feelings. I never knew it could feel so good to be bad until today. I will not be good only. You can do what you will. I would like just once to be your bad little child and to enjoy the fury in me. It would have been wonderful if you and father would have fought

with each other. But I was the only bad person in the family. Just a devil.

You let out all of your aggressions against me by calling me a devil. You played the good, good couple. It is so ironic. You were so wrong. I am BAD, and all persons are BAD. But it is you who were suffocatingly BAD towards me. You stepped on my soul with your morality of being bad. I could say nothing back to you. (She speaks loudly, with venomously inspired rancour).

Ugh! Ugh! Now you transform your badness into bodysickness. That's the only outlet you have left. You needed me to be your BAD child, and indeed I felt like a BAD child. I could never believe thereafter that other people could be BAD, only me, I alone was BAD. I couldn't accept that Ilsa could ever be BAD or WRONG. But sometimes she is BAD, really BAD and WRONG and MASOCHISTIC.

That comes from YOU, mother. I was always thinking that it must be my mistake... Ah, I see the devil that you have in yourself, and the devil that I have in myself, and I LIKE IT! I LIKE IT!... more than my good feelings at the moment. (Her face has a daemonic appearance, a triumphant expression that beautifully matches the venom in her voice).

I LIKE IT. I LIKE IT. I LIKE IT. I have no more to say to you other than that your morality has broken. It was your own aggression and bad feelings and with that you built up and fortified your morality. I spit out your morality, and the guilt feelings that you gave me. You can have them all back. Take THAT (She plunges her fist into the mattress as she speaks). Go away. I am finished with you.

This is Christa's most defiant encounter of the intensive. Her earlier ones were assertively phallic, but this was especially venomous, both in feeling and cognitive content. Her perceptions stamp its uniqueness as much as her feelings. This becomes progressively the case as a client moves into the last phase of the second stage of dearmoring. Now the direct confrontation of the armoring at the psychological level relates primarily to the confrontation of past and present interpersonal relationships from a perceptual perspective no longer mediated by the false self-system.

A new phenomenon emerges through the combined integration of all four of Christa's dynamic feeling capacities for here-and-now relatedness in their immediate confrontation with her mother's vindictively controlling posture. I call it the conquest from below and within of her intropunitive super-ego. Such a direct assault upon her super-ego would not have been possible if Christa were still enmeshed in a divergent collapse. This is because her split psyche still would have been sufficiently intact to prevent her from bursting through the internal barriers to communication between her head and her torso. Then she would be forced to live her fragmentation. But now, Christa is experiencing the opposite constellation of forces: feelings and perception are mushrooming from the organismic depths. They are sustained by a newly expansive fluid blood flow. The powerful flow pierces the deadlocked region between the primitive brain stem and the cerebral cortex. The opening of this region newly enables Christa to confront her intropunitive super-ego and its derivation from her mother's unacknowledged, but viciously tyrannical super-ego.

Another novelty is Christa's acceptance of her own demonically omnipotent attitude. She discovers joyous liberation in openly defying her mother. It feels good to provocatively flaunt her "bad" self in front of her mother's restrictive image -- no guilt, apologies or regret accompany her sheer delight. This new quality of self-acceptance signifies the interpenetration of her feeling center in her belly with her already awakened phallic feeling center in her lower back. Acting BAD IN FRONT OF MOTHER is tantamount to a final breakthrough into Christa's insidiously dominant super-ego. This breakthrough could not have happened until Christa's belly center had been awakened enough to permit her to remain centered in her own feelings while piercing the familiar rigid boundaries of her self-other capacities for immediate relatedness.

In summary, a synthesis of many different modes and levels of experience was necessary before Christa could enjoy her first significant confrontation of her intropunitive super-ego. One important ingredient is the creative convergence of both primary-process feelings and secondary-process perceptions which are both object-centered and subject-rooted. She combines two perceptions of her mother that have remained totally split off into separate internal persona: the distorted perspective of the false self-system and the more objectively accurate perspective of the combined natural feeling capacities for here-and-now relatedness. Christa's spontaneous internal synthesis marks a new plateau in the dissolution of her chronic character-muscular armoring.

Acting BAD IN FRONT OF MOTHER is obviously one-sided and partially dominated by a newly liberated complex of repressed emotions of rage and frustration. However, this is nearly always true of any freshly released psychic material. It is quickly brought into a more balanced perspective by the growing instantaneous interaction among the four primary feeling centers. Confrontation of chronic armoring in whatever form, including the intropunitive superego, is not complete until the very poisonous inner incongruencies have been eliminated. They must be objectified and felt at the surface. The objectification and feeling distinguish convergent creative encounters from a disintegratively divergent one. In convergent encounters, a person does not experience any real fragmentation of being or feeling ambivalence, because of the higher integration between primary-process and secondary-process capacities for subject-world encounter. Although the balancing of the polarities within has yet to stabilize, and despite the one-sided aggressiveness of Christa's encounter, her psyche is basically moving towards a convergent focusing of all her dynamic dimensions upon some objectified figure.

Christa's regression was feeling-filled -- she identified with the angry child within who was at last actualizing at the surface her negative feelings from the uncompleted feeling past. If she had remained detached from the restrictive parental image within and encountered it primarily from her Logos center, her encounter would not have been creatively regressive. Christa's passional defiance and self-satisfied omnipotence render it a creatively regressive experience. This was confirmed as Christa began to cry deeply and softly without tension ten minutes later, after further phallos-to-phallos bodywork. Christa had never cried with such total release in our presence. Her crying terminated as she asked me to hold her in my arms, another newly expressive act. Christa's crying stemmed from her lower front half and her desire to embrace me rose from her upper front half. She remained centered within herself, unencumbered by any self-torturing negations of her behavior. She had vanquished her intropunitive super-ego in a peak of self-actualization -- for the first time in her life, she enjoyed unreservedly sustained feelings of positive self-esteem emanating from her front half and traversing her diaphragmatic region unimpededly. Her longitudinal vegetative blood flow dominated her self-identity at long last, transforming the boundaries of her interior being, however briefly.

Chapter X

CHRISTA'S DECISIVE NINETEENTH SESSION

Christa begins the session with a dream from the preceding night. In the dream, she meets a Spanish man in Mexico and experiences unprecedented feelings of deep love: "It was a feeling I never had. It was coming from so deep within me as a total feeling towards this man. It was not like an ecstasy or an intense enthusiasm, but fuller". This theme pervades Christa's entire session -- her first taste of an integration of feeling response between her upper and lower front half, her Agape-Eros and her Hara intuitive sensibilities. Christa describes how this feeling stayed with her in the morning :

> This full love feeling continued. It went with a realization that this was the first real man that I have ever seen, and the first real feeling that I have had towards a man. What I have felt towards men until now was a complete surrender to the man, but it was fairy-tale-like and dreamy-like enthusiasm, and basically unreal. I have great difficulties to explain it.
>
> Maybe I can compare it with a feeling I had yesterday when I felt so sad but so good when I was crying during the session, and I said that it was coming from deep inside my belly. It was really coming from my belly. And I feel that something hardened inside myself is going away....
>
> And today I know that I had these new feelings before towards my students when I am working with them individually. Whenever I heard some positive remarks from them about me, I was always pushing those remarks away from consciousness. I actually felt ashamed to remember their positive opinion of me. Instead of letting some feelings of wanting to cry from coming up, I fought them down. So I have never felt to be a real woman.
>
> It is like as if there were a little hole here. (She points to the mid-point between her chest and abdominal cavities, directly over the diaphragm). And so now feelings can come up. The whole barrier there is not gone. I have to be careful that the little hole does not close up again. I would

be very sad if the little hole through the barrier would close again. I don't fully trust if the hole will stay open. I am waiting to see if it could stay open.

Asked if she experiences the hole as a path of openness, Christa continues :

> Yah, its a path. It's a little path. Not big. I feel that this block of mine here was in the past like energy coming up and then pushing together and making a tight knot and then exploding. I exploded into aggression, helplessness, and clinging. I could either hold my breath and become paralyzed or else go into a fury. It was the same in either case -- the same feeling of... of...

Me : Of collision ?

C : Collision, yah. Just here. (She points to her diaphragm). When I had these feelings I couldn't stay alone with myself because my feelings were always turned inwards self-destructively. I was always afraid that I could destroy myself during these moments -- only during these moments I lost all my controls.

> Now when I am sad it is different. Now it is coming from my own belly, but up until now it was like a power coming over me and possessing me, as if coming from outside. It was not, I know, but it was as if it were. But now I own it as my feeling coming from inside.

Christa's connection between her first real loving feelings towards a man and yesterday's crying from deep inside her belly indicate a higher level of congruency between her psychological and physiological levels of functioning. She has reached a new plateau of integrative functioning: from moment-to-moment her feelings towards others are beginning to match her awareness of their impact upon her organism. A more instantaneous connectedness is emerging between her ectodermal, mesodermal, and endodermal layers of receptivity to stimuli -- or, in other words, between her sensory, motoric, and deep feeling modalities of response. She implicitly senses with admirable accuracy how her former inability to experience love feelings (of inexhaustible depth and breadth) towards a man relates to her generalized inability to experience tender feelings towards herself. She also senses that both kinds of 'real' feelings emanate in some mysterious way from her tension-free abdominal cavity. I did not suggest these ideas. Rather she discovered these cause-and-effect connections within the texture of her own experience through spontaneous self-exploration.

Christa's enhanced congruency of functioning is further revealed by her explicit association of her new bodily sensation of a hole in her diaphragmatic region with her enhanced capacity for fuller feelings of positive regard for others and herself. She even senses that the former lack of this capacity has prevented her from feeling like a woman. Christa's cognitive experience of the psychodynamic causal interaction between these two distinct levels confirms unequivocally a notable loosening of her armored peripheral muscular sheath.

But Christa wins my highest esteem as she describes the difference between the movement and pattern of the fluid energy currents before and after the softening of her abdominal armoring. Her recognition that the opening of the barrier in her diaphragmatic muscle complex means that she will no longer have to fear the chronic collision of unreleased feelings that threaten to destroy her is a multidimensional insight. To be sure, the word 'collision' is mine, but I honestly believe that she was searching for this word to express the meaning she had already formulated. I never told her explicitly that her chronic emotional insecurity related to a collision of energy currents in her diaphragmatic region. She senses this herself. She understands that her hysterical attacks and craziest moments were a consequence of an inner freezing against energy moving freely in a longitudinal direction. She even senses how her previous alienation from her feeling and energetic depths caused her to project upon the outer environment the inner situation of imploded blockage.

Christa's direct reference to her energetic condition from moment-to-moment marks the beginning of her subsequent discovery of her autonomously functioning inner world. One of her primary faculties for staying in constant touch with this inner world is the blood flow. At last Christa can listen to her flow and correctly appreciate how it provides her with a capacity for having totally real feeling responses to her environment.

Christa makes further discoveries which result from the softening of her abdominal armoring :

> It's very strange when I lie in Ilsa's arms. I feel differently there too. Until now the hunger I had was always stronger than what she could gratify. She could never give me enough to satisfy me. I would stay hungry for more tenderness and affection from her. But now that has changed. Now I feel the need inside me first, and then I reach out for touch from Ilsa and I can feel the enjoyment and pleasure of being touched by her intensely. But the hunger is gone. The hunger is gone afterwards.

Christa's hunger is surely an expression of her Agape-Eros need to love and to be loved in a security-giving way. Her starvation for this kind of affection has made her need insatiable until her entire front half could shed its armoring enough to feel her heart's need for tender nurturing. Before, Christa never felt from her own depths her need for Ilsa's containing touch. Rather, she was compulsively driven to flee from her inner depths altogether in order to seek a short-lived security in the shelter of Ilsa's arms. Previously, Christa had been unable to identify her natural feeling need for being nurtured and contained through another's spiritual, emotional and organismic affirmation. She never could really believe that anyone else could really love her because she was internally cut off from both her heart feelings and her feelings of beingness in her belly.

Christa has finally unmasked her insatiable hunger for someone else to satisfy her need for an ontological sense of continuing security and well-being. Underneath lie the unmet demands of a tiny deprived infant. To the extent that she identifies with the primary need-tendencies of her chest and belly, she will be able to maintain an optimal balance between flight-propelled fusion with another and totally keeping her innermost real feelings from others. She will begin to creatively initiate a here-and-now realness with Ilsa, and thus begin to appreciate the limits that exist in any relationship in which another is expected to satisfy one's inner needs for emotional security.

Christa's awareness continues to expand during the session :

> When I am walking I also have different feelings. When I touch the ground with my feet, I feel a movement coming up from my feet through the body. There is no longer any split between my feet and my body. I also feel stronger throughout my body -- no cramping. I now can sense one single line of continuity from my feet through the back upwards... Before I walked mechanically and did not enjoy it, but yesterday I realized how comfortable it is.

These observations reveal how it is not the outer form and performance of the body's movements that matter so much as accurately sensing the inner feeling of kinaesthetic-proprioceptive unity of functioning. Christa is describing how unified her energy circuits have become, especially her voluntary and involuntary muscles operating from her toes to the top of her head. Another significant development is the striking improvement in Christa's sense of groundedness to the earth through her feet and her lower half movements since the release in her abdominal cavity.

I personally view these developments as icing on the cake, incidental to the real transformation process. I never structure exercises to alter the outer structure of the body. I wish to dissociate myself from body psychotherapists who emphasize such possibilities. I feel the same about will-induced vomiting and any kind of controlled muscularly coordinated movements. Ultimately, there are no right and wrong ways of moving if one relates to one's bodily actions primarily as a direct expression of one's primary-process feeling self. Feeling is everything when the individual soul is concerned, while actions are merely automatic extensions of one's innermost feelings and intentions at best, but more frequently than not they subserve the outer-world-conquering will centers of the closed, defended ego.

After discussing her new feelings of groundedness, Christa begins the first bodywork of the session. As she stands, I ask her to nurture the pathway of flow moving up the center of her front half between her belly and neck. She quickly begins to tremor evenly and softly. However, her mother's injunctions keep protruding into consciousness, preventing her from retaining contact with the thread of flow. I suggest that Christa stay centered in her body and find improvised movements which will allow her to feel the hole inside opening down the middle of her front half. She discovers a movement of her shoulders rotating in synchrony with a throwing backwards of the head -- her belly rumbles with drainage noises after each exhalation. Continuing freely, she vomits about four times over a period of ten minutes. Following each vomiting episode, she bends forwards from the waist with her arms and head dangling loosely. As she violently shakes her head in this position, her tremors pulsate more vibrantly, as she begins to throw her head up with each exhalation, and down with each inhalation. After she continues for several minutes without any further vomiting reflexes, I know that she has cleaned out whatever residue of tension in her front half is possible through do-it-yourself exercises. Without prompting, Christa moves into a pleasure-dominant circular movement of her pelvis, shoulders, head and neck that I call 'the going African exercise'. (see page 337) She does this until she falls with carefree laughter onto the mattress.

Christa begins to talk about her childhood enjoyment of the game of 'dying'. She now recognizes that the game genuinely released her nerves as she fell hard on the floor as if suddenly dead. I ask her to play the game. She stands on her feet and falls again and again on the mattress. After several falls, I ask her to remain collapsed while speaking to her mother. She begins to talk in the gentlest, slowest, and most relaxed manner of the entire intensive:

> You gave me the pleasure to play when I was little. You played with me a lot. But everytime I wanted to play with myself and for my own pleasure, you stopped it. You always broke it up then. You forgot that you had taught me how to enjoy playing. I learned how to phantasize with you. You were so different when you would play with me. You

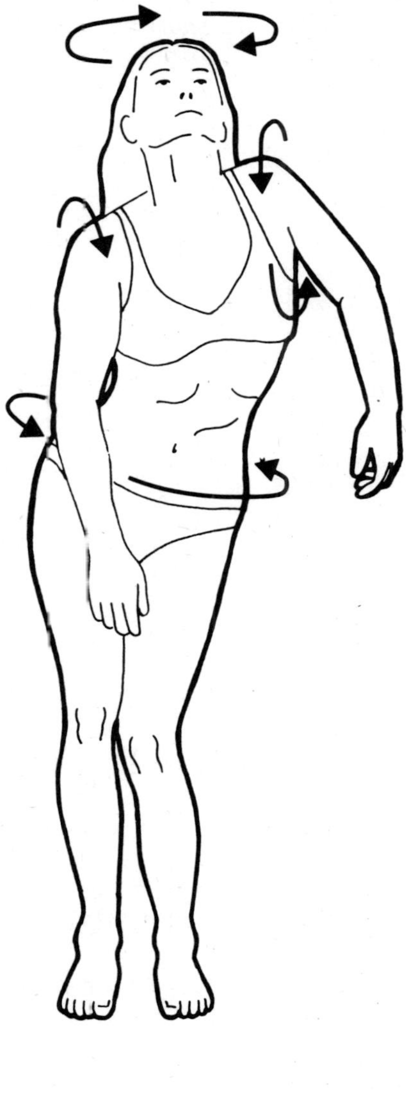

were neither tight nor stern. You forgot yourself, and I then felt so close to you. But when the playing was over, you were again this stern, tight mother that I am so afraid of...

You have broken up everything that I liked to do for myself alone. I was only permitted to do everything with you and under your control. Then I had to become as tight as you are, and I could not then really collapse -- never. Really fall down into my own body. Being tired. I had to be strong. Being helpless in front of you, I was tight -- so tight. Only when I was playing sometimes I could collapse. I needed to play in order to find any release -- to play for myself, with games, in order to be soft or weak.

I was afraid that you could see when I was sad and touched deeply with feelings. When I showed you my feelings I could be sure that other people would know about it in two or three days. You liked to exhibit my feelings to all people. I was so ashamed of this, and you didn't respect my reaction. Never.

So I could not show my feelings any more. Being simple, soft, or sweet I could never show you. I had to keep those feelings hidden away from your eyes, your hard-staring eyes, which were always controlling me. Controlling me and eating up my feelings in pieces, swallowing them up.

Owh! You are sitting on my stomach. You always have been sitting there... You have to go away from my belly. I have to take you out.

Very tenderly, Christa expresses the gratitude in her heart that her mother taught her how to use her phantasy in play. Christa could almost forgive her mother for her sternness and rigidity during their hours of games. But Christa's forgiveness quickly turns to bitterness and remorse as she realizes that her mother could be lighthearted only on the condition that Christa stay with her to feed her loneliness. Christa realizes a new dimension of her mother's needy possessiveness. Her bitterness arises as she newly realizes that she had to be out of her mother's eyesight in order to relax to the point where she could experience her own needs for feeling soft and weak. There was no possibility of satisfying her needs for sympathetic understanding and positive containment of her self-surrendering feelings in her mother's presence.

It is not accidental that Christa can face these objective realities from the distant past at this particular juncture of her treatment. She could not have done so earlier because her front half was too tightly held in stasis by a severe diaphragmatic block. A partial releasing of the block permitted her to experience directly by means of her kinaesthetic-proprioceptive sensations her inner emptiness and general absence of sympathetic feelings. She is at last able to subjectively feel how her Agape-Eros needs have remained essentially ungratified and nearly extinguished. She can face how her mother's vampire possessiveness became such a perverse model of any real expression of Agape-Eros that she had to close herself off from her mother's feeling vibrations in order to preserve her soul's integrity. What is new about this present encounter is Christa's object-centered discrimination of how her mother's alienation from any sympathetic, self-surrendering feelings contaminated Christa's development of any sympathetic feelings: "Being simple, soft, or sweet I could never show you". Her mother violated Christa's innocent unbosoming of her intimate feelings again and again before Christa vaguely sensed her mother's lack of positive regard for these disclosed intimacies. In her manic-compulsive restlessness and insatiable need to flee towards other people, her mother betrayed Christa's delicate trust and sense of privacy, or being-for-herself. Christa's severe armoring in her front half enabled her to remain wholly oblivious to the betrayal.

Christa is finally becoming able to feel the depths and breadths of her own unrealized potentialities. This would not have been possible before her entire front half began to expand internally at the endodermal layer. Her reference to the little hole that she feels in the middle of her torso is a concrete manifestation of this incipient expansion of her alimentary canal. Her reference to her mother sitting on her stomach is another manifestation of the same phenomenon. And her declaration that she must take her mother out of her belly is both symbolically and bioenergetically true. Her declaration is a manifesto of a yet-to-be completed exorcism of her mother's deadened body and soul from her own uterus.

Immediately following Christa's declaration that she must extricate her mother from her belly, Christa says with some relief: "I love my feelings, and therefore I cannot stay with you." This is Christa's first spontaneous self-affirmation of the intensive. Deeply moved, Katherine and I instinctively move to both sides of Christa, placing our four hands nurturingly on her belly. (see page 341) She drinks in our touch with unreserved pleasure. As her breathing deepens, her body begins to undulate in a slow involuntary rhythm, and gradually her two hands, which are lying extended to both sides, begin to twirl limply and mechanically, rising off the mattress from the elbows. They appear to be moving autonomously -- they are not obviously linked to the rest of her body, including her arms. As they twirl, Christa begins to whimper, progressively sounding like a little girl. When Katherine asks what her hands are saying, Christa responds with a soft but high-pitched little girl's voice: "I don't understand it. I just feel compelled to make these movements." She begins to cry deeply and haltingly from her belly, and then says: "They are turning around by themselves. They do not know why. They are sad -- like a flower that has wilted." Katherine asks Christa to let them talk, to give them a voice.

C : We are so sad and alone and sorrowful, and we don't know what to do. There is nobody. What could we give to anybody. We are so broken up. We cannot believe that we have something to give. We go unnourished like flowers.

Christa slowly becomes overwhelmed by loud, involuntary sobs, interspersed with coughing.

C : They don't know what they are doing... (Silence except for coughing)... I'm so sad, but I don't know about what.

Katherine says, "Don't close off your belly. Leave it open." This remark removes any resistance remaining in Christa's belly. She breaks into a poignantly vulnerable, slow-paced crying, which continues for a couple of minutes. And then she says:

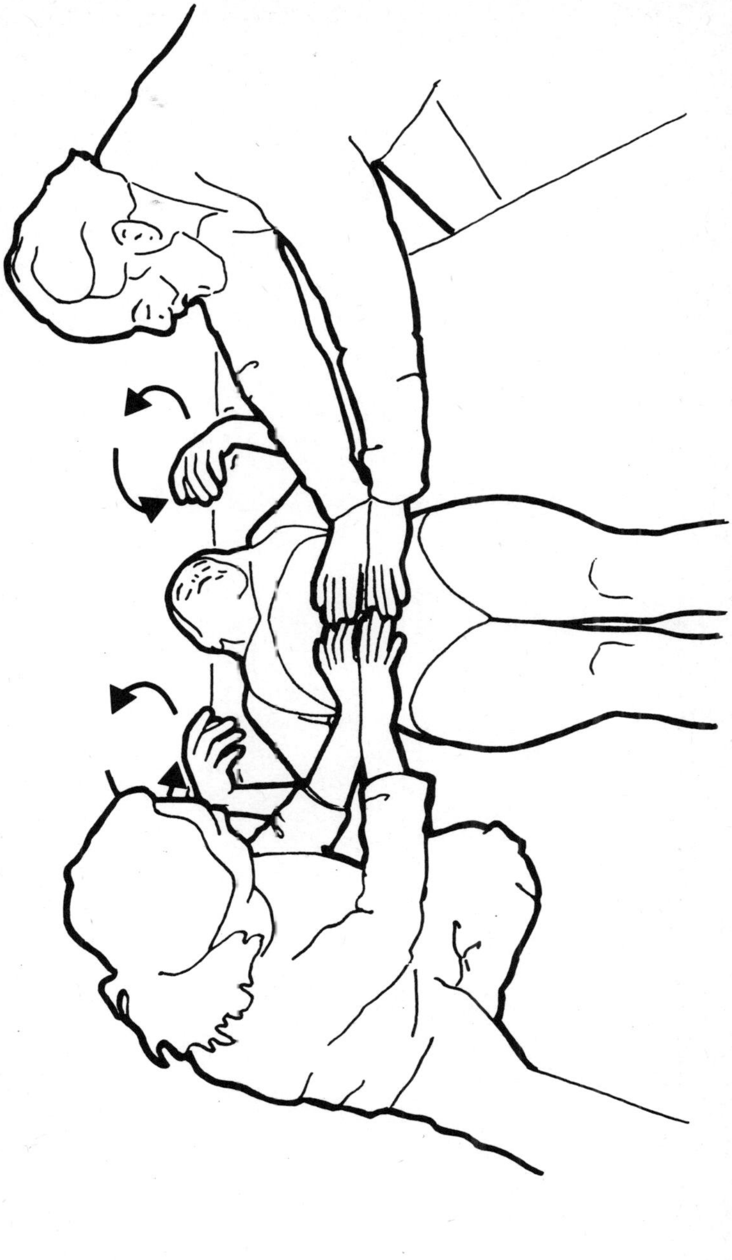

C : I am filled with so many sad feelings. I see myself and there are flowers around and I am breaking them with my hands. Just destroying them. Just poisoning my own feelings. All that was beautiful and deep I destroyed, not so much for others but for myself in my own feelings.

Me : Tell us an example.

C : Never could I read something I have written myself. I had to throw it away. It was not myself anymore. Or when good feelings were coming up, or sad feelings also. I killed them. Do you understand what I mean? So I felt broken up into two parts. In one part when I was doing something I felt good, but when it was over I felt bad.

At this point, Christa emits loud sounds of "Ow." Her belly suddenly spasms deep inside. We can feel it with our hands there. She exclaims :

C : Oh God........ I was in two parts and there was no connection between them. I was jumping from one to the other. So I never could enjoy my job. Only the time I was actually working it was all right, but afterwards the enjoyment was broken. It was like my mother would walk into my room and would see my feelings, I broke my own feelings in the same way... I do with myself what my mother did with me. I know it so well now... I cannot feel what I am doing to be a part of myself. There's the same split in here.

Christa slaps her belly several times. Removing our hands from her body, I ask Christa to talk to her mother, to tell her about the split. She begins:

C : You were a perfectionist with me, mother. You superimposed your perfectionism on me. I made myself into what you wanted me to be.

In the next second, Christa becomes possessed by a series of hollow, convulsive coughs which gradually develop into a vomiting reflex. The reflex is accompanied by full-throated sounds of her belly's reversed peristalsis. However, she does not vomit, but continues :

C : Her perfectionism is pressing me here... (She

points to her belly). I never was good enough. You never were satisfied with what I achieved. I never learned what relating to others was about from you. I learned such things later... (The hollow coughing resumes).

I would like to cough you out, together with all my own perfectionism, which is so inhuman, so inhuman. (She coughs some more). Whenever someone else is controlling my work, I function with inner stress. But when I can work freely on my own, then I am not so perfectionistic. When I am with my pupils and look upon these faces, I feel good and comfortable, but afterwards I can't believe that it is true.

Then I feel like a bad child, and I cannot accept that I can be right. With you mother I was not right -- never. You never knew what contact and relating are. There was always the stress to be more and more perfect. You never believed that I could become somebody, and I don't understand even now these two parts of you.

One part was your perfectionism. I had to be better and better, and the other part cut me down. As a little child you didn't believe me, trust me, trust my power and force. Nothing you trusted. You said: "Well we'll see. It will probably turn bad...".

And I feel sad that all the good feelings I could have had in the past I did not stay with. I became cold like my hands, which are like dead flowers. The work was like death, and afterwards was like death. Hands that cannot do anything. (She shakes her hands resignedly, starting to cry and cough.)

I could never enjoy myself. It's the same thing when my mother was keeping the split between pushing me more and more and not trusting me on the other side. I am the same towards myself. I can't bring myself together. I am so needy... I'm just a half human being, not a full human being.

I intervene at this point, asking Christa to take the position which Lowen calls the full bow: she places her hands underneath her heels, going back on the top of the head, while raising her pelvis as high into the air as possible. Her body resembles one huge bow, her head and feet representing the two ends. This exercise is especially suited to the rigid-compulsive kinds of armoring when they have reached a second stage level of dearmoring. As soon as she takes this position, Christa almost instantly begins to tremor all over her body. Her breathing increasingly deepens the longer she remains in this position. This indicates that her front half is continuing to stay expansively open all the way to her core layers. After falling on the mattress, Christa cries a little and then sighs deeply in despair :

> I'm sad because I'm feeling I lost a lot of opportunities to enjoy my life. Down there in my belly these good feelings are enclosed. It seems strange, but I think that I must allow myself to cry a lot in the future. Just cry for myself. I never could. I was afraid to be alone and to cry at the same time.
>
> I never was crying when I was sad. I was only crying when I was in a great tension. I was not crying when somebody was departing, or when it is natural to cry. I did not. All the natural feelings that human beings have I didn't allow. I just allowed my own tension. I think I have ahead of me to learn how to feel my own feelings.

The reappearance of Christa's unowned, amputated hands distinguishes this expression. The fact that they reappear after Christa has responded so yieldingly to our direct touch and allowed herself to descend totally out of her head suggests that they became severed from the rest of her body at a very early age. It remains inconclusive whether this happened before or after her birth. The precipitating event may emerge in her consciousness at some future time. However, it does seem clear that she killed her hands at a very early age in order not to have to use them to kill her mother or to keep her physically away. In Christa's first-stage primaling, she connected to the phantasy that her mother actually tried to kill her and that she would have died unless she actively fought back. It is difficult to know whether to interpret this phantasy literally or symbolically. Christa spent the first four months in an incubator because of a toxic blood substance which threatened her life. This may have been the way her mother unconsciously attempted to kill her -- by poisoning her bloodstream while Christa was still attached to the umbilical cord.

Whatever the truth, Christa's creative regression enabled her to relive the horror and pathos of having hands totally severed from her body's main river of flow. When Christa describes her hands as wilted, her metaphor suggests separation from any richly nourishing fluid blood flow. Their deadening is like freezing. Like all dearmoring, their return to life and vital wholeness presupposes a gradual thawing of their coldness and essential bloodlessness.

In contrast to Christa's earlier total alienation from the subhuman, disconnected behavior of her hands, she is now making connections in consciousness with their dissociated movements. By imaginatively projecting into their bizarre behavior and gradually imbuing them with original primary feelings, she demystifies their grotesque significance. At the same time, she begins to integrate their helpless and broken quality into a real appreciation of her deeper self. Imbuing them with total fragmentation and contactlessness, she compares them with her psyche's internal brokenness and fragmentation. They begin to symbolically objectify her own cutting off of her positive, life-affirmative feelings from finding natural gratification through interpersonal contact. In effect, she begins to link her severed hands with her similarly severed abdominal visceral circuits of self-affirmation and spontaneous enjoyment of being-for-oneself.

Christa's armored peripheral muscular sheath tried to murder her very soul in two distinct directions at once. It erected a wall against receiving the interpersonal primary feeling circuits emanating from other people's here-and-now energy vibrations. It also erected a wall against allowing the instinctual impulses coming from within to ever reach the surface of the skin and initiate interpersonal contact designed to gratify her own primary feeling needs. A total shutting down of spontaneous fluid blood flow from core to periphery and from periphery to core parallels the total shutting down of her soul's vitality and integrity of self-identity.

Katherine's request that Christa not cut off the energy currents streaming from her belly triggers Christa's warm outpouring of tears -- she cries softly out of sympathy for her fragmentation of essential being. Her crying is too unfamiliar for Christa to be able to identify her deep sadness as a passional sympathy for her soul's inner state of bleeding need. Christa has never experienced any kind of totally enveloping compassion for herself. And it probably would not have been possible for her to feel it on this occasion without Katherine and I touching her abdominal region in a blood-synergistic nurturing mode. The combination of nurturing direct touch to her belly, plus Katherine's affirmation of Christa's Hara center enabled Christa to imaginatively project into her severed hands. The direct touch polarized from within, while Katherine's words polarized from without the same constellation of dynamic forces. Now partially rid of her peripheral muscular sheath, Christa could respond more fully.

Christa is beginning to exorcise the Black Tower of her mother's negative image which was imprinted decisively upon Christa's chest and abdomen early in life. A muscular wall formed to shut down the primary feelings circulating from within and from without. The Black Tower would finally be exorcized and the chronic muscular wall finally dismantled when Christa could allow both her most extreme peripheral embodied parts, her hands, and her most extreme centrally located embodied part, her abdominal endodermal vegetative flow, to instantaneously polarize each other through the unarrested passage of the fluid blood in both directions at once.

Chapter XI

THE THIRD AND FOURTH STAGES OF CREATIVE DISINTEGRATION

I. The Dissolution of the Antilibidinal Super-Ego

We saw in chapter nine how Christa during her seventeenth session managed to encounter her mother with what seemed to be a daemonic-like abandonment of controls when she was able to behave as if she were a devilishly bad child. I subsequently hypothesized that Christa's daemonic-like manner of self-expression on this occasion represented the beginning of the conquest from below and within of her intropunitive super-ego.

I am further hypothesizing now that we have here the seed of what constitutes the essence of both the third and fourth stages of creative disintegration. Both of these stages are bound up with the final carrying through of the dissolution of the old, cerebralized false self-image and its nucleus, the antilibidinal, intropunitive super-ego.

The third stage of creative disintegration has in part to do with the awakening of at least three of the four dynamic primary feeling centers of the organism simultaneously. This simultaneous awakening permits there to be mobilized enough longitudinal endodermal vegetative flow from below and within upwards to directly threaten the still intact network of closed cortico-cerebrospinal energy currents and their psychic counterpart, the antilibidinal super-ego.

What we saw Christa doing during her seventeenth session was just the barest beginnings of this process of melting the antilibidinal super-ego within herself. She did manage to achieve at least a partial awakening of all four of her dynamic primary feeling centers for relatedness. She did manage to marshall a wholesale convergence of them on the figure of her mother and thereby establish an object-relationship which was fully liberated from perceiving her mother from the old perspective of her cerebralized false self-image - that is, from the perspective of a helpless, paralyzed, fearful, obedient child. She was able to bring together an integrated channeling of her energy in congruence with both her Dionysian divergent feeling capacities of her lower half and simultaneously with her Apollonian focusing feeling capacities of her upper half. This higher congruence permitted her to identify the destructive intropunitive super-ego in her mother and its introjection within herself:

> You could not understand that being a bad child was not only against her majesty, my mother, but that it was simply a child enjoying herself... You broke up my natural feelings. I never knew it could feel so good to be bad until today... You needed me to be your BAD child, and indeed I felt like a BAD child. I could never believe thereafter that other people could be BAD, only me. I alone was BAD... Ah, I see the devil that you have in yourself, and the devil that I have in myself, and I like it, I like it !

This brings us to a recognition of the importance of restructuring one's object-relationships from the uncompleted feeling past, and how such a restructuring forms an indispensable step towards transformation of one's self identity in the direction of core-centeredness. Christa's above remarks addressed to her tyrannical mother demonstrate how Christa as a child split the image of her mother into a good and a bad object. On the one side, she was totally good, totally accepted and idealized and introjected as a positive super-ego by Christa, and on the other side she was unconsciously rejected totally as some kind of terrible, libidinally seductive and perverse bad object. The differentiation in consciousness of the tormentors of one's childhood into good and bad objects forms an indispensable step along the path towards the dissolution of the antilibidinal super-ego, and seems particularly important during the third stage of creative disintegration.

The splitting of the object into a good and a bad aspect has been justly emphasized by the British neo-Freudian school of thinking of Fairbairn, Winnicott, and Guntrip. The reclaiming of this wholly unconscious and repressed splitting of the parental tormentors cannot occur until all four of the dynamic primary feeling capacities for relatedness have been at least partially awakened at the same time. We can appreciate this in how Christa resonates to her mother's bullying control from her head with disgust and contempt felt up and down the front half of her organism. Christa can feel how she has been poisoned in her front half by her mother's bullying morality. She can allow herself to playfully delight in exhibitionistically rebelling against the negative inhibitory parental will. An attitude of flambuoyant defiance and an acting out of becoming the BAD child she was never permitted to be in actuality is essentially an expression of her infantile omnipotence center, which is her primitive Phallos feeling need for relatedness towards mother manifesting itself.

Still another dimension to Christa's encounter that stamps it as intrinsic to the dearmoring process is the way it begins to shift its axis of valuing downwards out of the head, thereby isolating the antilibidinal super-ego still further, both within the tormentor and within oneself. A certain depth of wisdom appears in Christa's perceptual-conceptual restructuring of her mother as a synthesized object-relationship :

> You let out all of your aggressions against me by calling me a devil. You played the good, good couple. It is so ironic. You were so wrong. I am BAD, and all persons are BAD. But it is you who were suffocatingly BAD towards me. You stepped on my soul with your morality of being BAD. I could say nothing back to you.

Here we see the synthesizing and distancing functions of Logos beginning to be awakened inside Christa's embodied soul. Logos is usually the third of the four dynamic feeling capacities for relatedness to crystallize during the dearmoring process, with Hara following in its wake during the third stage of treatment. Logos must be distinguished from the games-playing analytical defensivness of the closed cortico-cerebrospinal circuits. During the middle and advance phases of second stage dearmoring its appearance as a mediator of subject-world feeling relatedness rests upon its flowering from within and below upwards. Logos becomes an extension at the level of cognitive consciousness of an internalized integration and unity of functioning of three of the dynamic feeling capacities for relatedness. Its crystallization, in effect, parallels the breaking down of any further dominance of the closed cortico-cerebrospinal circuits.

But it would be giving a distorted impression to

lead one to think that the third stage of creative disintegration amounts to a changing sequence of restructured and newly synthesized object-relationships primarily. It is a time of further upheaval, conflict, and chaos more than it is a time of cognitive restructuring of self and other. The fact is that the further there develops a descending of the boundaries of self-identity downwards out of the head into the organism-as-a-whole, the more sharply there becomes polarized a no-man's-land region of antagonistic and warring psychodynamic forces in the area of the upper back, chest, and neck. It is then that there begins to emerge the peculiarly irrational yet profoundly transpersonal voices of the primitive brain stem under attack from above and below: namely, the negative archetypes of the collective unconscious.

We are indebted to Carl Jung and his discovery of the universal existence of what he calls the collective unconscious for adding to our understanding of what I call the third and fourth stages of creative disintegration. Jung believed that the universal symbolic images that came from the deepest levels of our unconsciousness had the quality of 'archetypes'. For him archetypes consist of inherited thought-patterns of the mind that have a self-sufficient, pre-existent form at birth. They are fundamental categories of the imagination that are impersonal, collective and identical in all human beings. They are also the direct representation in consciousness of the animal instincts that we were born with. In his words, they are: "the instinct's perception of itself".

It is my own personal belief that Jung was forever switching his position about what archetypes are throughout his writings between conceiving them to be exclusively an expression of our animal instincts, on the one hand, and elsewhere as these primordial but essentially invariable and abstractly pre-existent forms of the mind. And in my opinion he unfortunately tended to conceive of them most of the time in the latter manner. I shall argue for the case that archetypes have a valid role to contribute to the healing and growth process to the extent that they are experienced as spokesmen of our animal instincts seeking to find satisfaction in the context of interpersonal relationships.

I am saying that I do not share Jung's belief that the collective archetypes are the ultimate mental categories or primordially pre-existent ideas of the mind-brain. This makes them too closely akin to Plato's rendering of those spiritual forms of the mind that remain laws unto themselves, things-in-themselves that have a mysterious sovereignty that permits them to exist in eternity independently of all human relations and natural influences. When Jung conceives of the collective archetypes to be the essence and substance of the collective unconscious, and sees the instincts to be mere compulsive drives towards concrete action, he has split the human psyche from the human soul in a very final way in my opinion.

I believe to the contrary that collective archetypes, in order to be authentic agents of healing and growth, are always direct expressions and refinements upon the animal instinctual impulses of our human organism. I say that it is our natural primary feeling capacities for relatedness that determine and regulate the emergence and assimilation in consciousness of archetypal forms, and not vice-versa. I say that archetypes serve always as facilitating agents of transformation of our raw instinctual potentialities for feeling relatedness into highly differentiated and individuated intuitive faculties of the core self. Archetypes are in no sense pre-existent forms of the mind that exist in some impersonal and abstract sphere of transcendental existence. They are always a reflection of how the primitive brain stem, as distinct from the cerebral cortex, registers changes and developments occurring among the instincts themselves.

Negative archetypes, as distinct from positive ones, are always a reflection of how the primitive brain stem registers the battle for supremacy between the antilibidinal super-ego and the primary-instinctual feeling capacities for relatedness. Their emergence in consciousness, in an armored or inwardly divided neurotic, usually precedes the emergence of positive archetypes. Generally speaking, the latter can only come into full flowering during the third stage of treatment when the dearmoring process has largely unfolded and expended itself.

The emergence of negative archetypes during the healing-growth-and - transformation process is the product of already achieved loosening and weakening of the character-muscular armoring. Negative or positive archetypes can break through into consciousness only when there has already been established a certain amount of fluid vegetative endodermal circulation between the abdominal cavity and the cerebral cortex. Although I cannot give scientific proof of this assertion, I can attest to its empirical accuracy in the light of all my clinical experience. The latter has consistently revealed how it is the fluid movement of longitudinal vegetative flow through and beyond the primitive brain stem itself from below upwards and from above downwards that parallels the appearance of negative archetypal imagery if armoring is still present. In fact, it is my belief that the actual triggering of negative archetypal forms in consciousness is caused by the fresh release from stasis and repression of an enhanced amount of fluid vegetative longitudinal energy flow. It is the threat to the closed cortico-cerebrospinal circuits generated by this fresh release that produces the negative archetypes.

Negative archetypes, which include every category of daemonic figures imaginable that suggest the ugly, the perverse, the forbidden, and the wicked, usually contain much fear of invasion, overflooding, and engulfment from below by animal instinctual impulses impinging upon the organized ego-system. The negative archetypal figure is, in effect, as much a defensive reaction as it is a spokesman for the instincts themselves. Its aim is to frighten the organized ego-system to cling to the status quo.

This is why all negative archetypal figures have a distinctly grotesque luminous-numinous daemonic quality to them. This unpleasant and often terrorful quality is an expression of an underlying situation of implosion and severe conflict within the very foundations of the psyche and soul. The quality of grotesqueness reflects an essentially imploded charge-discharge collisioning of opposed psychodynamic and bioenergetic forces that are playing havoc with the primitive brain stem itself. From a psychodynamic perspective, the grotesque daemons of the underworld have a secret and well-disguised mission, namely, to frighten into submission the organized ego-system with the view to reinforce the life-negative, anti-libidinal super-ego behind the ego.

This means that negative archetypal images represent a kind of ingenious synthesis on the part of the primitive brain stem and its brain-child, the primitive unconscious. I am inclined to give up altogether endorsing Jung's distinction between the personal unconscicus and the collective unconscious, and instead relegate both to the primitive unconscious, the brain-child of the primitive brain stem. Hereafter I shall refer only to the primitive unconscious, partly for reasons of logic but mostly in order to do justice to those aspects of the unconscious psyche that Jung first discovered and which I think fully merit the respect and reverence that he endowed them with.

To turn to the opening statement of the preceding paragraph, I think negative archetypal figures embody an ingenious synthesis on the part of the primitive unconscious to the extent that it distils and interpenetrates into a single image or essence ultimately opposite forces in the psyche and soul: instinctual impulses and rational resistances and inhibitions against those same impulses. They represent a complex blending of intrinsically disjunctive and intensely polarized forces that are in the midst of a struggle for survival. Hence their transient and temporary status as long as the dearmoring process continues until an enduring equilibrium that is relatively conflict-free is reached.

Let us take as an example of third stage creative disintegration what happened to Leslie. We cannot unfortunately continue with the eloquent example of Christa because she terminated her intensive just before negative archetypal figures could assume a dominance in her psyche and soul.

II. Leslie's Discovery of his Shadow Archetype

Leslie is a 45-year-old American clinical psychologist who came to us in Italy for a three-week treatment/training intensive during 1977. An abundantly experienced and fully committed professional psychotherapist, Leslie had from the beginning of his intensive the capacity to articulate his feelings and psychic reactions with greater differentiation than the average American male. It has been my opinion for a long time that the average American male is particularly alienated from any differentiated contact with his personal feelings and values, so Leslie made a welcome relief from this situation.

One of the psychological problems that still haunted Leslie a great deal and for which he had not yet found a solution and clearly wanted to work on during his intensive was a growing 'nastiness' in himself towards other people. He thought that his ongoing treatment in body psychotherapy with a colleague of ours who practiced in his city in the States and whom he had been seeing for two years had eroded his egoic controls. He found himself progressively falling prey to unexpected eruptions of inexplicable anger that were way out of line with the objective reality, and contradicted flatly his self-image of being a soft, friendly, patient and forbearing fellow with others.

He confessed to considerable confusion about this new 'nastiness' in himself. Yet when I confronted him as intellectually as I could manage with the idea that it might indicate a surface manifestation for an underlying Dr. Jekyll and Mr. Hyde syndrome, he immediately rejected the possibility with surprising assurity. Then in the next moment he diffidently offered the observation: "Except there are some people whom I've gotten angry with who do think I am a Dr. Jekyll and Mr. Hyde and even have told me so -- I didn't think I ever got that angry or mad. But that is often the case that I don't think I am ever angry or hostile".

Such an on-the-rebound set of remarks increased rather than diminished my suspicions that Leslie might indeed possess a Dr. Jekyll and Mr. Hyde syndrome. It was not until the third three-hour session with us three days later that psychic material became available to confirm my suspicion. The material unfolded while Katherine and I were administering a massive block pressure with the weight of our bodies and hands and arms to his upper back as he lay on his belly. (see page 355). We had been administering this massive block pressure to his entire upper back half for over ten minutes before he poured forth the following torrent of invectives :

> They were oppressive. They didn't believe anything from inside of me, so I kept myself tight. I kept it in. I kept a tight back. They were murderers.

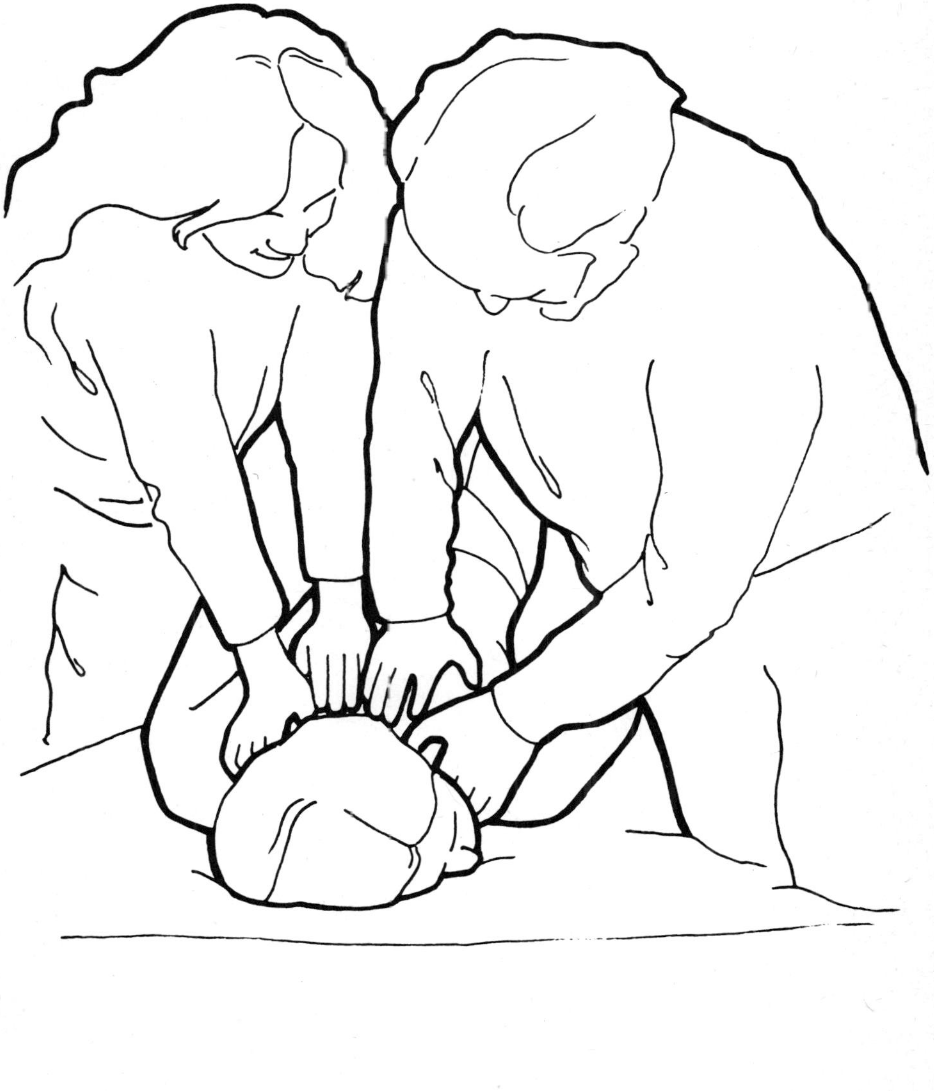

> They were horrible. OWOWOWOWWWOWWWO! OWWOWWOWOWWO! They can go to hell. They were impossible to stand. OWWOWWOWOWO! OWOWWOWWO! They were crazy bastards! OWOWWOWOWWWWOOOOO!

'They' refers to his parents and two brothers, or nuclear family unit. These invectives poured forth without explicit structuring or suggestion from us. They were purely spontaneous, rising from the pent-up tensions of an armored back. The OWOWOWOO sounds were expressions of pure but not very severe physical pain. The pressure we were applying was generating the pain. It had an alive, vital tone, indicating the deep release of affect behind the sounds and words. The release was also bioenergetic, facilitating a minimal expansiveness of the mesodermal wall in the back that amounted to a kind of decompression from within. It was this same decompression that opened his consciousness to negative feelings from the unfinished past.

Due to deliberate probing on my part following this spontaneous outpouring of feelings it became apparent how alive and compacted within the mesodermal wall of his back resided an enormous pool of negative feelings towards all the members of his primary family. We were a little astonished to discover how blackly embittered an attitude he possessed towards his parents and brothers to the present day. He described both of his brothers as having a "superior man complex". He attributed to his older brother a very neurotic character structure and to his other brother, who happened to be his twin brother, a nature which was "very cold, manipulative, and stuffy".

Further probing revealed that this bitter attitude towards both his brothers had much to do with their active distancing of themselves and emotional rejection of him over the past fifteen year period. Ever since Leslie's late twenties when he would travel some 200 miles in order to visit his parents for the week-end, and then make them feel miserable and guilty by angrily accusing them of having ruined his life, his two brothers had actively distanced themselves from maintaining any kind of close positive feeling contact with Leslie.

It then came almost as a shock to both Katherine and myself to witness Leslie draw a complete blankness of awareness when I asked him to remember what happened during those week-end visits at the home of his parents. After fumbling around for words to explain away and justify his inability to remember what happened, he then declared that it was a big puzzle to him why his parents had feared him so much during these week-end visits that they often threatened to have him placed in a mental hosital. And on other occasions they even threatened to call the police and have them take him away!!!!

The remainder of the third session after this exchange with Leslie consisted of a chase between him and me with me doing the pursuing and he the running away from my inquiries as deftly as he could. It became clearer and clearer to me from what he did not say but made at best offhand and oblique references to was that long ago he had hardened himself against feeling the pain of his estrangement from his primary family, and particularly from his twin brother. His ambivalent feeling attitude towards his twin brother was powerfully loaded and unresolved.

For example, at one point I asked him to yell aggressively out loud at his twin brother as he lay on his back on the mattress with his eyes closed a statement that he had spontaneously made a minute earlier: "I won't see you anymore". He repeated the statement in a diffident, monotone voice with not a trace of emotion. But then he begins to recall out loud the sorts of things that would take place between them whenever they met on rare occasions over the past fifteen year period. His voice becomes pungently sarcastic, conveying a heavily exaggerated loathing for these meetings between them. His hatred for them he does not realize he is expressing. Nor does he realize how painful they were for him to endure. But the more he talks about them at my encouragement, the more self-evident it becomes that it has been Leslie who has actively tried to cultivate a positive relationship with his brother. He blurts out in the midst of describing these meetings: "You hurt me terribly. Oh, my God, how you hurt me! I don't want to talk to you".

At a later point in the session during a time when we are applying more massive block pressure to his upper back, he says in a resigned manner to his twin brother: "I really don't have much to say to you. I don't want to hurt you anymore". But about three minutes later, during which time we have continued to apply the same block pressure to his upper back, there suddenly comes exploding out of his mouth with a voice venomously acidic in its rage and snarling harshness: "I want to get the hurt out of me, and I don't give a damn about you".

The latter outburst obviously comes from a deeper and more repressed layer of feelings embedded in his upper back region. The rapidity and the extremity of his oscillation between an attitude of resignation and one of rageful hostility tells us how severe is his underlying ambivalence towards his brother. Such severe ambivalence actively maintained in a 45-year-old man who also is a professional psychotherapist told me how distorted was Leslie's perception of his twin brother as a separate person. Leslie had split his brother into a good and a bad object without knowing it consciously. Having arrived at this conclusion about half an hour before the session was over, I decided to risk making a headlong attack on Leslie's perceptual framework. It was a gamble worth taking, I told myself, if the attack was launched early enough in the intensive to yield fruitful results before the end of the second week.

Openly to Leslie's face I questioned that his brother was the horrible, pompous, rigid, and impervious person that Leslie had portrayed him to be. Then I ventured the possibility that Leslie's behavior towards his parents during those week-end visits was the basic reason why his brother had pulled away from any continuing closeness to Leslie. I even went so far as to offer the interpretation that Leslie had depreciated his brother as some sort of inferior fellow unworthy of Leslie's attention or care as an unconscious device for killing his own inner heart feelings towards him. I ended by declaring that I suspected that Leslie in fact feels very inferior to his twin brother on account of the latter's far greater economic and social successes, but cannot stand the pain of facing this, and therefore has had to resort to psychological self-deception games to mitigate the pain.

Leslie's response to my Logos-inspired headon attacking of him was dead silence. The silence was so heavy that whenever Leslie looked me directly in the eyes, I could feel his truculent holding back of himself, as if he were determined to show nothing that would agree with anything that I had said, nor deny it. It was like he shut himself down from any further contact with me, positive or negative, and retreated behind a wall of inaccessible neutrality.

The session ended with me giving him the homework assignment of writing a letter to his twin brother in which he describes how he, Leslie, has been basically responsible for the emotional estrangement between them. Leslie showed a reluctant willingness to do the assignment, and kept a cool, diffident deadpan face as we said good-bye.

The homework assignment proved to be more fruitful than I had imagined it would be. He went back to his apartment immediately following the third session and wrote the letter to his brother. Then he placed himself on his back on his bed in the spreadeagle position with his arms extended over his head and his head extended over the end of the mattress hanging downwards. This particular position of energy release I had instructed him to do the previous day. He was supposed to move his head and pelvis spontaneously after tensions had accumulated from maintaining the position, but on this occasion instead of moving his body he found himself enacting a psychodrama in his imagination that related to his twin brother. He remembered how he used to enact the game of master and slave with his twin brother when they were between the ages of eleven and fourteen. Leslie usually took the role of the slave and his brother the role of the master, and an important feature of the ritual shared between them as boys was Leslie kneeling before his brother and masturbating his brother's penis in his hands while saying out loud: "I give in, master. I give in". Instead of repeating these same words Leslie substituted them with: "I give in, Martin, I want a relationship with you". He addressed these words out loud to the imagined presence of his twin brother as he lay in the spreadeagle position. Apparently the uttering out loud of these particular words proved to be deeply moving for Leslie, so much so that tears and sobbing for his brother's loving feelings from which he had become estranged filled his consciousness and simultaneously discharged his damned up feeling impasse.

As soon as Leslie had finished disclosing this incident to us at the beginning of his fourth session, he launched with what seemed to be a freshly uncovered enthusiasm into a rapid pouring forth of verbalized insights regarding his past relationship to his twin brother. He recognized for the first time in his life that he had always adopted a severely competitive and at the same time possessive attitude towards his twin brother. His competitiveness and possessiveness, furthermore, he had felt obliged to keep hidden from everyone in his primary family, including his mother. He recalled how he used to feel strangely euphoric and even joyously relieved whenever his twin brother showed evidence of any kind of weakness or failure to achieve some deed of conquest. This made him feel closer to his twin brother secretively. Similarly he recalled how inordinately miserable he felt everytime his twin brother succeeded at accomplishing some deed that went beyond Leslie's capacity to compete for or outrival.

As a ten-year-old boy he began to have a strong sense of loss and estrangement from his twin brother whenever the latter achieved something that Leslie could not compete for because he felt generally less well-endowed than his brother. A sense of foreboding of increasing separation between himself and his twin brother was the worst fear he had as a youth. The further his brother continued to surpass Leslie's capacity to actively compete with him, including scholastic activities as well as athletic ones, the greater became Leslie's secretive inner despair and sense of abandonment. The greater grew his despair, the more Leslie withdrew inside himself, tightened up his will-to-struggle-and-suffer-in-secret, and outwardly hardened himself in order to assume the false facade of a tough indifference towards his brother's triumphs.

I was glowing with a quiet kind of empathic positive regard towards Leslie and the breakthrough of important insights that he was sharing with us. I could feel his deep excitement at making the discoveries he was verbalizing. I was also feeling very vindicated and even self-satisfied for having taken such an aggressive stand with him during the preceding session. But the best is yet to come. After exploring his hitherto suppressed secret relationship of identification with his twin brother as a youth, he reported having had a dream the same night. Leslie prefaced telling us the dream by revealing that he seldom had night dreams, and even more seldom was able to remember them after waking up. He described the dream thusly :

> I had this strange dream in the morning after going back to sleep. There was this scene with a bench outside, like some of the benches in the Italian villages here. Suddenly in front of me there appeared this little fat man. Much shorter and fatter than you, Malcolm - less than five feet tall. He had a big black bristly beard. The hair on his beard looked almost like the hair of animal whiskers - very coarse and hard.
>
> He sat down on this bench, and I walked up and I sat in his lap. He was very ugly and scary to look at. I don't think I could have kissed him, but somehow my face got very close to his face. This made me very, very scared, and the anxiety or terror of it woke me up. I could not tell after I woke up what happened between this little man and myself. And I could not tell what this little man was.

It will take a presentation of what followed in subsequent sessions to prove it, but it is fairly self-evident that Leslie's fat little man is definitely a negative archetypal figure. Its highly luminous-numinous daemonic power is evidenced by its potency to penetrate Leslie's considerable resistances against having dreams or remembering them. The fact also that the figure of the little man was able to generate tremendous fear in Leslie, enough to drive him to take flight from the figure by waking himself up, is further testimony to its intensity of impact upon Leslie's psyche.

I think we can safely hypothesize that what happened during Leslie's third session with us had sufficient catastrophic effect to jolt, loosen, and certainly threaten his firmly implanted antilibidinal super-ego. The dream is sufficiently charged with both instinctual impulses and temporarily lifted repressions of those impulses to warrant hypothesizing that Leslie's cerebralized false self-image was being menaced by the third session and the events that followed immediately thereafter pertaining to his relationship with his twin brother. It is hard to pinpoint what it was that jolted and threatened his ego defense network. Was it the aggressive manner in which I directly attacked his whole object-relationship to his twin brother? Was it the aggressive catalytic bodywork that Katherine and I did together with his upper back? Was it Leslie's own creative unconscious at work in the afternoon following his third session when he reexperienced the sadomasochistic, sexually perverse game of master and slave that he used to play with his twin brother in their latency period of childhood? I don't think we have to pinpoint the cause and effect relationship of events with any accuracy. All perhaps contributed something.

What is more important is how we conceptualize these developments. I hypothesize that Leslie's fat little man had the grotesqueness comparable to that of a subterranean earth-polarized daemon, much like the figure of an antihuman, antilibidinal troll. I hypothesize that this fat little man is an exquisitely disguised personification, a kind of shadow disguise for Leslie's antilibidinal super-ego.

This interpretation somewhat conflicts with Jung's interpretation of what he regarded to be a shadow archetype. For Jung this archetype is usually among the first archetypes to emerge in consciousness at the start of the higher individuation process because it is conceived by Jung to reflect the least developed, most undifferentiated, and most repressed parts of the personal unconscious, as opposed to the collective unconscious. I find this interpretation too intellectually abstract and one that misses the essential point, which has to do with the breaking down and disintegration of the cerebralized false self-image. Jung is correct when he sees the shadow archetype as an expression of the most inferior and least developed dimensions of our dynamic primary feeling capacities. But it also denotes something more concrete in terms of the dearmoring-creative disintegration process of change and growth. This something more concrete has to do with the release of longitudinal vegetative currents of fluid energy flow in the region below the primitive brain stem and a corresponding marshalling of counter forces against this flow from above the primitive brain stem. But this is only the general bioenergetic precondition necessary for the emergence of the shadow archetype.

There is also the uniquely individualistic precondition, which varies with each human being during the course of his or her higher individuation process. In Leslie's case the fat little man is a personification of at least two severely repressed parts of his embodied soul: his Eros feeling capacity and his primitive Phallic feeling capacity. The repression of both these primary feeling capacities was finalized inside Leslie between the ages of ten to seventeen as he assumed a cerebralized false facade of willed indifference towards his twin brother's growing up and beyond a primary symbiotic relationship with Leslie. The emergence of the fat little man represents a kind of resurrection in consciousness from the uncompleted past in a highly disguised form of both the instinctual feeling needs themselves and the egoic defendedness against them when Leslie was a young teenager. In summary, the emergence of the shadow archetype signifies a multi-dimensional, essentially complex series of events occurring at a largely unconscious level.

Jung expresses the matter thusly :

> The meeting with oneself is, at first, the meeting with one's own shadow. The shadow is a tight passage, a narrow door, whose painful constriction no one is spared who goes down to the deep well.
>
> But one must learn to know oneself in order to know who one is. For what comes after the door is, surprisingly enough, a boundless expanse full of unprecedented uncertainty, with apparently no inside and no outside, no above and no below, no here and no there, no mine and no thine, no good and no bad.
>
> It is the world of water, where all life floats in suspension; where the realm of the sympathetic system, the soul of everything living, begins; where I am indivisibly this and that, where I experience the other in myself and the other-than-myself experiences me. (*)

Precisely correct, both psychodynamically and bioenergetically, although Jung himself did not fully

(*) The Archetypes and the Collective Unconscious. Bollingen Series, pp. 21-22.

appreciate the implications of his own words. Jung did not appreciate, for instance, that the narrow door, the tight passage has a direct unconscious reference to the chronic collision and build-up of an impasse of antagonistic energy circuits in the region of the neck and the primitive brain stem. He did not realize explicitly in his own differentiated consciousness the wisdom that the emergence of the shadow archetype presupposes a breakthrough of vital vegetative energy currents in the endodermal layer in the region of the neck from below upwards. He did not realize how with this bioenergetic breakthrough there is also ushered in a revolution within the psyche itself amounting to a resurrection in consciousness of feelings and events that have been encapsulated and isolated off in a state of chronic repression since childhood and adolescence. Nor did he realize explicitly how the passage through the narrow door of painful constriction is a fully embodied one which involves a fullscale descent downwards out of the mind-brain into the oceanic and subterranean realms of the dynamic Being centers in the front half of the body. What he depicts as the boundless expanse of wateriness he is correct to perceive in terms of the dominance of the autonomic nervous system and its flourishing in the endodermal depths, but he could never admit to it explicitly enough in terms of embodied organismic processes to be able to truly affirm an equating of both the repressed and collective unconscious networks with either the primitive unconscious of the primitive brainstem or the primary dynamic Being centers of the body. In the last analysis, Jung stays locked in the realm of the transcendental psyche.

Jung fails to appreciate that the shadow archetype represents a kind of shadow disguise for emotionally damned up positive libidinal forces struggling for active expression and completion in the present. Leslie's fat little man, like nearly all negatively loaded archetypal images, points to what has been twisted and repressed and locked up inside the psyche from the emotionally uncompleted past and wants to find release in the present. Its abnormally exaggerated psychic power, as reflected in its luminous-numinous visual grotesqueness, is the consequence of a high amount of energy implosion and psychological conflict intertwined as one. And hence the general tendency of shadow archetypes to pursue, torment, and haunt the psyche of the armored person in the midst of creative dearmoring and regressive disintegration.

We see the latter phenomenon operating with Leslie during subsequent sessions. Throughout the fourth session of his intensive he consistently non-confronted, or refused to confront, anyone of his three statements made at the beginning of the session; namely: "This made me very, very scared, and the anxiety or terror of it woke me up. I could not tell after I woke up what happened between this little man and myself. And I could not tell what this little man was". In spite of my deliberate efforts to force him to face these statements and explore their hidden and not so hidden implications, he refused to explore the significance of the dream in any manner or at any level.

However, it was another story during his fifth session, which occurred three days after his fourth session because the week-end intervened. I quote verbatim his account of the inner psychological highlights of his week-end, which he spent for most part in a hotel in a nearby Swiss city.

> I got to begin to feel I was this man in the dream with a long, bristly, steel-wool sort of beard. And a terrible big mouth and belly. A big ugly nose. The skin of his face was abcessed and had a nasty reddish color.
>
> He was following me all week-end in my waking phantasy. I said to him: 'Go away. Go away. You're so ugly that nobody wants you. No use you following me. I don't know what to do with you except to lock you up'.
>
> I had phantasies of locking him up, tieing a ball and chain around his neck, and putting him down inside some dungeon-like, rock-enclosed jail. I finally did this in my phantasies, but then I found that I could not fall asleep for many hours afterwards.

This quoted passage sums up in a kind of exquisitely succinct manner what Leslie has done to himself unconsciously his whole life. With his defended ego and its unconscious accomplice, his masochistic character-muscular armoring, he has successfully managed to conquer his primary natural feeling needs for relatedness in just the same way he fought with the haunting figure of the fat little man throughout the week-end. The "dungeon-like, rock-enclosed jail" is synonymous with his masochistic muscular armoring, particularly that part of it which encompasses the lower half of his body from his diaphragm down. He had learned how to tie a ball and chain around his own neck and put his embodied primary dynamic feelings of Eros and primitive Phallos that he once extended exclusively to his twin brother down inside a rock-bound, dungeon-like jail within his own psyche and body. The ball and chain that he projects on to the fat little man is his own trapezius muscle complex encased in a transverse band of chronically hypertense armor. The dungeon-like jail is his own iliopsoas muscle complex conjoined with the anal-sphinter muscle complex that forms a solid ring of armoring around his body front and back at the level of his anus and lower abdomen.

The daemonic figure of the fat little man also is a personification of opposite but dialectically interrelated feeling needs and libidinal impulses: those of Eros and those of primitive Phallos. Since his adolescence Leslie has learned how to conquer his needs for libidinal fusion, both spiritual and sensually perverse, when he hardened his will against his twin brother. This would explain the rather strange behaviour exhibited in the dream when Leslie walked up to this fat little man sitting on the bench, sat in his lap and put his face so close to the face of the little man that he may have kissed him. Leslie has managed to kill most of his spontaneous hetero-sexual and homosexual impulses since adolescence as part of the price of maintaining his egoic integ-rity and pride. Similarly, he has managed to conquer, repress, and kill most of his primitive Phallic ag-gressive impulses since adolescence until in the past few years a streak of irrational nastiness began to show itself in his makeup.

It was against his twin brother - rather with him more that against him - that he had been able to exercise unrestrainedly a kind of primitive Phallic aggressiveness within a fraternal competitive ambience that also was repressed and forced into the dungeon-like, rock-bound fastnesses of his upper and lower muscles and upper legs. To be sure this same repressed

Phallic aggressiveness resurfaced in his late twenties when he used to harass and torture his parents passive-aggressively during week-ends, but this was a more perverted secondary expression of what originally was a more innocent and libidinally positive kind of competitive aggressiveness that he exercised as a youth in his relationship with his twin brother. Once he made the secret vow to withdraw from any further active engagement on a feeling level with his twin brother, his natural development of a natural primary Phallic aggressiveness was aborted.

This same secret vow to withdraw inside himself, to willfully withhold in and back down inside himself, his most uninhibited instinctual impulses of loving attachment and negative rage and disenchantment in relation to his twin brother became the essential cause for his development of a masochistic character-muscular armoring. At the nucleus of the masochistic character structure is a highly compressed and over-charged ambivalence of feelings between libidinal Eros and Phallic anger towards the one person from one's early childhood who became the most important object-relationship at a feeling level. With Leslie it was not his mother who was this important object-relationship, but his twin brother.

Another feature of this highly overcharged ambivalent object-relationship in the masochistic structure is often an egoic competitive dimension. It is this competitive dimension that generates, when the Eros aspects of the relationship begin to deteriorate, a neurotically compelled drive to always keep a superior position of control over the other by distancing oneself and withholding oneself from them. The masochist seldom wants to engage himself closely with another, either to manipulate or dominate, so much as maintain thickly protected walls of distance between himself and intimate others. He prefers to withdraw inside himself introvertively if he possibly can rather than engage the other actively in order to manipulate. He hates to manipulate others as much as be manipulated by them.

Leslie's fat little man is a disguised representation of his masochistic passive-aggressiveness as much as it is a representation of all the other psychic and bioenergetic elements mentioned thus far. It is a representation of Leslie's twisted and secondarily elaborated rage, frustration and hostility carried over from childhood. Leslie himself realizes this when he said nearly at the end of his fifth session :

> The ugly old man of my dream is the nasty part of me who wants to keep me from getting very close to people. He gets very scared then. He's nasty to people. He makes me try to turn people away. I don't think he's the devil because he's too scared.

And towards the end of his sixth session, Leslie states :

> That old man has a lot of self-contempt. He despises my heart feelings. He gives me a lot of shit when I even feel jealous, angry, or hurt.
>
> I developed a false sense of superiority. It's very clear to me that this old man represents a compensation for inferiority.

In summary, the ugly old man emerges as a daemonically self-destructive figure which functions simultaneously at least in three distinct forms, all of which are unconscious within Leslie. At the feeling level of interpersonal relatedness he kills any libidinal inclinations towards opening himself trustingly to others from his heart center. In the psychodynamic sphere he communicates to egoic consciousness in the head anti-life directives and injunctions designed to maintain a false self-image of self-sufficiency and a will-to-suffer-and-survive-as-secretively-as-possible. These are two of the most characteristic traits of the masochistic character structure and here they function as Leslie's anti-libidinal super-ego. In the bioenergetic sphere he feeds upon and clings to a massive rigidity and armoring in the mesodermal voluntary musculature across the back at several points. The latter is usually so severe that the transverse rings of armoring serve as a clamp at both ends of the torso against allowing any feeling resonance between the front half dynamic Being centers and the outer world. It is this clamping from behind at both ends of the torso that sustains a condition of total withholding of positive tender feelings, both towards others and towards oneself, that is peculiar to the passive-aggressiveness of the masochistic structure. Loosen either one of these transverse clamps too quickly and there will invariably ensue an unexpected outbreak of archaic and hitherto repressed Phallic rage and hostility, which brings us to Leslie's seventh session.

Throughout the fifth and sixth sessions, we had continued to give massive quantities of diffused pressure to Leslie's lower back through various catalytic methods, including the use of the Lowen stool. The latter method is particularly penetrating to the thickly armored mesodermal wall of the back, and Leslie was showing during these two sessions at an organismic level an enhanced capacity for surrendering his body when laying on his upper middle back on the stool. His head could fall further and further backwards, and his pelvis fall further and further forwards and downwards simultaneously.

Perhaps he overpushed his body unknowingly with his powerful will, and stretched his musculature, both voluntary and involuntary, beyond a comfortable threshold of toleration. I say this because he arrived for his seventh session looking worn out and in a truculent, ashen-gray disposition akin to a depressive stupor. He laid out on the mattress and began whining about how horrible he felt and what a miserable day he had had yesterday. He complained about how cold he had felt all day, and wanted a little emotional food and warmth from us. And he felt too exhausted and generally out of sorts to want to do any hard, active body work. He wanted to be taken care of gently and softly like a baby by us, and be permitted to remain absolutely immobile and passive. We accepted his verbalized wishes and proceeded to administer direct touch methods that remained soft and nurturing.

But this did not placate him. After about forty-five minutes of administering nurturing touch to his whole body, which ached all over, he began to mumble and moan out loud in a manner that indicated he was regressively disintegrating. He then clasped with his closed cortical circuits on to a single phrase, "I need food and warmth", and he repeated it again and again monotonously and without affect or feeling. Then suddenly he began to yell the phrase with such intensity of affect that it caused his whole body to suddenly shoot up into the seated position on the mattress. He then turned his head towards me who was still giving nurturing touch to his neck and upper shoulder regions, and accused me with vehement ferocity of not giving him enough food and warmth!!!

His face had transformed itself into a snarling twisted contortion of daemonic proportions. He looked like a mad dog who was preparing to attack me, and he spoke with such eloquence and hostile savagery that he frightened us both, and we disengaged our hands from his body and withdrew to an emotionally safe distance about six feet away from the mattress. He accused me of having no heart and no tenderness for him, of having no warmth of soul or consideration for his needs for feeling warmth. He declared that he himself had far more warmth and consideration for the needs of others than I did. He roared at me like a wounded wild boar whose ferociousness served to keep me at a safe distance and gave no space for me to respond or defend myself against his viciously nasty accusations, which went on and on and on.

The ugly man inside Leslie had, in effect, finally revealed himself in all his damned-up sadomasochistic nastiness. How powerful and omnipotent Leslie became in his fuming, blustering rage and carthartic pouring forth of invectives against me! His omnipotence resembled that of a three-year-old child in the middle of a temper tantrum, but with the additional force of an adult brain that could conjure up the vilest choice of gutter language to express its thoughts. And although we both realized in the midst of its happening how utterly inappropriate to the outer immediate reality and infantilely archaic was the whole performance, we did not risk relating to Leslie at a feeling level or even a defensively egoic one for fear it would plunge him into further irrational excesses of cartharsis against me. We kept our distance for the remainder of the session until he eventually quieted down and withdrew inside himself into a stony silence. I dared not probe or provoke him to anything.

We were witnessing in Leslie what we have witnessed so frequently before in trainees and patients with a masochistic character structure; namely, the emergence of an omnipotent Tyrant Prince species of behavior. Tyrant Prince behavior is characterized by a quality of hostile rage that unfolds as if from out of nowhere all of a sudden, much like a sleeping volcano may erupt with great force and overflood the mountain with burning, life-destroying lava. Precisely the same kind of bioenergetic principle applies to the character-muscular armoring of the masochist. The erupting of both the volcano and the tyrant-prince-like behavior are triggered off by a loosening of the subterranean foundations deep down inside the cone and its connection to the earth-center, the belly center in human beings. In Leslie's case there probably occurred a loosening of the transverse ring of armoring that encircled his lower abdomen on account of the excessive energy mobilization work during the fifth and sixth sessions of his intensive. This loosening, however, met with a counter movement of resistance at both psychic and bioenergetic levels that eventuated in a tightening up and contracting of his entire diaphragmatic region, causing an almost complete shut-down of longitudinal energy currents flowing either from below upwards or from above downwards. This stalemating of energy flow in the region of the diaphragm caused Leslie to collapse into an emotionally neutered, cortex-dominated, passive-aggressive morass during his seventh session. The only way to liberate himself from this morasslike state of being was to unconsciously mobilize a Dionysian-divergent style of totally irrational, contact-destroying Mr. Hyde-like tyrant prince behavior, using me as the decoy.

Sadomasochistic tyrant prince behavior is always designed to hurt and wound the other as destructively as possible in order to temporarily neuter and depotentiate their emotional or spiritual capacity for closeness and feeling contact. It is something like the stinging wound of a porcupine quill thrust into the flesh of another living organism who has reached out to touch it directly. It wants to shock the other into a kind of paralyzed contactlessness and withdrawal from any further direct engagement. Its volcanic aggressiveness is really more defensive than offensive although it does not give the appearance of such. Its underlying motive remains disguised, except to the really sophisticated recipient of sadomasochistic passive-aggressive rage, just as disguised as the ego-super-ego-legislated defensive maneuvers of Leslie's fat little man against his vital primary feeling centers.

Throughout the eighth session Leslie continued to neuter and depotentiate us both by remaining firmly bogged down in his heavy swamplike depressive-paranoid morass. This was his best way of maintaining a kind of defiantly stubborn stand against facing in consciousness squarely the haunting background presence of the life-killing fat little man inside his psyche. He brooded, moaned, and complained throughout the session about the hopelessness of going on with the intensive, and how badly and despicably our therapy had failed at helping him to feel better. In other words, he continued to obliquely attack and invalidate our efforts to contact him at a feeling or intuitively penetrating level, so much so that I assumed a totally client-centered non-directive stance and let him have as much distance from me as he both needed and verbalized. I gave up any attempt to confront him with his defensive tactics at the psychic level, and at the bodily level refrained from superimposing any kind of willed do-it-yourself energy mobilization exercises or catalytic direct touch methods. I totally let him wallow in his defensive suffering. I even let him persist in his illusion that it was his twin brother who had persecuted Leslie over the past fifteen years, not vice-versa. And most significantly of all, I let him entertain the still greater illusion that the ugly little nasty man of his dream had stopped pursuing and persecuting him simply because he had not been actively festering his consciousness for the past three-day period.

My attitude of letting Leslie be, including a deliberate letting him have and remain circumscribed by his defensive maneuvers, during both the seventh and eighth sessions had its rewards. I have increasingly found this to be the case with all our clinical work with patients and trainees, namely, the wisdom of assuming a client-centered, non-intrusive orientation whenever the dearmoring process has exceeded a comfortable threshold of toleration, either at the organismic or psychological levels. The competent humanistic body psychotherapist has to develop a delicately attuned nose for sensing this exceeding of the thresholds of comfortable toleration in the patient precisely because the patient does not know this to be the case himself as long as he has not arrived at advanced second stage dearmoring. It is the therapist's responsibility, I contend, until arriving at this stage to permit the egoic and bioenergetic defenses within the patient to have their freedom to be and express themselves, unchallenged and non-confronted. It is also the therapist's responsibility to continue in this permissive, non-directive stance towards the client long enough to allow the psyche and organism of the latter to fully integrate, assimilate, and digest the novelties of change and discovery accomplished during previous sessions. Otherwise, the treatment becomes therapist-centered rather than client-centered, and quite without realizing it the therapist is transformed into a goal-directed, one-dimensional bully obsessed with de-armoring the patient at any price to the neglect of respecting his innermost needs for security and safety within the relationship.

Between the eighth and ninth sessions of Leslie's intensive there fell the week-end. My only structured homework assigned to Leslie during the last few minutes of the eighth session was the task of going 'into the pit', as I like to call it. This entails spending six to ten hours consecutively in one's bed underneath the sheets in the darkness during the middle of the day in order not to fall asleep and by virtue of not falling asleep nor being permitted to leave the bed except to go to the toilet, to be required to face one's deepest layers of consciousness, from the emptiest cerebral chattering to the profoundest, feeling-toned illuminations of the repressed or creative unconscious. Going into the pit can be extremely productive with manically energy-overcharged, strong-egoed neurotics who possess a sizeable amount of mesodermal armoring which is pressuring unconsciously from within for release and dissolution. By being forbidden to discharge their manic charge through immersion in outer-world activities and sensations, they often become seized while in the pit with wave upon wave of internal messages and energy rebellions that generate anxieties and insights galore.

This is exactly what happened to Leslie. Leslie arrived for his ninth session exhibiting what was for him bizarre mannerisms. He seemed clearly incapable of walking in a straight line: instead of maintaining his habitual overly willed control over his actions while walking, he tottered along and stumbled into the consulting room with weaving-like movements, as if he were dead drunk. Immediately upon reaching the center of the room he collapsed on to the mattress without bothering to remove his outer garments, including his leather jacket. He seemed disoriented and bewildered, and after he laid out flat on the mattress we could better see the extent to which his four limbs were rapidly shaking. Then when he began to speak, which was as soon as he laid out and before we ourselves had time to sit down on the couch besides each other, his voice revealed tremendous uncertainty, hesitation, and an unmistakeable quivering in the sound. It was quite obvious that his organism was undergoing severe anxiety and loss of normal controls, and he was helpless to change it.

The following is what Leslie said, word for word, during the first half hour of his ninth session:

> I've been very anxious and frightened about coming to this session and having to see you both. Ahhh... Mmmmmm. .. ... Ahhh-h-h- I am having trouble to get started because I don't know where to begin. Ahhh - ahhh - I guess I've seldom felt so unsure of myself for a long, long time - certainly not in recent years.
>
> Ahhh - Friday when I left here I returned to my apartment, and after I got there it suddenly hit me what I really wanted to do, and it came as a big surprise that I did want to do it, and that was - - let's see at first I just wanted to lay out on the bed and imagine going into the pit, but then it hit me that what I really wanted to do was to become the old man in all his nastiness. Then it was that I crawled under the sheets in the dark and put all the lights out. And I was off on - ahhh - on what was something like a nightmarish journey - ahhh - back into my past.
>
> I went back into all the times in my life I had been hurt by others and would react by becoming the nasty old man. There were plenty of such times - ha, ha, ha, ha - plenty of them - and it took a long, long time to remember half of them - and I felt worse and worse - I felt awful - terrible just remembering those events - and how I reacted in them - but - I - - - - - went on with the painful stuff; I felt it pulling me

somehow.

At some point later - I can't say when - maybe after an hour and a half or more - Ah h -h-h- I realize I don't want to tell you - I phantasied choking Roberta Geist around the neck with my bare hands (Roberta was another trainee of ours as well as a colleague of Leslie's and one of the few women Leslie had ever met who had had the courage to tell him his outbursts of rage were like Dr. Jekyll turning into Mr. Hyde) mmmmm - ahhhhh - and - ahh - I - ahhh - loved it.

(Along the sides of Leslie's right arm and face there appears an involuntary jerking movement that occupies his own attention enough to stop his stream of words for a couple of minutes. He obviously is confused by the jerking movement, but says nothing, and neither do we. My conjectures to myself at the time were that Leslie was so overwhelmed by what he had just reported in a monotone, affectless voice that conveyed not one nuance of the slightest feeling that his body, outside and in defiance of his own cortical-cerebral approval, was expressing the excitement mingled with anxiety that his flat, monotone voice could not express.)

Ahhh - I then - after some minutes of getting completely lost and crazy as if I were some kind of fiendish monster who took delight in killing others - phantasied choking my brother.

(At this point his voice breaks down completely for the first time, losing the capacity to intone words. His voice seems to spasm and become strangulated inside his larynx, and all he can do is allow rapidly intermittent sobs of physical pain, half muffled and held back inside his throat. He is obviously enmeshed in a struggle to withhold showing any feelings or emotions through sounds or words. I do not actively intervene, but let him writhe and twist his body with his self-conquering will into further pain in his throat. After winning the struggle with his rational will, he then allows his breathing to emit these enormous sighs that reveal during the exhalation a halting arrestment of breath every quarter of a second. It's as if his chest cannot handle nor tolerate the depth of the exhalation and is rebelling against it.)

I could not leave off staying with the grotesque feelings of delight I got from murdering my brother - again and again and again - like a compulsive impulse to do it again and again and again and again and again. I felt diabolical. I felt fiendish. I felt inhuman. - I felt just like the nasty old man that I have never really allowed myself to feel !!!!! And I loved murdering with my bare hands. I loved it!!!!!

You two were standing with all of your weight on my thighs some of the time. You were also holding my arms behind my back so that it prevented me from moving. Then I would plead to you: 'Please, please, please let me go so that I can kill him again'.

(His voice now does not break completely, but alters into a strange, not to say, weird kind of pseudo-human voice, half-human and half-inhuman, as if it were one's phantasied image of the voice of Mr. Hyde himself, but a half-convincing, half-emasculated Mr. Hyde, not a truly potent one. It rasps and gasps for air and sounds like a hollow, half-embodied empty reed.)

I enjoyed feeling evil - - evil - - - evil. . . . I realized after a while that I had a deep inner desire - impulse - no, desire - to kill all happy people. I realized how often I had thought to myself that they had no right to exist. Only those who suffered had the right. I began to perceive myself with greater focus of consciousness to be a murderer underneath the facade I have of kindness and gentleness. That the facade is just a bullshit reaction formation to the reality that I am underneath evil - nasty - a vicious person like that nasty old man of my dream. Uhhh Ugggg !!

Then I returned to my actual past again and was able to remember how I was a kind of murderer - a psychological one - when I went home to my parents when I was twenty-eight. I went home on week-ends in order to take revenge on them by making them feel as miserable as I could. I tortured them psychologically anyway I could think of. And if I couldn't succeed in torturing them, I had secret phantasies of wanting to kill them both. I was so miserable myself that I guess I wanted them to be too. . . . And then I remembered how I always resented my mother ever being happy. (He is becoming calmer and more emotionally collected and taking greater and greater cerebral distance from his subject-matter.) The result was of course that the whole family went away from me - cut themselves off from me, including my two brothers. I didn't blame them the other night when I was in the pit. I could see how it was the evil old man in me they could not stand and who drove them all away from me.

(He now has become still less anxious, has stopped his bodily trembling, and is beginning to invest some energy in the here and now relationship to Katherine and me. He looks at us directly for the first time.)

I didn't like Katherine standing up for you when I attacked you for having no feelings. (He is referring to his Tyrant Prince tyrade against me during his seventh session.) What I wanted you to do was to feel shitty and miserable and unhappy with yourself. I wanted you to beat yourself mercilessly.

On Saturday I went back into the pit for another long time. I knew I was not finished with the nasty old man inside me, and I had to deal with him once and for all. I felt like a very vicious black dog often during this second time. I wanted to attack people with my mouth and bite them to pieces like a nasty black mad dog. . . . . . I can't go on with it. Enough shit. Enough embarrassment.

(We remain silent, sensing that he needs distance from us and freedom to say what he wants. We wait in silence until he starts speaking again.)

This morning I went into the pit a third time. I didn't want to suppress anymore this nasty old man inside of me who is really as vicious as that black murderous dog. On this morning's pit trip I could finally identify myself on a feeling level with that nasty old man. More intensely than Friday night or Saturday I could experience myself to be that nasty old man. He was a dominant part of me this morning. I could vividly feel his lurking fullness and murderousness.

Yesterday morning - Sunday - I didn't go into the pit. I was too freaked out from Friday night and Saturday's pits to be able to face it again. I needed a rest. But I could still feel my huge rage against my brother on Sunday, but this morning I did not feel angry with him anymore. This is because I finally understood why he moved away from me. I also understood this morning why my mother's refusal to feel my pain and hurt made me go inside and then this nasty old man started to permeate and poison my insides. . . . I really feel this evil guy has dominated my life underneath until I got married ten years ago.

We see here a still completer and even terminal carrying through of what emerged during Leslie's seventh session as his sado-masochistic tyrant prince eruption against me personally. Now his tyrant prince behavior has been able to progress still one stage further in the direction of a Dionysian-divergent style of creative disintegration and regression, namely, to the stage of a full investment in and embodied acting out of the Dr. Jekyll - Mr. Hyde split that has characterized Leslie's armoring. This Dr. Jekyll - Mr. Hyde species of splitting is unique to the masochistic character-muscular pattern of armoring, I should like to point out, and until it can emerge in all its Dionysian - divergent ferocity and anxiety-generating chaos within the patient, whether during clinical sessions or outside the sessions, there can be no final dissolution of the masochistic armoring.

From a bioenergetic standpoint we see from Leslie's experiences in the pit how critically important it was for him to spontaneously mobilize his uncompleted acquired perverse secondary needs for primitive Phallic aggressiveness. Until he could enjoy and affirm with a kind of daemonic, diabolical delight the perverse pleasure of becoming a killer who could murder a professional colleague - Roberta Geist - and his twin brother with his own bare hands, he could not, I contend, bring to further completion those repressed dark negative forces within that are symbolized by the nasty old man of his dream. To be able to enact this daemonic psychodrama presupposed the mobilization of an enormous quantity of fluid longitudinal endodermal energy currents that moved upwards from his lower abdomen and back regions through his upper back and across his upper arms into his forearms and hands. By enacting this twisted melodrama of perverse Phallic destructiveness he not only exorcized the secondary armoring acquired from his repressed primary Phallic need, he also gained the objective possibility of irreversibly weakening the tenacious grip of the nasty old man over his unconscious psyche.

This brings us to the general clinical phenomenon of how best to work creatively with negative archetypal symbols when they surface in the consciousness of the patient. It is my theoretical position that it is always insufficient to be content merely with an intellectual or even intuitively guided feeling-charged understanding of the meaning of the symbols themselves. It is always insufficient to remain embedded within one's feeling-oriented Apollonian focused consciousness when trying to confront the meaning of negative or positive archetypal symbols. Negative ones even more than positive ones demand a further uncovering of their damned up and hitherto chronically repressed ontogenetic causes and instinctual foundations. Nothing less than their Dionysian-divergent acting out and endowing them with a concrete sensory-motor-affective embodiment provides a sufficient prerequisite to their being fully understood and fully digested and absorbed into the integrated core self. To say it more precisely, I believe that until all four dynamic primary feeling centers are awakened and permitted, each in their own way, to converge psychodynamically and bioenergetically upon the negative archetypal symbol itself, the latter cannot be adequately or fully objectified in consciousness to be creatively depotentiated and reintegrated into the unitary psyche.

In the case of Leslie's experiences in the pit the second week-end of his intensive it became such an apocalyptic experience of death and rebirth of his very soul only because his two most severely repressed dynamic primary feeling centers were liberated from the yoke symbolized by the nasty old man of his dream. How apocalyptic a death and rebirth experience this was for him is conveyed by his phantasy that Katherine and I were standing with our full weight on the front of his thighs during the time when he was most actively engaged with the repetitive murdering of his brother with his bare hands. We obviously were functioning as deterrents or inhibitors or super-ego-like impulse-restrainers to his indulgence in his perverse acting out of his destructive impulses. His creative unconscious must have informed his own psyche, in the interests of protecting the latter, that he was exceeding his psychic and organismic thresholds of toleration by projecting forth the image of me and Katherine standing on his thighs and simultaneously holding his two arms behind his back. This image of us functioning in this peculiar role was really a phantasied projection of his own Eros and Hara centers informing his creative unconscious that he needed to exercise internal restraints against overzealously skyrocketing the mobilization of his destructive impulses. The masochist, even more than the rigid types of character-muscular armoring, has a tendency to skyrocket the dearmoring process once it is liberated from the internal chains of repression. Yet I also believe that we can trust the psyche and organism of the patient, if the two are functioning together even weakly, to provide a certain autonomous self-regulation and self-protection in the midst of second stage dearmoring.

Another way of saying the same thing is that by opening up to the limits Leslie's primitive Phallic instinctual powers, there was also partially awakened and opened up his other three primary feeling centers, those of Eros, Hara, and Logos. The latter came together to form the externalized image of me and Katherine functioning as his inner restrainer against overexceeding his psychic and organismic thresholds of toleration. In this conjoining of three primary feeling centers to form a kind of self-regulatory internal check and balance against the excesses of the fourth feeling center overindulging its uninhibited carthartic expression of itself we find still deeper evidence for my earlier statement that the shadow archetype represents a kind of shadow disguise for positive as much as negative repressed libidinal-instinctual capacities.

Leslie could not have discovered the many implications and wider significances contained in actually identifying himself fully with and becoming the figure of the nasty old troll if he had dealt with the latter the way a Jungian psychoanalyst would have. Jung was never able to recommend to either therapist or patient a full and total identification with a negative archetypal figure for fear it would drive the patient psychotic. Jung seems indeed to me too complacently content with a largely rational Apollonian intellectual analysis and interpretation of archetypal symbols as an adequate means for understanding their meaning. I am sure that this can be explained in part by his general tendency to overlook how bound up archetypal symbols are - especially the negative ones - with the uncompleted personal feeling past and what this past presupposes, namely, the repression of our natural primary instinctual needs for relatedness and their secondary conversion into perverse and distorted instinctual needs. Jung tended to regard the latter and not the former as being characteristic of the true nature of instinctual needs and impulses unfortunately, much like Freud in this particular regard. For this reason he could never endorse or encourage the kind of total descent out of the rational transcendental spheres of the psyche into the darker, lower, and what I believe to be core instinctual layers of the psyche that I have conceptualized to be synonymous with the creative regression and disintegration process and so indispensable to authentic transformation of the personality structure. Jung feared the psyche's need to regress generally because he did not realize how trustworthy is our instinctual heritage at the level of the primary dynamic feeling centers.

Therefore Jung and I must firmly part company and disagree with each other when I contest that what he called the various unconscious complexes of the integrated psyche, together with what he called the more positive archetypal constellations - vis. the anima, the animus, the Wise Old Man, the Puer Aeternus, the Unus Mundus, the Mysterium Coniunctionis, the figure of Jesus Christ as personifying the archetype of wholeness, and the various pagan Gods and Goddesses of primitive cultures as reflecting these psychic complexes and archetypes of the collective unconscious - are all, each and every one, Apollonian-like transcendental mirrorings of our instinctual primary feeling needs for relatedness. It follows from my point of view that we must dispense with the concept of the collective unconscious as the ultimate repository of the psyche and substitute in its place the discovery and actualization of the primary instinctual needs. Part of this process of discovery then becomes that of allowing our primitive unconscious to have dominance during the third and fourth stages of creative regression and disintegration, especially to the extent that our primitive Phallos and Eros life-affirmative libidinal needs have been crushed and distorted. The phenomenon of regression then emerges as absolutely imperative to the healing and growth process. Until patients can return to and reexperience that period of their early ontogenetic development when their primary instinctual needs were either twisted into something distorted or else invalidated and squashed out of existence completely by the manner in which their parents related to them, there is no real possibility for appropriation and a claiming of full identification with the many instinct-determined positive archetypal masks of Godhood within.

To return to Leslie, his week-end in the pit represented the high point of his three-week intensive. For his remaining four sessions he filled in with his flowering Logos faculty the apocalyptic changes that he had concretely experienced during the preceding week-end. He consolidated and digested, in other words, with rational focus what he had become initially overflooded and overwhelmed by on a feeling and cognitive level during the week-end. He reexplored openly with us all his past intimate relationships from the revolutionary new perspective of that of blaming himself and not the other for his alienation from and disillusionment with the other. For the first time in his adult life he could honestly admit and feel how he himself, under the unknown spurious domination by the nasty old man within, had unconsciously poisoned all his intimate relationships with ambivalence, distrust, and hostility.

This revolutionary new perspective included the enhanced bodily sensibility of having direct sensory sensations coming from the region of his chest and heart. He could directly sense the battle for supremacy always going on in his chest region whenever he began to have tender and loving feelings towards any of his intimate relationships, past and present. This new proprioceptive sensibility confirmed how severely armored he had been in his entire mesodermal layer against having strong Eros feelings towards another human being. One of the most essential features of a Dr. Jekyll - Mr. Hyde split is a total cutting off and permanent isolation of any direct internal exchange between the chest region and the lower back region of the body. This total cutting off of internal energetic communication between these two regions had been penetrated and weakened in Leslie's organism during his week-end in the pit, we can safely conjecture. Consequently he was able because of this energetic breakthrough to take a revolutionary new perspective towards himself at the psychological levels. By loosening and dissolving further the bands of transverse armoring across his upper and lower back regions, he no longer felt so compelled to contract his back half whenever his chest region became filled with enhanced endodermal vegetative flow. The discharge of severely imploded passive-aggressiveness that had occurred on the week-end had undermined the armoring in his back at both ends, permitting him to sense and feel directly his previous bodily habit of tightening his entire back into a defensively paranoid, passive-aggressive stance whenever he experienced positive feelings of Eros in his chest.

His week-end in the pit permanently transformed his feeling attitude towards his twin brother. He could give up entirely his previous passive-aggressive stance towards his brother and feel his newly liberated Eros need for tender loving relatedness with him. This change of fundamental soul-attitude towards his brother is evidenced by the objective fact that about a week after Leslie finished his intensive with us he wrote a long letter to his brother. In this letter he acknowledged fully how he, Leslie, had actively contributed to why their relationship had gone so sour and had progressively deteriorated over the past fifteen years. The letter must have been an inspired one because it produced a very positive reaction in his brother. Four months later the two men met alone for several days, during which time Leslie was able to confess still further how he had unconsciously sabotaged their hitherto intense emotional closeness to each other. They passed those several days together for the first time as adult men without feeling compelled to passively compete with or try to invalidate the achievements of the other.

III. The Fourth Stage of Creative Disintegration : The Flowering of the Eros-Phallos Libidinal Circuit

The second stage of treatment is distinguished generally by the emergence of the importance of the primary feeling centers in the upper front half and lower back half of the body, of the Being centers of Eros and Phallos. We have just seen this born out in the example of Leslie's discovery of these same unsatisfied feeling needs in himself. His experience is prototypical of what happens during the second stage of treatment to nearly all of our trainees and regular patients, regardless of the type of patterning of character-muscular armoring that they have started with.

The third stage of treatment is distinguished generally from the second stage by the emergence of the importance of the primary Being centers of the lower front half and upper back half of the body, of the Hara and Logos feeling-intuitive soul faculties. The transition from the second to the third stage of treatment, a stage in which the dearmoring process has largely been completed already, will be dealt with in the next chapter.

The essence of the fourth stage of creative disintegration is the further flowering of Eros and Phallos, but this time wedded to the sexual instinct directly. This is a stage of personality transformation, therefore, that takes place primarily outside of the clinical consulting room in the privacy of the bed chamber. The competent humanistic body psychotherapist who has him or herself passed through this stage already will know best how to guide and facilitate its unfoldment within the privacy of the bedroom. Otherwise the patient will be required to discover alone and largely without the guidance of the psychotherapist how to go through this fourth stage. This section of the chapter is written more for the latter category of reader, because it has been my longstanding observation that the majority of body psychotherapists, or any other style of psychotherapist, practicing professionally today has not discovered nor passed through experientially the fourth stage of creative regression and disintegration. The many good reasons for this reality will not be discussed in this book, but they all relate to the kind of social pressures and restrictions superimposed upon the primitive and creative unconscious networks of the members of our modern Western urban-technological, future-shock civilization.

If there has been a moderate to severe amount of armoring in the patient, and the antilibidinal super-ego is still actively fighting for its survival, then sexual lovemaking will be plagued by considerable inhibitions of a moralistically negative character. This psychic state of affairs makes for the appearance during the midst of lovemaking of new kinds of negative archetypal forms and forces, and usually more terrifying and powerful in substance than those that appear during the third stage of creative disintegration. Nevertheless, if these negative archetypal forms can be openly tolerated and lived through in consciousness, their terrorfulness and power will eventually become atrophied, and the rewards on the further side will be so magnificent that they will be worth the pain and terror of the journey. The rewards will include having embodied sensory-motor-affective experiences of oneself and one's beloved that possess a sacred-profane, numinous-luminous awesomeness and mystery about them that transcend and surpass in end-state fulfillment any other peak experiences of self-actualization hitherto encountered. The single most outstanding achievement of such peak experience during sexual lovemaking is the uniting of two separate human beings into a mystical Oneness and Union with the ultimate creative forces in the universe, within and without.

I will use my own personal history of development and dearmoring to illustrate this fourth stage of disintegration. I do so not for exhibitionistic or narcissistic reasons, but simply because no-one can know better than oneself the infinite nuances and subtleties of one's inner experiencing during sex. What I am going to describe from my private sex-life happens to be the least flattering material I could possibly select to share openly with the reader.

Like Eldridge and Leslie of this volume, I too once possessed a substantial neurotic split in my psyche and body which could be classified as masochistic in nature and structure. My masochistic armoring had prevented me from discovering my Eros-Phallos libidinal circuit of flow until I was forty years old. Furthermore, it prevented me from totally embracing and accepting this particular circuit of flow as an intrinsic part of my core self for another eight to ten years after once having found it. Not until I arrived at the mellow middle age of fifty can I conscientiously admit myself to have become relatively free of my character-muscular armoring and its elusive accomplice, the anti-libidinal superego in my head. What will follow as true excerpts from my personal sex-life occurred during the latter period, between my fortieth and fiftieth years, when I was still unquestionably hounded and persecuted from within by my own armoring during the midst of lovemaking.

Even as late as my early forties I was still burdened by a heavy Promethean-like false self-image that I was self-actualizing in my work but a very unhappy martyr in my love life, and that I had to suffer and resign myself to this discrepancy between my public and my private life. I accepted this discrepancy less and less, however, and the more I actively sought to eliminate this discrepancy, even though it meant taking greater and greater risks in terms of my intimate man-woman relationships, the more dearmored and growth-motivated I became in the sphere of sexuality.

I had separated from my first wife when I was thirty, and after a moderate amount of sexual experimentation with different women between the ages of thirty and thirty-five, moderate because I was still very involved unconsciously with my first wife, I finally started living with a French woman who was the absolute antithesis to my first wife. This French woman was nine years younger than myself, and very split neurotically when we started living together. I became - unconsciously - her father substitute and unofficial psychotherapist combined, and after a marriage contract entered into when I was forty because of purely pragmatic considerations, our mutual inability for passional lovemaking began to catch up with us. With my second wife I played victim to her role of tormentor-persecutor as much as she did precisely the same thing with me. We regularly took turns at it. I was still quite alienated from core self to be able to face or identify my underlying passive-aggressive perverse need to provoke her to rage, although I could accurately sense these same elements in my many masochistic patients. And although our sex life was better than that which I had known with my first wife - a totally undifferentiated American child-woman - it lacked many important dimensions to make it fulfilling or soulfully contactful. She was too hysterically split inside to be able to risk falling in love with me, and I was still too alienated from my lower half Dionysian libidinal needs to be able to fully face and acknowledge our mediocre sexual rapport.

In contrast to my first wife, there prevailed a very sophisticated understanding with my second wife regarding extramarital affairs. They were totally acceptable on her part, whereas I had a much lower toleration of them if it was she who had been the one to defect. I was often very embarrassed at feeling so jealous and possessive of her sexually, and could never give myself a rational explanation for my intense jealousy. She was of little help because she tended to ridicule and caricature it. It was therefore with strongly ambivalent self-assertiveness whenever I tried to inform or convince my second wife that there was something seriously wrong with out intimate relationship as sexual mates. She always dismissed my opinion as off the wall, and blamed me rather than herself for any inadequacies at the sexual level. In effect, she was even more estranged than I from her Eros-Phallos libidinal circuits.

Finally at the age of forty-one, after we had been living together for six years, out of an increasing but still nebulous feeling of sexual frustration, longing, and general psychological malaise and resignation, I embarked upon an extramarital affair with an older woman. This affair lasted eighteen months. It provided me with a sexual rapport so marvellous and fulfilling to my still suppressed

Dionysian-Phallic needs that it showed me how sadly lacking had been the sexual rapport with my second wife. It also gave me the renewed faith in myself to continue a more active searching for a woman who could reciprocate the kind of passional and beatific fusion that took place between this older woman and myself. Such an ideal woman, I now knew, had to be at least ten years younger than the woman with whom I was having the affair, and free from the many psychological hangups that still possessed my second wife.

After separating from my second wife and sado-masochistically hanging in with the affair with the older woman, out of sympathy to her deep love for me, I started again experimenting with new man-woman relationships. I knew I could never fall in love with the older woman in spite of our marvellous sexual contact. I could never give her my heart, as much because of my own armoring as for the fact that she was too old to be for me a desireable mate for the remainder of my life. She gave me her heart and soul as well as body, and it became an increasingly impossible situation between us, exacerbated by a growing sense of guilt and shame within me for continuing to see her at all. Partly in order to disentangle myself from this truly decisive, growth-enhancing and soul-opening relationship I plunged into another with the impulsive impetuosity of a twenty-five-year-old. This new affair also lasted about eighteen months, and she lived with me in my house. I will not speak about it here except to say that this new heavy affair provided me with the opportunity to express whatever dormant passive-aggressive anger and rage still lay coiled inside. This new lady could not only stand her ground against me, but fan the fire significantly enough to permit us both to work through our unresolved Aedipal fixations at the expense of abusing the other's soul ruthlessly. We were well-matched as fighters, and bad lovers, both spiritually and sexually, and the whole eighteen-month marathon of battles and revenge-takings were just what I needed to prepare myself for appreciating a woman like Katherine.

It is with Katherine, now my third wife and professional colleague, that I finally discovered my Eros-Phallos libidinal circuit. She was in reality the most emotionally mature American woman I had ever met before I asked her to come and live with me. It was her emotional maturity that attracted me to her, not her physical beauty or sexual compatibility. She was not perfect. There were still many scars discernible from earlier heart wounds. Yet her Eros, Spiritual Warrior, Hara, and Logos intuitive faculties were alive and sufficiently in touch with each other internally to make her the first third-stage lady in my life I ever fell in love with.

To be more accurate, her third-stage level of individuation permitted her to fall in love with me before I was able to actively reciprocate her love. She seemed to have few inner defenses against letting herself fall in love with me even though throughout our entire first year together my deep-seated distrust towards women and my determination to be honest with her obligated me to tell her that I could not reciprocate her love feelings from my heart as yet. I knew that I wanted to, but I also knew that I could not. After having lived through four primary-commitment, long-term intimate man-woman relationships, I wanted this new liaison to evolve slowly and cautiously. I had reached that point in my own internal evolution where I could no longer afford to allow myself to make another big mistake regarding the choice of the right woman for me.

My departure from throwing myself headlong into a new amorous adventure was the beginning of wisdom. I had suffered too deeply and with increasing consciousness from the failures to make passional contact in all my earlier man-woman relationships. I had suffered too deeply to have arrived at the hardened cynical position, now so prevalent among so many social circles of Western capitalist society, that men and women are doomed to eternal competition and conflict and consequently it is basically an illusion to think that they can find happiness or fulfillment through each other, that there could exist man-woman relationships of mature mutual dependency that provided a supreme kind of wholeness within the relationship. I had had a taste of such wholeness and fulfillment during my affair with the older woman. We had had some beatifically supreme, self-actualizing moments together. These moments had revivified my belief and hope at finding the right woman for me.

It was this very belief and hope that was in part responsible for my uncharacteristic cautiousness with Katherine during that first year. I had to test her again and again within myself and for myself without disclosing to her what I was doing. Never before, with the exception of my first wife, had I so deliberately and consciously withheld large parts of my feeling capacities for relatedness from my intimate man-woman relationship. Yet this withholding was correct in terms of my own soul's development. The American psyche is so incredibly naive and impetuous when it comes to matters of sex and the heart, and so anti-rational because so much of the time it is excessively calculating, egoic, and rationally survival-oriented. I needed to learn how to feel my feelings with full cognitive, rational awareness of them as they emerged and subsided inside of me, rather than remain stuck in my former pattern of becoming intermittently possessed by them and then intermittently turned off and alienated from them, killing them with my inexhaustible cerebralizing resources.

Our sexual life from the beginning of our relationship had been excellent, and certainly as good as it had been between me and the older woman. In fact it was so good in every other respect as well as the sexual that it seemed to me personally too good to be true!!!! This is a common disbelief and skepticism in anyone with a masochistic background from which one is finding liberation. It has to do with a fear of falling into a truly ego-disintegrating passional Eros-Phallos libidinal circuit with another. Reich called it pleasure-anxiety, and everyone who has been neurotically split must pass through a period of pleasure-anxiety. For Katherine, on the other hand, it was just the reverse perception that she frequently shared with me, namely, that if you find it so beautiful, true, and good between us now, you haven't seen anything yet because it's going to get better and better!!!! Her assurity and self-confidence about our sexual potential, it should be pointed out, sprang in part from she having gone through two extensive former marriage relationships, as well as an unknown number of more casual sexual affairs. Yet she never paraded these former sexual relations in front of me in order to manipulate me into believing she knew more than I about sexual matters. To the contrary, she was extremely tight-lipped and wisely discrete about ever mentioning her former intimate relationships in terms of their sexual dimension.

Even for her, however, we began to have shared experiences during lovemaking from the first year onwards that transcended in beauty and depth anything she had ever known before in her former relationships. I am referring explicitly to our mutual discovery of archetypal visionary objectifications of oneself and the other that extended the horizons of our perception of the other each time it happened. These archetypal visionary objectifications were embued with such numinousness as to fill us with feelings of reverence and awe and gratitude to the natural universe each time it happened. They permitted us to worship each other as Gods and Goddesses, Kings and Queens, sacred and at the same time frightening transpersonal creatures, half-animal and half-human.

All of these archetypal visions had in common a pre-Christian content. They were all pagan in character by Christian standards. That is, they came from the mythological legends and stories about the Gods and Goddesses of primitive, ancient pre-Christian cultures. This was their most important objective visual quality, and one that astonished us both again and again and again. They were either Egyptian, Greek, African, Polynesian, American Indian, East Indian, or totally non-modern-Western-world in their visual presentation. The one and only exception was when I became the figure of the Devil, the anti-Christ.

Let me describe in some detail one of these experiences of pre-Christian sacred-profane archetypal rituals that became perhaps the most repetitive motif of all our archetypal experiences throughout our first six years together. I refer to me becoming the Greek God Pan and Katherine a Positive Great Earth-Mother Archetype. Each time it happened, I felt both lured and in fear, even after it had already been happening for several years. There was always a fairly regular, set sequence of events that happened, involving a gradual descent from my mental head-consciousness into altered states of being that became progressively body-centered.

During the first phase Katherine and I would lay relatively immobile side by side with our limbs touching the torso of the other or the autoerogenous zones specifically. The pregenital stimulation would be very, very slow to unfold. If either one of us were feeling tense and manicky, this would prohibit the possibility of us being able to lay quietly long enough side by side before we both could sense a general massive retardation and deceleration of our energy metabolism. Usually, even when not feeling tense and overexcited by the day's events, we would have to hold one another chest to chest for an extended period lasting between ten to twenty five minutes before our energy metabolism could reach a condition of massive slowing down and a deep subterranean circulation of our core endodermal longitudinal energy currents. The latter, we have already seen, is a necessary precondition to the emergence of regressive psychic states governed by the flow of the blood throughout the organism as a unitary totality.

It made little difference which parts of the body were in direct touch. It was not even necessary to directly touch the erogenous zones themselves. In fact it was contraindicated whenever we were on the tense, nervous side for then there would be too rapidly escalated a localized genital sexual high that remained mesodermal and ectodermal in its charge-discharge flow. If we wanted to sink down into an endodermal energy flow, we had first to slow down throughout the organism without overexciting the erogenous zones. What we were guiding ourselves towards half-unconsciously was a magnetic field of energy flow that emanated and circulated between our chest and abdominal regions. This same horizontal magnetic field seemed to pull us not only towards each other but also downwards out of the head into the earth. The more powerful the magnetism of this energy field, the more our blood flow seemed to begin to vibrate in single unitary synchrony with that of the other, particularly in the front half regions of the body.

During the second phase I would regularly pass into a psychosomatic stage in which every muscular tension still remaining in my mesodermal wall would claim the foreground of awareness. It was a time of aches and pains, usually disconnected from each other at first, but progressively becoming interconnected with each other at both ends of the spinal column. They were often so unpleasant that they occupied all my energy, and my body would be forced involuntarily from within the mesodermal layer to twist, writhe and move. I forgot all about lovemaking and became engrossed with a kind of do-it-yourself de-armoring process whose high point was the release of my middle back mesodermal wall, which was always announced by an enormous belching of gas from below upwards across my diaphragmatic muscle complex. The loud, not to say grotesquely obnoxious, sounds of my belching were like a volcano erupting forth its imploded gases. This went on from five to ten minutes, depending upon how much pressure I continued to apply with my right hand to the back of my neck on either side of the center position. Katherine found this phase anything but romantic, although she never made me try to stop or inhibit it because we both knew it was an indispensable step towards my letting go my cerebral controls.

Once the belching subsided and I could relax again into a deep, slowed-down state of relative immobility, whenever we resumed direct touch with each other there was not only the magnetic field generated between our bodies, but also an enormous heat in the regions of my belly, lower back, and genitals. This heat came from deep inside these regions, clearly from the now fully eroticized or libidinalized endodermal vegetative flow, and from below upwards the heat finally melted my diaphragmatic area, bringing me thereby out of my upper half completely into my lower half. From this point onwards there unfolded a psyhological metamorphosis.

As my phallos grew spontaneously erect, it also felt and sensed as if it were growing in size to gargantuan proportions. Simultaneously I felt and sensed my ears becoming elongated and tapered to a fine edge, my feet changing from those of a human being into a goat-like animal being, and sometimes even a tail extending forth from my anus. By the time my penis had become fully erect, I had lost my normal egoic identity and had assumed the embodied and psychic identity of Pan. I have described the embodied transformation, but there was also a distinct psychic transformation. It entailed a complete change of attitude towards Katherine. When I looked at her or initiated any kind of direct touch with her, she became illuminated into a highly desireable sexual being whose pulsating blood flow seemed to fill me with a desire to worship her!! Normally when I look at or touch Katherine it is without the slightest element of sacred-pagan worshipfulness or mental idealization.

This was especially the case during our first five years together, when I had the greatest difficulty to enjoy her sexually in an uninhibited and at the same time tender manner. Yet as Pan I could do both with unselfconscious ease and sublime delight.

The final phases of our sacred-profane ritual were always the most unpredictable. It had to do with my becoming further transformed into a younger and younger Pan-like son-lover and she into an All-Powerful Great Queen-Mother-Earth-Goddess. This phase would not begin until I reached out and touched her generously proportioned breasts with my hands or mouth. In our earlier years together I would regress to infancy once I started suckling at her breasts with my mouth. But in later years I would retain my identity as a young Dionysus or Pan and regress to that of an adolescent youth. With either possibility I would become intoxicated with her ample breasts and as I allowed my whole body to embrace hers, it felt as if I were becoming absorbed by her oceanic and earthy vastnesses, so hugely large and boundless in her organismic proportions she increasingly became. I could vividly feel myself shrinking and becoming smaller and smaller in size as she grew larger, fuller, and more powerful in every sense.

Then it was that she would assume for me any different number of possible images: that of the ancient Greek Goddess Demeter, the Egyptian Queen-Goddess Isis with me feeling like her son-lover Osiris, an Incan High Priestess with an American-Indian-like beauty and nobility of both appearance and being, or a more impersonalized and elemental Mother-Goddess who gives sustenance and nourishment from her whole body and not just from her breasts. During these latter experiences of visionary and psychodynamic transformation she might assume the dark, vital form of a huge, earthy black African negress, or a Polynesian peasant woman, or a softer, more watery and oceanic sea-goddess who gradually incorporates me inside of her inexhaustible depths and currents.

Once anyone of these archetypal images emerged of her as a Divine Female Being whom I felt compelled to adore and worship, I could dimly sense the very boundaries of my own body becoming more and more nebulous. It was as if I ceased to identify with the proprioceptive messages that ordinarily were transmitted to me from my voluntary musculature and skeletal networks. Instead I found myself becoming metamorphosed into a shapeless and undifferentiated ocean of fluid lava flow which included us both together in a Single Unitary Whole. We lost, in other words, all sense of our separateness as organisms and totally fused with the endodermal, blood-mediated energy flow of the other. This loss of all sense of familiar boundaries at the bodily level usually occurred shortly before orgasm, and with this death-like loss of our normal physical boundaries we also gave up our archetypal objectifications of self and other. In their place superceded a still more embodied image of ourselves as an animal-like, serpentine Unitary Uroboros with my phallos entering her vagina and extending through her torso upwards and coming out of her mouth. No longer did she feel all-powerful and larger in size than myself, but simply the sacred-pagan Other Half of myself, communion with whom permitted us both the sublimely beatific experience of mutual death and rebirth.

What I have just finished describing seldom happened as smoothly and so logically ordered as presented. Very much to the contrary, this whole sequence of phases usually was interrupted or completely shut down by fears stemming from my still intact character-muscular armoring. These fears could appear at any moment during the whole sequence, and continued to intrude themselves during our sacred-profane rites of initiation into the realms of the Old Gnosis, or, if you like, the realms of a regressive and transpersonal Mysterium Coniunctionis, until I reached my fiftieth year.

The many masks of Godhood available to us cannot be gained without first purging and exorcizing from ourselves all remnants and reverberations of our old cerebralized self-images of identity. In my own case I had to purge and exorcize from my character structure all remnants of my life-negative, anti-libidinal rigid Christian upbringing. Until the advanced young age of twenty-two I had but one vocational objective consistently in mind: to become an Anglican priest in the Protestant Episcopal Church of America. Having been brought up by a mother and father who adhered to a Puritanical hierarchy of values which both ensnared and enchained me from a very early age during my adolescence, I had no choice but to make my peace with their counterfeit, pseudo-religious belief system by introjecting it intellectually and emotionally. I lived in terror of girls as sexual beings throughout my teens and twenties largely because my parents shared a Christian-inspired deep-seated terror of sexuality. A Christian-Puritan hierarchy of values so totally dominated the consciousness of both my first wife and myself that our sexlife for eight years resembled that of two lost children groping for glimpses of Eros in the darkness under the bed sheets while being engulfed by feelings of anxiety, shame, disgust and an incredible alienation from our animal instincts that neither one of us could ever openly admit to ourselves alone or share with the other.

Given such an early religious background, I had indeed some just objective reasons for becoming seized with fear and anxiety time and time again within seconds after my embodied transformation into the figure of Pan while making love to Katherine. In spite of the fact that it became an increasingly familiar and even regular happening, it took me more than five years to face Pan fully in the light of rational consciousness to the point where I could mentally digest and emotionally accept Him as a repressed but vital and real part of myself. And until I could and did integrate Him into my embodied self-image that continued to persist after having made love to Katherine, he continued to haunt me like a shadow archetype. I often would become paralyzed with fear inside when Pan emerged during the first five years together with Katherine. The paralysis would extend to a total arrestment of both my sexual longings and feelings of spiritual tenderness that were being freshly awakened within me towards Katherine. I would withdraw my five senses from engagement with her and become as if suspended in immobility while there ensued inside of me an energy-consuming Titanic battle between my repressed instinctual tendencies and my Christian-prescribed anti-life inhibitions against those tendencies, between my Eros and primitive Phallos instinctual impulses and my anti-libidinal super-ego. And so great was my anxiety, confusion, sense of guilt and shame whenever this battle engulfed me that I never once dared to reveal to Katherine what was happening. I kept it an absolute secret for over three years !

The archetypal figure of Pan represents more than a negative shadow of my repressed libidinal desire carried over from a Puritanical upbringing. I had had no problem whatsoever getting my phallos erect with all my previous sexual relations, both with my wifes and during my extramarital affairs. I had never been lacking in either phallic desire nor potency. What had been lacking until Katherine, however, was a capacity to open my heart simultaneously while making love. The soul power of Eros had always been missing in my lovemaking. This is the power to surrender one's core self so totally to one's beloved in passional ecstasy that the boundaries which define her separateness of eing and my separateness of being are temporarily obliterated and transcended, and a kind of apocalyptic, Phoenix-like death and rebirth fusion between us becomes the final achievement, not orgasm. Like most other people I knew, I did not even have any idea that such a possibility of single unitary fusion between a man and a woman was psychodynamically or bioenergetically conceivable until I started living with Katherine. Passion-inspired uroboric Fusion was merely a romantic if not somewhat frightening illusion until meeting her.

Pan, to the extent that he symbolized a breakthrough of my hitherto repressed soul's capacity for experiencing Eros towards another, was a kind of primitive manifestation of my core self's anima finding its disguised flowering. According to Jung the anima is the feminine nature within the male whose incorporation into our core self identity is indispensable to higher individuation. I fully agree. Pan was for me an hermaphroditic archetypal figure whose primary significance was his feminine-like tendency to worship and celebrate Katherine as some kind of goddess. Whenever I became Pan I exercized a feminine-like sensibility and slowness and delicacy of response when touching Katherine sensually that surpassed my usual libidinal lovemaking abilities. Her body and my body became transfigured into luminously numinized entities when Pan presided, and for the first time in my life, under Pan's tutelage, I was able to become totally absorbed in the concrete realm of immediacy - sensory-affective-motor immediacy - and share with Katherine a spontaneity and innocence of mutual appreciation of the sacred beauty, goodness, and mystery of her feminineness of being.

For several years I could not face the hidden anima aspect of Pan. During these years I tended to perceive him purely as my resurrected and long-suppressed primitive phallic libido. This was indeed his masculine side, and I had been during my teens, twenties, and even thirties severely alienated from my primitive sexual instincts. Pan was in actuality in his pure satyr-like phallicism a kind of shadow disguise for his other aspect, his embodiment of my feminine anima and heart feelings of Eros. But my Puritan saturated consciousness and unconsciousness could not grasp this at first. I was still too dominated, both consciously and unconsciously, by a false self-image that can best be portrayed as that of an intellectual and morality-bound Prometheus. I was still too much of a priest in normal clothes in my role of a psychotherapist whose self-identity hinged upon his soul-saving abilities. Like Prometheus saved man from being destroyed by the Gods by his superhuman determination to persevere and suffer against overwhelming odds, I too was zealously committed to my Christ-like role of saving others with a will-to-persevere-and-suffer-through the psychopathological twistednesses and follies of my private patients, while masochistically neglecting my own personal needs. Foremost among those needs was my phallic sexual need. What I could not recognize then to be also a neglected need was that of Eros, or that of my heart. My Promethean-Puritan false self-image prevented me from perceiving with any intuitive accuracy how much my Spiritual Warrior, Agape, and Logos faculties tyrannized my private relationships as much as my professional ones. As long as my Promethean false self-image prevailed, I would remain blinded to how badly I had neglected and suppressed my Eros as much as my primitive phallos needs.

It was not only the phallicly libidinalized figure of Pan that I feared revealing to Katherine out of a sense of guilt and embarrassment. I had far greater anxiety about revealing to her the intense pleasure I obtained from the more advanced phases of our sacred-profane ritual. I was profoundly ashamed for over eight years by my tendency to metamorphose into a child, infant, or adolescent much younger in psyche and body than my actual age!!! I was often filled with unambiguous fear whenever I found myself obtaining a Dionysian kind of pleasureable abandonment from suckling at her breasts. Any kind of erotic enjoyment of her breasts during our earlier years together would always evoke a double-edged reaction within me, comprising both positive pleasureable excitement and negative unpleasureable anxiety. This was particularly true when I regressed to the ontogenetic level of full infancy and felt myself to be no longer a phallicly potent and tenderly sensitive Pan but a deprived, grasping and voracious infant. However, I could not continue except for a few brief moments - perhaps as long as half a minute at most - in this extremely regressed infantile mode before I throttled the process with my anti-libidinal super-ego telling me: "Stop this at once! It's too infantile! It's too incestuous! Stop using her to satisfy your infantile greed! She's not your mother! You have no right to use her like your mother! You are disgraceful! You are perverted! "

I would withdraw my mouth from her breasts and nuzzle against her body passively, shortly after receiving any one of these relentlessly persistent self-critical messages from my brain. I would also withdraw away from her back inside my head and say nothing until I had recovered from my over-indulgence! Once having done so I might renew a more conventional kind of lovemaking or just drop off to sleep. It was not until I was able to find the courage to risk sharing with her verbally the intoxication and sense of abandonment that suckling her breasts gave me that this particular pattern just described changed between us. This had much to do with the acceptant nature of her response, namely that she enjoyed, fully as much as I, my enjoyment of her breasts. She affirmed how my erotic pleasuring of myself with my mouth at her breasts - or my hands - it made no difference to her - awakened her genital longing for me to enter her. At first I would not believe her. I refused to believe that she was speaking the truth. She just wanted to placate me, to spoil and indulge me, I told myself. I had to ask her again and again and again over a period of several years what she really felt and thought about my delirious, Dionysian delight at suckling or fondling her breasts, and hear her reply again and again and again essentially the same way, before I could begin to believe and accept that she obtained as much libidinal pleasure as I did from our hand-breast and mouth-breast contact. The doggedness and the tenacity of the anti-libidinal super-ego !!!!

But even when I ceased regressing to total infancy and ceased to feel like a polymorphously perverse needy-desperate baby, and remained merely a youngish - about seventeen-years-old usually - Pan or son-lover-like figure, who did possess a gigantically potent phallus and could and did make love to her with it, I continued to feel moderately ashamed of the fact that she became so all-powerful and so Queenly and I felt so clearly subordinate and inferior in both size and psychic maturity. I was ashamed to reveal to her that psychologically as much as physically I felt myself to be younger than her. I felt embarrassed to openly acknowledge to her that she had assumed the numinous aura of a Positive Great Mother Archetype while I felt like her heathen, profane son-lover. As late as my late forties my anti-libidinal super-ego would send me the message that I was worshipping her as if I were her slave, and that I was giving her too much power over me. In other words, I was becoming too subordinate, and could I trust her not to take advantage of this situation? Would she not try to exploit my growing dependency upon her for passionally Dionysian sexual fulfillment and our discovery of the many dark Gods and Goddesses within? I asked these questions secretly to myself nearly every time we attained to the advanced archetypal phases described earlier. It was not, once again, until I risked sharing with her openly my doubts, ambivalences, reservations, and fears about imbuing her with so much power over me and hearing her unconditionally acceptant response again and again that I could finally, once and for all, bury my old fears and dissolve my anti-libidinal super-ego by the time I reached fifty !

I could finally bury my old masochistic character-muscular armoring when I could believe in her love and respect for me to be enough to quell within her any unsatisfied need to bully, manipulate, or dominate me as a consequence of our emotional dependency upon each other. Not until I could permit myself to depend emotionally upon at least one other human being so completely that I became as vulnerable to her whims, needs, and impulses as I was to those of my mother when I was between the ages of six months and four years old, and not be used or humiliated by the will of the other, could I shed the last vestiges of my masochistic distrust and paranoia regarding my fellow human beings, both male and female.

In this context - the psychopathological - to fully love another presupposes the opening of the front half primary feeling centers to a level of vulnerability that once prevailed between the young child and its mother, and until both adult lovers risk this vulnerability they can transcend neither their character-muscular armoring nor their Judaic-Christian Western cultural backgrounds.

The crucial truth we are brought to at this point in our argument is that the flowering of my Eros-Phallos libidinal circuit within signifies not only a surpassing of my Promethean false self-image and its subtly intropunitive, anti-libidinal super-ego, but in addition, a surpassment of our Christian religious tradition and culture. Not until Katherine and I together could transcend the Procrustean-bed-like rigidities of the Christian faith and its cultural legacy of sin, guilt, shame and fear regarding the sacramental ultimacy and sacredness of pagan sexuality could we discover the Hidden Wisdom of Great Mother Nature within us both. Not until we could transcend a fear of regressively creative disintegration back to earlier religious traditions and mythologies could we discover the counterfeit, intrinsically anti-life and anti-nature polarization of Christ and the Devil.

The devil or Satan, Lord of the Wicked Underworld, is unquestionably the supreme negative shadow archetype of the Christian religious tradition. It is no accident that he is frequently portrayed as animal-like in nature, and grotesquely instinctual and libidinally perverse. This portrayal follows from the fundamental Christian idealization of moral purity, which amounts to a perpetual striving for moral and rational perfection within oneself, a striving for a kind of imitation of Christ, whose incarnated perfection is a reflection of the more supreme perfection and self-sufficiency of the monotheistic Supreme God. This idealization of moral and spiritual purity unfortunately in my opinion has been achieved at a great cost, namely, a complete betrayal of the human body and its mediation of the primary feeling instincts for relatedness between real human beings. The whole Christian tradition revolves around a striving upwards towards self-contained perfection and spiritual purity within oneself, not downwards into one's animal Dionysian propensities of the lower half or even outwards towards the immediate human-centered orbit of other people which is the orbit of Eros.

It follows from such an abstract idealization of the spiritual will to perfection and moral purity, a product of the cerebral cortex from beginning to end, that whatever we have come in this book to regard as embodied soul is the province of the Devil himself. For radical Christians the experiencing of the many masks of Godhood within oneself by means of instinct-regulated, life-completing individual human relationships is forbidden because it is the work of the Devil. According to radical Christianity the path to self-perfection necessitates a surpassment of the satisfying of fundamental human soul-needs by means of interdependent completion of those needs through other human beings. One must learn to deny, renounce, and sublimate such interpersonally field-dependent soul- needs and turn to Christ the Savior for salvation and self-completion. A kind of direct object-relationship with Christ is encouraged as the only acceptable path to self-perfection.

It was against such a cortex-dominant religious upbringing and tradition that I was rebelling the night on which I made love to Katherine as if I was the Devil himself. It happened one evening after I had spent the week-end skiing. Perhaps for the latter reason I felt more restless and manically overcharged in my pelvis and lower back than normally. I felt impatient to enter Katherine with my phallos in order to penetrate her aggressively and to 'fuck' her with total abandonment. I shall never forget the uprush and overflooding by contradictory feelings that besieged me from the moment I entered her with an atypical amount of pure animal desire to 'fuck' her. On the one hand, I experienced my entire spinal column as if it had become inflamed with tongues of red fire that came from below upwards on both sides of my back. The tongues of red fire felt like primitive phallic animal desire to overwhelm Katherine as a sexual object. They were absolutely heartless. I also felt strangely light rather than heavy, yet highly male-potent and vividly aware of the new-found power in my legs and phallus simultaneously.

It was from the midst of these novel body sensations and abnormally intensified animal desires to conquer Katherine as a sexual object that there suddenly emerged as if from nowhere an image of myself as a naked, red-and-black-colored daemonic Lord of the Underworld, Satan himself. I was astonished to find myself suddenly becoming the Devil with a huge phallus, like Pan, but, unlike Pan, a powerfully authoritative tail and horns and a face that felt tyrannically omnipotent. The image also included a phantasied vision of me and Katherine riding together in open space across the boundless black Heavens of Hell in a tornado-like spinning and whirling that propelled us towards the distant horizon. The surface of the earth remained far above us as we were whirled across the dark subterranean regions below.

But, on the other side, I felt panic-stricken in the same moments that I felt astonished at becoming the Devil. However, the fear did not reach the paralyzing consequences of outright anxiety, so that it was not necessary for me to withdraw from Katherine's vagina. And the anxiety quickly subsided as soon as I could cognitively recognize that my fear of the Devil was a clear legacy from my Christian-Puritan upbringing. My Logos intuitive faculty enabled me to face the forbiddenness of the vision for what it was and, furthermore, to eliminate the fear and continue with the archetypal experience. The latter could not have happened, however, without Katherine's help. She was expressing in unusually loud tones sensual sounds of delight that indicated she was enjoying my enhanced aggressiveness and primitive phallic thrusting deep into the bowels of her.

As soon as it was self-evident to me that she was indeed enjoying herself, I summoned my voice and called out to her with an attitude that was both playful and profound: "I feel like the Devil and I like it, and I want you to be the Devil's wife." She responded at the non-verbal level by immediately accelerating the rhythmical rolling and undulating of her pelvis and total body, and these accelerated sensual movements were accompanied by cries and groans of ecstasy that sounded louder and more uninhibited. She had always been extremely inhibited about emitting spontaneous sounds of delight during our lovemaking, so when I heard these unusually loud sounds of carnal pleasure coming forth from her this was all I needed to escalate our rite of initiation into Hell to its logical consummation, namely, one of the biggest and most explosive orgasms of my life !

I have never felt even slightly inclined to romanticize the figure of the Devil as some kind of a hero rebel, or ever wanted consciously to become like him. He represents for me too absolute an authoritarian phallic position of supreme power over another person to gain my esteem. He seems too heartless to me, although he can be a wise spokesman for Logos at best on some occasions. Christ for me is a much more appealing personification of self-actualizing virtues than the Devil. But Christ too has his faults. To be sure his virtues are tremendous. In his public life he radiated Agape, a dedication to spiritual soul values that distinguish a Spiritual Warrior, and the wisdom of the Hara-Logos soul polarity to be discussed in the next chapter. But he was a kind of innocent Prometheus who appealed to the worship of magic, mystery, and authority in the masses of people. And most importantly, he undersold the healing power of Eros and the Eros-Phallos libidinal circuit. I am sure that my own Promethean self-identity in the role of a dedicated psychotherapist was in part inspired by my incorporation of Christ into my unconscious psyche, and this did not change in the slightest when at the age of twenty-three I consciously repudiated the beliefs of the Christian faith.

I also have no doubts that it was basically a good thing that I could finally become the supreme negative archetype of Christianity, the Devil himself, within the context in which it happened: making sexual love to Katherine after living together for six years. It was a good thing because it permitted the further uprooting and dissolution of my previous fixation to the Puritan moral belief that a purely phallic aggressive taking of a woman sexually is both evil and forbidden. I have no doubts that becoming the Devil while making love to Katherine loosened any residues of repressed libidinal impulses that may have lingered over from my adolescent and young adult years, and consequently lowered if not completely extinguished any further inhibitions against asserting my primitive phallic libidinal capacity with Katherine. My passive-aggressive masochist character structure was also further undermined by my expression of pure phallic desire with an uninhibited lower back aggressiveness. This was evident from the way in which the ring of armoring that encompassed my lower back at the level of the anus retaliated vindictively for a period of several days after becoming the Devil and caused me much pain in the iliopsoas muscle complex innervating my groin.

Becoming the Devil with Katherine was also a positive achievement because it enabled me to affirm one new visage of Dionysus without freezing up into shame or sadistic domination but, to the contrary, infusing a sense of erotic fun and play into the lovemaking. I actively made her a co-partner who shared my phallic ecstasy as soon as I found the Logos-inspired voice to tell her verbally where I was and to invite her to participate with me in a new archetypal ritual of contact. Together, then, we advanced one step further along that road towards a death of the old, narrow Christian morality and an opening up of consciousness and soul towards the new, universal trans-Christian polytheistic morality of ancient religious cultures.

This brings me to the more detached reflective realization that becoming Pan was for my personal evolution along the path to self-actualizing functioning far more important and transformative than becoming the Devil. This is corroborated objectively by the hard and simple fact that my repressed need to become the Devil was fully satisfied after two experiences - the second experience happening a year later when the metamorphosis amused us more than jolted us to the foundations of our beings. In contrast, my becoming Pan occurred again and again and again an innumerable number of occasions spread over a period of at least six years.

How can we explain the striking discrepancy between the number of times I became the Devil and the number of times I became Pan before I could conclusively digest and assimilate each archetype as an intrinsic part of my ongoing core self? The most obvious initial answer is that Pan represented a part of my core self from which I was far more alienated than the Devil. I was far more alienated from my front half primary feeling needs than my back half ones, and Pan belongs more to the former and the Devil more to the latter. The Devil personifies the Great Anti-Christ, or Anti-Spiritual Warrior. He is a product of the Will, the pure Will to Conquer and Rebel, whereas Pan is a product of the Heart and a mediator of Love in the male, a spokesman of the anima.

This brings me to the somewhat astonishing revelation that the Christian emphasis upon a belief in the ultimacy of the polarity between the archetype of Christ and the archetype of the Devil rests upon a huge denial and distortion in consciousness of the fundamental importance of Eros and Hara to all personal religious experience. Christian belief and practice affirms exclusively the kind of spiritual love of God and others that I have hitherto referred to as Agape. This is a mode of love mediated more by the back half will centers than those of the front half, stemming as it does from a morality bent upon individual self-perfection and cerebralized spiritual purity. What has not been sufficiently appreciated even by the most enlightened and liberal-minded of contemporary Christians is the appalling extent to which Christianity unawarefully encourages both a repression and a distrust of the feeling capacities of Eros as much as Hara. The Christian unconscious is in fact heavily burdened by a masochistic fear of total surrender to anybody else but one's mentalized relationship with Christ and God-in-Christ. The Christian dichotomy between Christ and the Devil has so overinfiltrated our Western capitalist conscience and unconscious psyche that it has poisoned our belief in Eros and Hara, and in this latter sense it has given subtle support to a set of acquired perverse secondary needs to invalidate the sacred-profane religious ultimacy of intimate interpersonal human relationships. The Devil is in his psychodynamic grassroots the Supreme Shadow Archetype of Western Christianity whose hidden function is that of concealing the sacred-profane ultimacy of the universal Dionysian-Apollonian sexual polarity : the Eros-Phallos libidinal circuit. It follows that he and she who dares together, hand in hand, to pass through the gates of Hell will find Heaven on the other side !

To return to my personal experience, I was far less afraid of becoming the Devil than of becoming Pan. I was also far less afraid of perceiving the dark, satyr-like masculine side of Pan - the side mediated by my unsatisfied primitive phallic sexual desire - to be a repressed but intrinsic part of myself. Not until I had shed a good deal more of my character-muscular rigidities after I started living together with Katherine was it possible for me to begin to differentiate the other, more important and more repressed side of Pan within myself. For this same reason I could not share with Katherine a word about what was happening inside me whenever I became Pan during our first three years together! The feminine or anima side of Pan nearly terrorized me for its extreme openness and reverential-like surrender to Katherine's power. It was this surrender of my very heart and soul to her that freaked me out far more than any kind of surrender of my genital to hers. It is the more total surrender of one's very primary will centers that is what makes Eros so far more frightening to actualize than surrendering to a completed genital embrace and fusion during orgasm. The latter never requires a dissolution of the will centers in the back, whereas it is a precondition for the realization of the former.

The fact is that I needed to become Pan in order to discover what Eros is all about. I had to completely transcend the hero figures of our Christian culture in order to explore how to do this. This relates to the illuminating recognition that our Western Judaic-Christian traditions are latently organized against the religious essence of one human being worshipping another human being, particularly when that other is of the opposite sex! The unconscious fear of sexuality - what Reich called pleasure-anxiety so justly - goes less against the grain of our Western consciousness today than the fear of total individual obliteration that envelopes one whenever one loves from one's heart and consummates that love with one's Eros-Phallos libidinal circuits. Yet this is the hidden, long-range goal of the creative regression-disintegration process described in this book. To say it another way, that goal is to learn how to worship, adore, and become one with one's beloved at the same time during sexual lovemaking. It is Eros, and not primitive Phallos, Agape, or Logos, that mediates this supremely sacred-profane but holy-of-holies event, and orthodox Christianity and orthodox Judaism would rather we never found this out!

There prevails throughout our Western consciousness to this day a taboo against regressive dedifferentiation of one's individual boundaries of egoic identity. This is doubly true of the male ego than of the female ego. This taboo distils essentially down to a fear of succumbing to the two Being centers in the front half of the organism. The male ego's fear of this yielding is directed as much inwards towards his own front half primary feeling centers as it is directed outwards towards those of his primary sexual partner.

In my own case it took me eight years of becoming various embodiments of Dionysus and she a Great Positive Mother Queen-Goddess before I could accept the numinous archetypal bliss and wisdom of total regressive dedifferentiation of my back half will centers. I actively fought losing my will centers for eight years because my Western consciousness, reinforced by the anti-libidinal super-ego of my character-muscular armoring, could not permit Katherine to become the protectively nurturing container of my embodied soul and Beingness and I the contained one. I felt too profoundly threatened to the deepest foundations of my Being at the prospect of losing myself in mystical sacred-profane interpenetration with her. Yet until I could accept this most sacred of all communion of the natural opposite forces in the universe - a man and a woman - I could not become transfigured into my own godhood or Holy Ghost within.

The fascinating thing is that once I gave up this struggle within myself, I ceased to need to identify with the archetypal figure of Pan, or any of the other faces of Dionysus, and now I can allow my own embodied intuitive soul faculty of Eros to guide me during our sexual lovemaking. I no longer need the unconscious creativity of my primitive brain stem and its Apollonian invention of archetypal images to guide me into the sweet love-death of passional Uroboric fusion. Now I can remain centered within my four intuitive soul faculties and their moment-by-moment polarization of each other internally. I am saying here that once I gave up struggling from my egoic cortico-cerebrospinal circuits against the inevitable descent into the dedifferentiated blood-consciousness of my lower half below the diaphragm during lovemaking I no longer needed my primitive unconscious to act as a mediator between the cortex and the viscera. I can go with and fully accept the regressive disintegration that a progressive fusion of one's endodermal core self with the endodermal core self of one's beloved necessarily terminates in.

Passional Uroboric fusion is not to be confused with a giving up and a kind of betrayal or sacrificing of one's masculine identity. I have deliberately excluded from this chapter describing those countless occasions while making love to Katherine when it was I who became the worshipped one and she the worshipping one. Whenever this happened it was I who was the protectively potent container of her and she the contained one. She would then project onto me some archetypal image of a Lord-God-Great Positive Father Figure who was also her very phallic male beloved. This would usually happen during our pre-genital rites of initiation prior to my entering her vagina with my penis. However, whenever I did enter her, regardless of what particular archetypal rite we might have been immersed in, from the moment I would enter her it would always be my phallus that became the dominant energetic source of enhanced endodermal blood flow. My entering of her would almost instantly dissolve whatever archetypal projections that had existed before entering her, and these projections would be replaced by a more human-centered and totally here-and-now embodied enjoyment of the organismic totality of each other, including the ectodermal and mesodermal layers as much as the endodermal. Once my phallus began aggressively polarizing her vagina from inside it is as if we become transformed together, indistinguishable from each other, into a perfectly balanced unitary fountain of flow, she being neither greater in potency or psychological dynamism than I, nor I greater in potency or psychological dynamism than her. We both become reduced to two halfs, equal in every respect, of a single two-in-one mandala-like circle of pulsating undifferentiated flow in which the final orgasm unfolds with or without dramatic overtones.

Armored, egoic masculine man has yet to fully confront how much he fears and defends himself actively against seeing or accepting the naturally greater superior magnetic energy field of woman's front half. Her ability to generate from her endodermal depths a magnetic field of vital energy flow than can reach out horizontally across the empty space that separates her from her beloved and draw him to her body irresistibly tends to threaten the great majority of males more than is generally acknowledged. Yet until he can risk yielding to her superior horizontal magnetism, he cannot let go long enough of his own egoic self-identity and its close affinity with the will centers of his back half to begin to obtain a glimpse of the instinctual power of Eros within. He needs her superior and more natural groundedness in Eros and Hara to guide him towards these same feeling capacities and soul faculties within himself.

Until he can bring himself to risk trusting his beloved's greater front half flow not to take advantage of her more powerful position when he becomes opened to her, he has no possibility, I submit, for ever discovering the boundarylessness of passional, archetypal lovemaking. When women love their man from their Eros center as distinct from their cerebralized love-will, whether Christian or Judaic in background, they do indeed possess both the soul power and libidinal magnetism to become metamorphosed or simply elevated to the position of Queens, Goddesses of various kinds, Great Positive or Terrible Mother Creations, or erotic sirens. The primitive unconscious of the male will imbue them with such pre-eminence once the horizontally polarized vital contact between them is established. Men must learn to trust their women unconditionally during the most vulnerable stages of pregenital lovemaking when the descent out of the cortex is actively taking place. If they do, they can be reassured that once they arrive at the genital stage itself, after he has entered her with his phallus, he will have the power once again available to him to bring about through his phallus a sublimely just equalization and harmonization of their endodermal imbalances of magnetic flow. His greater vertical energy flow up and down his back half will beautifully, spontaneously counterbalance her greater horizontal energy flow up and down her front half.

Chapter XII

THE FIVE UNIFYING POLARITIES OF THE CORE SELF

I. The Deeper Significance of the Four Stages of Creative Disintegration

The four stages of creative disintegration are not ends-in-themselves. Rather, they represent indispensable transitions to the emergence of an enduring personality structure. Ecstatic visionary experiences of Pagan Eros infused with Libido represent a way station along the long journey to wholeness.

Each of the four stages of creative disintegration facilitates the movement out of neurotically split modes of functioning. They are distinct stages of partial death and rebirth of the personality structure. After the neurotic passes through each of these stages, the five unifying polarities of the core self begin to emerge. And it is these polarities which make possible a relatively stabilized psycho-organismic structure which possesses end-state Being and Substance.

The core self is distinguishable by its integrated differentiation of functioning. It possesses continuity, unity, solidity -- qualities unavailable to the defended egoic nucleus as it passes through the four stages of creative disintegration. The core self is synonymous with what Jung calls the inner self. It is composed of both transcendental and embodied soul aptitudes. Its penchant for maintaining a centrally internalized stability keeps it allied with the conservatively self-preservative inclinations of Great Mother Nature. In short, the core self is distinguishable for its individuated integration, not its facility for creative disintegration.

Before describing the nature of the core self, I will render a religious interpretation of the deeper significance of the four stages of creative disintegration: 1) primaling, 2) the feeling discovery of the primary unsatisfied feeling needs for relatedness within the endodermal depths, 3) the anxiety-ridden encounter with the daemonic and shadow aspects of the collective unconscious, and 4) the sacred-profane religious-mystical fulfillment of Yin-Yang lovemaking between an unarmored man and an unarmored woman.

Five distinct categories of personality change occur during the four stages of creative disintegration: 1) cognitive-perceptual, 2) modification in the hierarchy of values, 3) changes in the boundaries of inner and outer worlds, 4) bioenergetic changes, and 5) changes in the psychodynamics of the personality structure and psyche.

1. <u>The Cognitive-Perceptual Changes</u>

The cognitive-perceptual changes occur as the total organism becomes the essential agent of perception, thus surpassing the modes of cognition structured in the isolated mind-brain. The movement is away from an analytical dissection towards a mode of perception which is richly felt throughout the organismic totality and gradually distills into a single intuitive essence. In other words, the emerging cognitive perception is influenced by the creative unconscious far more than by mental consciousness. Not only can this level of consciousness make higher syntheses of heterogeneous elements, it can execute the synthesis largely outside of rationally focused consciousness.

This mode of perception interpenetrates the five senses, the creative imagination, and the natural instincts. Gradually, these three distinct spheres of cognition converge upon the perceived object. The convergence is mediated by the endodermal depths of the longitudinal energy flow. The endodermal depths provide the root of the whole synthesizing process, enabling a perception of others, oneself in relation to others, and certain human social situations as Divinely transfigured and imbued with Holiness. The creative unconscious is a kind of sophisticated blood-consciousness, if you will. It penetrates to the essence of an object or situation to establish a structured core-to-core contact through the intuitive concentration of the Logos faculty.

An individuated adult who passes through the four disintegrative stages becomes able to cognitively apperceive reality both in terms of its sensory-motoric aesthetic immediacy and, alternatingly, in terms of its synthesized Apollonian intuitive essences. For example, when I see the pristine beauty of Katherine's face in its bare visual configuration, I sometimes feel within myself the enormous spiritual and animal vitality glowing from within her, especially through her bottomless eyes. On certain occasions, I recognize a timelessly serene goddess composed of eternally feminine human elements, whereas on other occasions, I see a mountain lioness with a long sensuous back and the fire of desire exuding forth.

2. Modifications in the Hierarchy of Values

The modifications in one's solitary hierarchy of values is the religious dimension in its most intrinsic form. The heart of religious experience is the metamorphosis from an outer-directed, egoically struggling and survival-motivated mode of valuing to one which is instinct-directed, soul-sustaining and transpersonally growth-motivated. The dominant ego's adaptive orientation to the outer world is always either compulsively deficiency-motivated or conquest driven. Such drives prevent real contact, either at the level of aesthetic immediacy or of the objectification of intuitive essences. The same is true for the average man's so-called religious commitments and sentiments because they are completely prescribed and structured by the social milieu of collective mental consciousness. Beliefs, injunctions and faiths are adopted without the creative discernment of Logos or any kind of internalized instinctual valuing process. Hence, they comprise a valueless valuing process because they occur exclusively within the boundaries of the cerebralized collective consciousness.

Such is the prevailing valuing process in our Western religions. The hidden goal is absolute conformity to the group. With the exception of mysticism, Western religious movements incorporate a massive and deceptive brainwashing. They do not guide the individual down into the unconscious creative depths of Logos, Hara, Agape-Eros, or the Spiritual-Phallic Warrior. Rather, their movement is up and out into the social realms of group allegiance, family obligation, national-cultural identifications, and materialistic prosperity for group members. Hence moral motivation remains superficial and always group-dictated.

By contrast, individuated religious depth begins as a movement downwards into the primary-process-regulated front and lower halves of the human organism. This descent must precede the emergence of the core self. Western religious beliefs have an unmistakable bias in favor of the intellectually illuminated psyche as the proper locus of spiritual values. Consequently, they neglect what I call the embodied soul as the intrinsic source of spirituality. And it is the pagan Apollonian and Dionysian Gods and Goddesses of ancient religions and Eastern religions which alone can claim the sacred function of liberating the figure of Christ as the grand inquisitor of humanity.

Perhaps it is for this very reason that the four stages of creative disintegration lead gradually to the emergence of the light and the dark Gods and Goddesses within. Because of our Western enculturation, they represent the most repressed parts of our soul. Therefore, they cannot enter fully into consciousness until the armoring has reached its final stages of dissolution. A greater mobilization of vital energy flow must be awakened before these repressed instinctual psychic forces can be actively polarized before consciousness. I have not made an arbitrary hypothesis that numinously imbued sacred-profane lovemaking between an unarmored man and an unarmored woman brings the dearmoring process to the very threshold of a higher individuated wholeness. Such lovemaking presupposes a richness and vitality of embodied soul-power that can bring about a meeting of the most supreme spiritual opposites -- masculinity and femininity at the level of the embodied collective unconscious.

The ultimate spiritual polarity is masculinity and femininity. Therefore, an awakening of almost any constellation of the four intuitive soul-powers of the creative unconscious (Logos, Hara, Agape-Eros and the Spiritual-Phallic Warrior) involves some sort of polarization of the masculine and feminine intrapsychic dimensions within each individual. We shall call this phenomenon the hierosgamos principle of Yin-Yang complementarity. I personally believe the core self is essentially founded upon this principle. Jung was the first to recognize this principle at the crux of the medieval alchemical vision of human wholeness: the union of opposites in a single image. What Jung depicts as the sacred quarternity of wholeness is best understood as the balanced integration of the four intuitive soul-powers of the creative unconscious. In other words, it is not pagan-profane lovemaking which alone reflects the sacred ultimacy of the Yin-Yang complementarity. It is reflected in every core-to-core spiritual or final feeling instinctual contact between a self-actualizing adult and some objective reality.

Once a person becomes almost fully dearmored and fully individuated, his or her capacity for totality of investment spontaneously polarizes at least two of the four primary dynamic energy fields which mediate the four intuitive soul-powers. It now becomes possible to experience on occasion end-state religious experiences which are much quieter and emptier than those described during archetypal sexual lovemaking at the end of the last chapter. For example, the whole range of end-state religious experiences that the Eastern religions describe in terms of various paths towards enlightenment which bring us to various kinds of unbounded fusion with the cosmos as a unitary whole represent for me the consequence of a slow but sure awakening of the Hara-Logos spiritual circuit within the embodied soul. The majority of our own patients and trainees who have arrived at advanced stages of both dearmoring and higher individuation have been propelled by inner instinctual necessity to allow themselves to surrender to religious experiences guided by their Hara-Logos circuit.

Many different modalities of subject-world religious experience become possible, as I shall outline in the next section. They all hold in common a paradoxical hierosgamos quality, by virtue of the temporary union of spiritual opposites. But more importantly perhaps, they all have in common the crystallization of a numinously felt pleasureable fusion and communion between the core self and the objectified universe. A sacred experience occurs whenever a spiritual-passional communion is established between the core self and some other part of the natural universe, and this communion is differentiated into individuated and transpersonal meaning.

I am allying myself here with the occidental nature romanticists of the past and present, with the more sophisticated and less freakish psychedelic-enlightened hippies of our modern Aquarian age, with the quest for humanistic understanding and fulfillment which typified the medieval alchemists, with the practices and symbolism of the various mystery religions of ancient Greece and the Middle East, with certain practices and traditions of the Far East, especially Tantra Yoga in the Indian Vedic system and Zen Buddhism in the Chinese and Japanese traditions, and, finally, with the more pantheistic of the Western Christian mystics.

3. <u>Changes in the Boundaries of Inner and Outer Worlds</u>

The process of progressive creative disintegration gradually annihilates the tightly constricted boundaries of self-identity which characterize the neurotically defended ego. As the id-dimensions of the psyche begin to dominate consciousness, the horizons of a tenable psychic identity become wider and deeper. The neurotically-infested Freudian rendering of the secondary-process reality principle gives way to increasingly id-like boundaryless states.

For example, the catastrophic shock of primaling produces a total withdrawal from both inner and outer worlds. Truly spontaneous primals bring the first glimpse of what it means to live totally in the present moment of felt immediacy. They reduce the boundaries of subjective identity to the most primitively dedifferentiated perimeters possible. Utterly immersed in the present moment of organismic catastrophic shock, the subject becomes disconnected from both the felt living past and the anticipated future. Everything seems to stop as the usual boundaries between inner and outer worlds become obliterated. However, if not truly spontaneous, primals merely become another clever maneuver on the part of the compliant patient to convince himself and his therapist that he is reexperiencing childhood trauma, and his cerebralized self is hiddenly resonating to the unconscious and conscious wishes of the therapist.

During the three subsequent stages of creative disintegration, consciousness begins to open. Consciousness becomes filled, but never overwhelmed, with intensely alive archaic feelings as the uncompleted past presses upwards for recognition. The discovery of each one of our unsatisfied primary feeling needs is like a river pouring through a narrow channel which has been wedged in the defended ego. As the mesódermal walls of the closed cerebro-spinal circuit are broken through at certain points, they become significantly weaker, yet not destroyed. And, as the vital currents flow back from above to their origins, the egoic boundaries of self-identity loosen to the extent of plunging the client into dissociative or highly regressed and scattered states of being. As the familiar boundaries crumble, time past and time present become intertwined during the equalization process. The disorientation of chaos reigns until the ego's defenses can resume dominance, although less effectively than before.

The further opening of consciousness to the archetypal depths continues to destroy the chronic egoic tension between inner and outer worlds. Altered states of consciousness become substantially real for the first time in a neurotic's life. These altered states have enough form and vividness to prevent the defended ego from discounting them as sheer phantasy. In other words, instinctually-charged synthetic images replace the vague feelings which characterize the second stage of disintegration. Focal consciousness and the repressed unconscious become polarized in the psychodynamic process. This process partially explains the emergence of a synthesized image in the form of a collective archetypal symbol. Although still elusive, these archetypal symbols are so loaded with damned up vegetative energy that they at first express themselves in a largely undecipherable fashion during dreams and waking phantasies. However, as the armoring dissolves further, they are eventually identified and lived out at the embodied expressive interpersonal level.

I am convinced that as the vegetative blood flow infiltrates every cell and muscle grouping of the total organism, the psyche becomes compelled to descend into the impersonal cultural and phylogenetic past as part of the animal-spiritual equalization process. The more fully we can for brief periods obliterate the boundaries which maintain a rational, coping ego, the more we are able to penetrate the barriers which divide modern socialized man from his ancestors, both human and animal.

The descent into the front and lower halves of the organism continues as a regressive descent backwards in time which transcends the usual constricted boundaries of time and place. The regressive lure towards the ancestral past is a lure towards a greater internal unity between inner and outer universes. Then one's identity becomes simpler, more whole, more natural and more innocent in substance and structure. Such are the numinous psychic qualities mediated by the instinct-regulated embodied soul.

In contrast, the qualities mediated by the transcendental psyche are more complexly individuated. When the two realms come together in one archetypal experience, differentiated Divinity within and without is realized. With this experience, we pass beyond the third stage of creative disintegration to discover the transformative rebirthing process that accompanies regressive descents into ancestral rituals and patterns of interpersonal relating.

The final stage of creative disintegration is far more metaphysically significant than an ecstatic Yin-Yang sexual coupling. It enables an individuated person to totally surpass the armored mesodermal boundaries which are so imperative to life in a modern Western urban-technological socity which is soulless, machine-dominated, nature-alienated, and patriarchal. As described in the previous chapter, Katherine's and my fusion with the totality of the natural universe represents a kind of religious transcendence of the limitations and imbalances inherent in our modern Western culture and society. The patterns of interaction created between us were too apocalyptically Dionysian, too universally intrinsic, too profanely but profoundly passional-sacred, and too pristinely God-like to be reconcilable with modern Western life dominated by grim survival realities.

Regressive descents into ancient myths and archetypal rituals permit us to actualize at the embodied level of waking interpersonal contact the transcendent function -- Jung's name for the higher balancing function between consciousness and unconscious instinctual need-tendencies. This function serves to counterbalance the overdeveloped excesses of one's contemporary culture and society. A higher law of compensation enables the psychodynamic polarities of the core self to affirm any soul-faculties which have been either underdeveloped or totally ignored due to the pressures of the culture and society.

For example, through archetypal lovemaking with

Katherine I discovered how to creatively disintegrate my neurotically Promethean will by affirming my underdeveloped Eros and primitive Phallic Warrior dimensions simultaneously. The awakening of the latter spiritual polarity had the power to dissolve the last remaining remnants of chronic armoring which kept me from realizing my own Godhood within. My back half core faculties were still too chronically dominant. Therefore they could only be extinguished by a total submission of my will-power before a power totally alien from myself and will-less in its essential nature. Hence the turning point was when I could totally surrender to Katherine in the form of a Great Mother Goddess. This surrender had nothing to do with a repressed desire to make love to my real mother, or even with a wish to regress to childhood and obtain from Katherine a sensual satisfaction of my unsatisfied primary need for maternal love. As a very young child I was in fact deeply loved and contained by my real mother.

Different people may well enact a whole gamut of archetypal rituals which emerge in accordance with this higher law of spiritual-animal-cultural compensation. For example, if one has already actualized his primitive Phallic Warrior-Eros polarity, he may well discover his Agape-mediated core-to-core contact with the integrated Sophia-like animus of his beloved woman - a much quieter, less libidinalized mode of relating - to be his way to actualize his own inner Godhood. Or in discovering the enormous gulf between the masculinity and femininity of essential Beingness, he might become more softly incarnated as an ascetic Divinity which reflects Hara, Logos, or the Spiritual Warrior, such as God the Father, Moses, Jesus Christ, or Sir Galahad. In place of fiery sexual ecstasy, the experience might be a Logos-to-Logos interpersonal relating which permits the Western focal consciousness to assume priority. Once again, the transcendent function of spiritual-animal-cultural compensation would facilitate an instinctual movement towards wholeness and completion. The perfection tendencies of the individuated soul operate in a mysterious, half-conscious or largely unconscious manner.

In summary, the creatively regressive descent inwards and downwards towards the endodermal regions of the core self catalyzes a progressive destruction of the ongoing boundaries of embodied identity as maintained by the voluntary musculature of the mesodermal layer. Leaving our conventional will and musculature behind, we become transported down into the center of the natural universe. We even shatter all familiar boundaries which maintain a constant tension between inner and outer worlds. And if we are fortunate as Yin-Yang lovers, we surrender to direct touch which enables a magnetic pull of the blood to merge us in oceanic Uroboric wholeness.

Uroboric wholeness is the final beatific experience of creatively disintegrative regression. Thereafter, both lovers intuitively know how to reparent themselves by calling upon the Divine Mother and Divine Father within the other and within oneself. They no longer need a parental substitue outside of themselves to find inner wholeness. All they need is each other as embodied soul-powers waiting to be resonated with according to the need of the moment. The experience of oceanic Uroboric wholeness through the embodied presence and Being of the other reconciles the lovers with all of humanity, past and present. It provides ultimate containment within the natural universe.

4. Bioenergetic Changes

Since the many bioenergetic changes which underlie the creative disintegration process have been accentuated throughout this book, I will merely summarize them at this point.

From a bioenergetic perspective, primaling thoroughly jolts the congealed character-muscular armoring. For a few brief moments, it violently uproots the chronic split between the two antagonistic energy networks, the cortico-spinal and the vegetative. The result is a primary-process equalization of the impasse between them. Of necessity, consciousness cannot acknowledge the impasse itself. It can only register the fleeting harmony which follows the shake-up.

Underlying the chaos attending the discovery of the unsatisfied primary feeling needs is the gradual dissolution of pockets of static energy encapsulated within the mesodermal musculature. The chaos is not generated by sudden breakthroughs into repressed affects or quantities of previously encapsulated energy. Rather, the chaos results as an aftereffect of such breakthroughs upon the energy economy. Each breakthrough is followed by a period of dearmoring which in turn is followed by a period of rearmoring. The transition between these two periods involves an energetic metamorphosis between a world-open convergence-equalization patterning and a closed, imploded charge-discharge patterning. This subsequent reversal of the energy patterns is responsible for the tremendous confusion, ambivalence, loss of identity, and anxiety at the psychic level. This is partially because the energetic metamorphosis produces a dichotomous splitting of the perceived objective reality. The afflicted perceiver views the same reality from an opposite perspective and with a totally irreconcilable difference of attitude.

Only when the convergence-equalization patterning becomes stable enough to prevent retrogression to an imploded charge-discharge energy pattern can the neurotic find the sustained focal concentration of consciousness to allow him to establish real contact with his internal world. And then, as the tendency towards energetic equalization grows progressively stronger, more and more channels of internal energetic discharge increasingly open. This process eventually enables the core longitudinal energy currents to polarize by way of the blood flow the dormant archetypal knowledge located in the primitive brain stem. Then, for the first time, the neurotic can explore from a feeling level of differentiated consciousness the personally uncompleted past, and later, move into the transpersonal realms.

As the Hara-Logos polarity emerges, the core self becomes able to sustain an internally differentiated balancing of the various excesses of Apollonian and Dionysian consciousness, as well as of the various spiritual polarities. Even the archetypal revelations which distinguish the fourth stage of creative disintegration become admissible to the integrated core self only to the extent that they can be assimilated into the ongoing personality structure by the Hara-Logos polarity. This polarity functions as the wise reconciler of every differentiated subject-world encounter. Usually, apocalyptic or mystical experiences of archetypal revelation continue to occur during the third stage of treatment, the stage of higher individuation. However, such experiences occur less frequently, less dramatically, and with a greater inner centeredness. Furthermore, they are more evenly balanced between rational awareness and unconscious possession as compared to those which happen during the advanced phases of the dearmoring process. Because they now have surpassed any need to release repressed psychic material, they lose much of their frightening intensity and paradoxical form.

Even more than the crystallization of Logos, the emergence of Hara is the development which guarantees a self-actualizing life which contains peace, unity, and simplicity. Now it becomes possible for a person to obtain natural spiritual pleasure from states of being characterized by minimal energy mobilization and dedifferentiated emptiness. This arises from the greater plasticity and motility of endodermal energy flow which becomes available to the self-actualizing adult during Hara-dominant states of dedifferentiated emptiness of Being. Stillness in the silence of one's solitude can now bring the most supreme but quietly fulfilling reveries, insight, and feelings of well-being as Logos and Hara play and interpenetrate with each other.

5. <u>Changes in the Psychodynamics of the Personality Structure and Psyche</u>

The transformation of the enduring personality structure that results from the passage through the four stages of creative disintegration is the emergence of the core self. Critical to this emergence is the slow crystallization of the Hara-Logos circuit. This crystallization process occurs primarily during the third stage of personality change after the four stages of creative disintegration have been completed.

The slow crystallization of the Hara-Logos polarity runs parallel to the gradually increasing third-stage capacity to find as much intrinsic value and fulfillment in energetic equalization as in energetic mobilization. This same development parallels the natural aging process in terms of years. The more the capacity for energetic mobilization and equalization becomes centered in the endodermal layer, the less necessary it is to mobilize large quantities of energy for experiences of creative encounter. This is because the blood-mediated circulation of the core longitudinal energy currents remains core-centered and facilitates an embodied soul grounding that is in constant circulation between the endodermal, mesodermal, and ectodermal layers.

This is particularly the case with the crystallization of either side of the Hara-Logos polarity. The emergence of essence-making Logos as an intuitive faculty of individuated cognition requires but the smallest quantities of energy mobilization. This capacity is closely affiliated with the subtle synergizing capacities of the cerebral cortex, while only distantly allied with the gross world of action. Similarly, the emergence of harmony-bearing Hara requires even less mobilization of biological energy. Its cultivation presupposes a continuously dedifferentiated state of equalization throughout the endodermal depths. This state is noteworthy for its absence of any kind of energetic mobilization or differentiated encounter with the outer world.

Hara-Logos revelations and feelings rise up aimlessly from the creative unconscious. They reflect an already assimilated set of data gained from encounters with objective novelty under the tutelage of the other intuitive faculties. Hara becomes their final vessel, not the mind-brain. Like a gigantic, slow-moving whirlpool, Hara draws the differentiations of objective novelty back inside itself, magnetically absorbing the fruits into its bottomless embrace. It reconciles the various possible conflicts betwen Agape-Eros, Logos, and the Spiritual-Phallic Warrior by incorporating them into its inexhaustible receptivity.

The other side of this sublime receptivity is a wise non-attachment to the conflicting forces absorbed. Hara is extremely self-protective in the most profound meaning of the term. Especially when polarized with Logos, Hara has the power to keep a person rooted within his soul rather than fixated to superficial realities. Logos provides the boundaries and rationale by which to keep the outer world separated off in consciousness. More unconsciously, Hara keeps one's attention centered on the internal frame of reference. When balanced and in harmony within the same circuit, Hara-Logos states of being permit a rational-irrational self-regulation which remains independent of all objective realities except the threat to survival. Even one's sexual mate becomes temporarily non-existent.

II. The Five Important Psychodynamic Polarities of Higher Individuation

During the third stage of treatment, the stage of higher individuation, the various spiritual polarities become differentiated into distinct personal traits of adult character. This development entails a fresh reorganization between the vegetative endodermal flow and the cortex-regulated central nervous system. During this reorganization, the two energy networks become congruently matched, especially during periods of creative subject-world encounter with inner or outer universes.

Higher individuation in my understanding revolves around living out all the important spiritual polarities at some time or another. For this reason there must be a flexible dialectical balance established between both poles which can easily evolve and just as easily dissolve, to be replaced by the dominance of one of the other spiritual polarities. Since the primordial psychodynamic polarity is between masculinity and femininity, a man must find his anima, or Agape-Eros and Hara capacities, and interiorize them in dialectical balance with his naturally dominant back half masculine soul-powers. Similarly, a woman must find her animus within, or Logos and Spiritual-Phallic Warrior capacities, and interiorize them in dialectical balance with her naturally dominant front half feminine soul-powers.

The masculine/feminine polarity is biologically and archetypally predetermined at birth. It is different from the individually created instinctual-spiritual polarities of the core self. The same is true of the primary-process-autocentric versus the secondary-process-allocentric polarity. It, too, is largely predetermined by virtue of the fact that man is half animal and half spiritual in his essential constitution. The primary-process-autocentric pole is closely bound to the animal side, while the secondary-process-allocentric pole is closely linked with the spiritual side. This polarity must also become dialectically balanced during any individuated creative encounter, regardless of which of the five polarities is dominant. The same holds true for the polarity between Being-in-the-World and Being-for-Oneself. The individuated adult learns to incorporate all three of these predetermined polarities into every one of his core-self-mediated experiences.

Finally, the actualization of each creative act of becoming can best be defined in terms of its internal movement towards unification between each side of the five core polarities. Self-actualizing creative acts always involve a dialectic of movement from total indeterminacy through a middle phase of meeting of opposites towards terminal unity of process and satisfaction. Therefore, both ends of any single polarity do not move in dichotomous opposition or negation. A creative tension and balanced interpenetration of both poles is always maintained when creative encounter develops.

We turn now to these five polarities. Each mediates the foundations for a complex constellation of personalized virtues, abilities and idiosyncracies of character.

1. <u>The Self-Assertive-Self-Surrendering Polarity</u>

The self-assertive-self-surrendering polarity defines the degree of dynamic psychological health and fluidity of balanced responsiveness in any individual. It serves as a dialectical centering of will needs and love needs. Self-assertive tendencies express the healthy volitional need for freedom, self-determination and autonomy. In contrast, self-surrendering tendencies express the healthy need for pleasurable sympathetic contact, meeting, and fusion with others.

This polarity defines whether a creative act of becoming reflects a movement towards separateness from or a movement towards fusion with something outside of oneself. They are spiritual dialectical opposites in the same way that the back half need-tendencies and the front half need-tendencies are vital psychodynamic opposites.

For example, an individuated adult may move from a position of initial indeterminate openness to a stranger to one of progressive withdrawal from and even active opposition. In this case, the individual withdraws from the sympathetic feeling vibrations in his front half towards the other. The withdrawal is enabled by a retreat from the centrifugal circulation of soft, fluid, blood-dominant energy currents moving in the front half of the body. Concurrently, the back half of the body hardens to stiffen the will in polarized opposition to any continued contact with the stranger. The hardening is determined by an uppacing and temporary rigidification of the energy currents moving up and down the spinal column in the mesodermal and ectodermal layers. Despite the desire for separateness, the compassionate individuated soul cannot so totally withdraw from his front half sympathetic need-tendencies to establish a hostile barrier against the stranger. Therefore, he allows his Logos and Spiritual Warrior faculties to interact sagaciously with the stranger just long enough to relinquish him.

This is an extremely simplified example of how this polarity is always in operation in human relationships. When this polarity dominates, a creative encounter can crystallize through the guidance of Eros that permits a wise balancing of positive and negative responses to another human being. Such a balancing is both spontaneous and deliberate. Nevertheless, it is essentially facilitated by the back-half soul-powers and the front-half soul-powers finely balanced in relationship to each other as much as to the other person.

Another way of describing this polarity is to see it in terms of a control over oneself and others, on the one hand, and a surrendering of any control over oneself and others on the other hand. The more one moves towards surrender, the greater the mobilization of sympathetic vibrations emanating from the front half of the organism which reach out to actively resonate with the alien Being of the other person. Moreover, the resonance arises from an attitude of letting the other be just as he is. Subsequently, a pleasurable reciprocity becomes possible. In the place of willful opposition, non-manipulative caring for the other person may slowly evolve. Love has many different forms, but if authentic, all are front-half dominant. Nothing is more insidiously destructive to real love than the willed love of the idealized egoic self-image. It emanates from the volitional centers in the back under the rigid control of the closed cerebrospinal circuit.

2. <u>The Agape-Eros-Spiritual-Phallic Warrior Polarity</u>

One side of this polarity is the spontaneous immersion in a carefree, child-like enjoyment of living reality from moment to moment. Such naive freshness of appreciation of the living moment is the quintessence of the anima in man, and the eternal youth in both man and woman. The other end of the polarity is a disciplined and purposeful engagement of the other at an adult level of responsible confrontation. Such is the quintessence of the Spiritual-Phallic Warrior. The Warrior represents a secondary-process, masculine seriousness of orientation. Thus, soft, light, innocent sharing of the Puer Eternus in us stands in polar opposition to the somber piety and heaviness of the Spiritual Warrior, which reflects the more heroic aspects of our nature. The latter only functions well when a task requires a dense concentration of will, energy and determination in the face of uncertainty.

This is the polarity of extroverted depth and happiness since both poles are primarily outer world directed, but when interpenetrated, they always succeed in achieving the goals being sought after. When the poles are balanced, they make things happen in the immediate environment with optimal perfection and competency of execution. Our modern Western civilization was founded and continues to thrive upon this polarity of self-actualization. It has enabled us to conquer the threats of an indifferent natural environment, but more importantly, transform creatively the social and cultural horizons around us.

This is the Westernized individual growth polarity par excellence. At the higher individuation stage, its dominance propels a person to expand his horizons of communal influence and to actively continue to perfect and evolve all of his positive virtues. This polarity motivates us to continually open ourselves to unknown novelties in the interest of expanding our boundaries of world identifications. It gives us the active phallic desire and moral courage to face the boundless possibilities that life holds each day and to embrace the adventure of pursuing the exciting and the challenging for its own sake.

Given such properties, it is not surprising that this polarity requires an enormous generation and long-term sustaining of spiritual energy. The best character traits of most Americans and Europeans hinge upon the actualization of the action-centered, pragmatically effective, and, at the same time, joy-affirmative capacities embodied in this polarity. This explains why Americans in particular possess so many youthful and perpetually self-renewing characteristics -- an immense reservoir of vitality, a tremendous drive to accomplish tasks which other cultures perceive as superhuman, an earnest investment in immediate happenings which spontaneously arise from moment to moment. Anyone who believes in the primacy of action, as Americans instinctively do, tends to cultivate the character traits centered in this polarity. But it is not until the eternal child and struggling adult hero find within a profound adjustment to each other can there emerge a quality of extrovertedness that is truly self-actualizing, even for the most charming and successful self-made American or European.

3. The Hara-Logos Polarity

The Hara-Logos spiritual polarity is the polarity of quietude and introversion. It functions as the great guardian of continuing wholeness of the core self. It provides the locus for a self-actualizing person's innermost citadel of creative death and rebirth during periods of absolute solitude. This polarity usually does not crystallize until the third stage of treatment because it embodies some of the most complexly individuated and feared dimensions of higher functioning for the former neurotic. The fear arises from the fact that the Hara side of the polarity is the furthest removed in substance and process from the structuring activities of rational consciousness.

Even the Logos side of the polarity is removed from rational consciousness, but Hara is thricefold more so. The genius of Logos is its capacity to synthesize conscious and unconscious elements in the midst of forming a concrescent creative encounter with objective novelty. But it is in between such encounters, when chaos or emptiness and a total absence of structure prevails, that Hara always returns the soul to undifferentiated states of diffuse and labyrinthine modes of being. Hara returns the soul to a Buddha-like fertile void in order to dismantle the rational brain and the modern outer world's demands for a constant tendency towards dominance. Only the Hara-Logos circuit, when allied along a continuum of spiritually enlightened emptiness and desirelessness, has the potency to maintain an inner thread of continuity by which the embodied soul can thrive as an internally stable entity. All self-actualizing Mothers know what I am talking about instinctually. Maintenance of an inner fertile void is our most trustworthy source of a quiet and relatively self-perpetuating contentment.

Western man in general is severely threatened by this polarity -- especially those Westerners who live primarily an extroverted, outer-directed life style, like the majority of American males. The American male has been brought up to believe that only his intellect harnessed to his will to achieve in the outer world can provide any kind of ongoing contentment and emotional security. Modern technology, industry and science have moulded this mistaken illusion. It is an illusion because it largely, if not wholly, dismisses the priority of safeguarding the instinctual-spiritual imperative for solitude and doing nothing in order to maintain any sense of inner peace and identity. The action-dominant extrovert has a horror of falling into undifferentiated feeling states which are characterized by a sense of formlessness, emptiness, quietude, and absolute passivity. The typical American male and female finds it utterly self-annihilating to spend as few as six hours alone in total solitude while doing nothing in the way of productively coping outer world activities. To do nothing threatens to plunge him or her into interior spaces and nebulous introverted states that have a frighteningly menacing significance. I have known very few American men or women who could remain inside themselves long or deeply or free floating enough to discover any of the multitudinous jewels of the Hara-Logos polarity.

I have found that only the centered, dedicated artist in the Western world knows how to drop out of the outer world long enough to attune himself to the Hara-Logos polarity's unique capacity for contemplative fulfillment and the generation of intuitively inspired revelations that surface into consciousness from the endodermal Being centers. Only the most individuated souls among us know how to transcend the immediate outer world and to quietly enter those archetypal realms of the imagination that tap our transpersonal visionary resources. Understanding and evoking essences then alone matters.

The sweetness of such a non-utilitarian enterprise remains accessible only to those who have found within a subtle balance between Eastern and Western religious values and capacities. This polarity, above all the others, reconciles the Eastern adulation of Hara with the Western appreciation of individuated, meaning-making Logos.

4. <u>The Dionysian-Apollonian Passional-Sexual Polarity</u>

The Dionysian-Apollonian polarity is between the back-half-dominant animal sexuality of the male and the front-half-dominant animal sexuality of the female. The two poles are arranged in pure complementary opposition to the body and soul of the Absolute Alien Other. At the animal-sensual level male sexuality is piercing, omnipotent, phallicly aggressive and self-aggrandizing. Female sexuality is equally absolute in its front-half receptivity and sacrificial-like self-surrendering. His Phallos-libidinal circuit and her Eros-libidinal circuit instinctually resonate to each other from the beginning of physical lovemaking. But it is never pure sexual drive that permits two individuated lovers to traverse the huge abyss that separates them naturally and eventually meet in the hierosgamos union of spiritual transformation into beatific oneness.

Passional sexuality is generated from the direct maximal polarization of soul contact between intrinsically Wholly Other Alien Holy Beings. This is one of D. H. Lawrence's most precious teachings. He knew how passional sex could thrive only if a pure Dionysian-Apollonian alchemical-spiritual intermingling were first realized between the embodied soul of the man and the embodied soul of the woman.

Such naked soul-to-soul polarization during lovemaking is impossible if there is much character-muscular armoring in even one of the partners. As long as repressed emotional energy is pressing for liberation and recognition within the psyche, this very pressure for recognition tends to overinvest any archetypal images which do manage to crystallize with an exaggerated power and possesiveness over the psyche and soul.

It follows that lovemaking during third stage full functioning tends to be less possessively dominated by archetypal instinctual forces than during the fourth stage of creative disintegration. Permanent elimination of the repressed and the forbidden permits an upgrading in importance as well as ease of access to awareness of embodied feelings and sensations at the surface of the skin. It simultaneously increases the reciprocity of fluid magnetic currents streaming between the endodermal depths of both lovers. As these two species of libidinalized flow, sensations at the skin surface and the deeper magnetic currents between the two lovers, increasingly move into the foreground of awareness, the archetypal forms recede into the background. In other words, the Apollonian-convergent aspect of the lovemaking becomes relegated to a secondary role while the Dionysian-divergent aspect assumes a more important role during third stage lovemaking.

This conclusion is consistent with my general impression that archetypally-dominant lovemaking results in part from a temporary upheaval of the body-soul-psyche axis of identity during the advanced stages of dearmoring. Once the characterological rigidities are dissolved, archetypal images recede into the background of awareness. As the egoic false self dissolves, the Apollonian-convergent aspect loses its possessive, semi-dissociative hold over the psyche. Thereafter, lovemaking becomes a more undiluted experience of the Dionysian-divergent depths -- Pagan Eros and Pagan Phallos emerge as the Lords of Existence and assume many diverse cultural forms, including those from our modern Western world. Archetypal imagery is still present, but without its former occult-like darknesses of semi-forbidden intensity.

The majority of lovemaking in Western cultures does not belong either to the fourth stage of creative disintegration nor to the third stage of full functioning. In contrast, it is either intellect-controlled or action-and-performance dominated. Exclusively back-half-oriented, it tends to be will-calculated, passionless, and casual. Any variety of rationally controlled sophisticated lovemaking has these same spurious qualities.

A powerful set of unconscious forces, both cultural and psychological, are at work in contemporary America which are organized against the cultivation of passional sexuality between a man and a woman. This cultural-psychological denial of the instinctual healing power of passion underlies most of the enormous rage, frustration, cynicism, hatred, contactlessness and mutual castration which prevails between American men and women. The unconscious forces are too many and complex to be examined here. But in one way or another, they all relate to America's extrovertive, action-oriented, will-to-conquer, competitive lifestyle. American women as much as American men are so constantly encouraged to affirm only their back half will centers that they are generally suspicious of and distrust the front half feeling capacities for relatedness. Hence, there is an enormous proliferation of popular ideologies which postulate the non-existence of innate sexual differences and capacities. The very fact that so many American men and women seriously question these innate instinctual-psychodynamic differences between the sexes demonstrates the culture's desperate degree of alienation from Dionysian-Apollonian passional sexuality.

In opposition to this soul-destructive set of unconscious forces at work in contemporary America, I take the explicit position that the hidden religious significance of the four stages of creative disintegration is the gradual discovery of the spiritual fulfillment inherent in Yin-Yang passional sexuality. Furthermore, Americans will not cease from pursuing self-and-soul destructive forms of sophisticated sexuality until they realize that their extrovertive lifestyle alienates them not only from the peace and inner centeredness of the Hara-Logos polarity, but also alienates them from the barest possibility for experiencing passion in their lovemaking. Passion presupposes a massive slowing down and shedding of one's adrenalin-charged libido. Passion presupposes an abandonment of the performance principle and a gradual submergence below the water and the earth into the realms of non-action and boundaryless passivity. Passion presupposes a total loss of the will centers and their engulfment by the front half needs for full horizontal groundedness.

American women especially are suffering from a denial of full horizontal groundedness as indispensable to their self-actualization. Their alienation from the feminine soul-powers of their front halves is sustained by the ideologies of the femininist movement. Women are erroneously believing that any kind of submissiveness towards the male, even in bed, is an expression of weakness and sick dependency. In other words, women should be just like men in every way imaginable. Such a perspective has already wreaked almost irreversible destructiveness between American men and women. If it continues, it will strangulate the deepest wellsprings of endodermal life flow within each female breast and belly. And without this flow, neither she nor her man-woman primary relationship can be whole. It is woman who must teach man how to love passionally, and never vice-versa. Passion is the antithesis of phallic performance.

5. <u>The Transcendental Psyche-Embodied Soul Polarity</u>

On one side of this polarity is a higher synthesis between the intuitive faculties of Agape, Logos, and the Spiritual Warrior in league with the mind-brain. On the other side of the polarity resides a higher synthesis between the more instinctual forces of Eros, Hara, and Phallos in league with the sexual genitals. This is the polarity of supreme balance in the individuated adult. It involves every one of the important polarities which compose the enduring core self.

Since this is the polarity of higher idealized perfection, let us be a little wary about emphasizing its possibility. Only the rarest among self-actualizing persons can ever hope to live according to this polarity. It is almost perfect, while man is never perfect. Perhaps even the rarest among us can actualize themselves according to this polarity only for brief periods in their adult lives.

After this polarity has crystallized, it mediates a process of alternation between higher differentiation and higher integration. This alternation transcends the rapid oscillation between psychodynamic extremes which characterizes all psychopathology. This alternation is much slower and totally congruent with the two poles of the polarity, the Transcendental Psyche and the Embodied Soul. The Transcendental Psyche regulates periods of productive encounter with objective novelty which defines higher differentiation. The Embodied Soul regulates the periods of productive non-encounter characterized by undifferentiated Beingness which defines higher integration. One might call this the higher creativity alternation of the creative unconscious because the rhythm and pattern of alternation is totally in the service of preserving the creative unconscious.

The preservation of the creative unconscious is more important to the core self than any kind of compensatory reconciliation between consciousness and unconsciousness, as Jung would have it. This is because the unconscious as defined by Jung is too circumscribed by the Transcendental Psyche and insufficiently grounded in the Embodied Soul. The creative unconscious hinges upon the five unifying spiritual polarities. These polarities are far richer in substance than bare consciousness and unconsciousness. I would even claim that Jung's postulation of the compensatory relationship between consciousness and unconsciousness is an expression of an oscillation process between extremes which is akin to the isolated shifting between figure and background that is caused by psychopathological isolation of psychoorganismic functioning.

The higher creativity alternation safeguards spiritual wholeness. While the Dionysian-Apollonian Passional-Sexual polarity safeguards a higher integration between soul and body, the Hara-Logos polarity safeguards the more introvertive dimensions. In contrast, the higher creativity alternation of the creative unconscious safeguards the spiritual totality of the core self. The alternation involves a productive disequilibrium at all times between the transcendental inclinations and the instinctual tendencies. This productive disequilibrium involves a creative tension between the two poles of each polarity and also between each of the five polarities as well.

The more creative an individuated person is, the more he can sustain a greater degree of productive disequilibrium among the various soul centers. He can maintain a resiliency in the manner in which any one of the five polarities might assume dominance over both the psyche and soul. A perfect equilibrium between psyche and soul would enable great internal and external order and stability, but very little growth in the boundaries of the ego or the core self. For growth to occur, the creative person must always take risks and tolerate the accompanying internal tensions and external uncertainties. Such a person must always have experiences of inner spiritual disequilibrium as long as he experiences deep pleasure in remaking his own internal boundaries and/or external environment. Only a vegetable longs for perfect and unending inner harmony and balance. What makes man human, in contrast, is his will to keep creating in the face of inner and outer challenges.

Spiritual wholeness is too delicate to be one-dimensionally determined by even the higher creativity alternation between periods of differentiation and periods of integration. Its foundation is as much organismic in nature as it is spiritual, and this implies in particular a resilient, relaxed, but nevertheless, well-coordinated diaphragmatic region. Every one of the five unifying polarities must traverse the diaphragm energetically before a creative encounter can be marshalled. This relates to the fact that spiritual wholeness involves the finest cooperation between the ectoderm, mesoderm, and endoderm regions of the metabolism because of the importance of subjective-objective interaction between inner and outer worlds.

The diaphragmatic region in the self-actualizing unarmored adult functions as a central stabilizing nucleus of interlinking pathways of vital energy currents. The diaphragmatic region is always the center for an optimal dialectical tension between upper and lower, front and back halves, and between horizontal and vertical groundedness. In the last analysis, I must reject the shakra theory of spiritual wholeness and its localization near the spinal column. Only the diaphragmatic region is spatially placed as the literal instinctual center of the core self's functioning, regardless of which of the five unifying polarities is currently dominant.

Each of the five unifying polarities generates a characteristic pace and quantity of energy flow across the diaphragmatic region during the course of its realization. The highest quantity as well as the most intense pace is the Dionysian-Apollonian Passional-Sexual polarity. The next highest quantity and rate of acceleration is the Agape-Eros-Spiritual-Phallic Warrior polarity. Then follows the Self-Assertive-Self-Surrendering polarity. In order of diminishment, the two polarities which generate the lowest quantities of energy as well as the slowest rates of acceleration across the diaphragmatic region are the Transcendental Psyche-Embodied Soul polarity and the Hara-Logos polarity.

The diaphragmatic region, when it encompasses the endodermal, mesodermal and ectodermal layers, functions as both a barometer and safety valve in the determination of ongoing spiritual-instinctual wholeness. At the endodermal layer, various imaginal forms and intuitive voices communicate regarding the adequacy of the pace and quantity of energy flow in the innermost depths. If the pace and quantity are too great, the core endodermal flow between the abdominal cavity and the primitive brain stem becomes too busy and one-sidedly dominant. This then makes immediate contact with the sensory motor world in the here and now by way of the mesodermal and ectodermal layers too subordinated. The self-actualizing subject listens to this excessive endodermal busyness and returns to his or her senses until equilibrium is reestablished. At the mesodermal layer, messages of overcharging or undercharging of the voluntary musculature and the cortico-cerebrospinal circuit warn of an excessive fixation to any one of the five polarities in the midst of forming a subject-world creative encounter. The self-actualizing subject then stops his concentration and convergent style of functioning and gives time for equalization. These warning messages come in the form of muscle pains, tensions, and pressures on both sides of the mesodermal wall moving either outwards or inwards. And at the ectodermal layer, concrete sensations at the skin's surface communicate chemical imbalance in the fluid blood and lympathic flow in some localized parts of the body. This is translated by the transcendental psyche reflectively or by the embodied soul impulsively as indicating the desirability to change over to another pace or mode of being-for-oneself and being-in-the-world.

Any one of these three types of messages functions as a safety valve. They directly warn an individual's consciousness, or his creative unconscious, that he must shift gears to either the opposite side of the polarity or to a completely different polarity, or else back off from any kind of creative encounter altogether. If consciousness is directly warned, the appropriate shift is clear. But if the creative unconscious is warned, which is more usually the case, the message is more complex. If the transcendental psyche has been overstimulated due to excessive periods of higher differentiation, there must be a shift to a polarity whose rate of expenditure of energy flow and acceleration of flow is less than the previously dominant polarity. But if the transcendental psyche is understimulated, then the indicated shift is toward a polarity which requires a greater mobilization of energy flow in the region of the diaphragm. The new polarity will be self-regulatively affirmed until the imbalances registered in the endoderm, mesoderm and ectoderm layers of the metabolism have been corrected. This in turn restores the more complete interiorized centering of the core self according to the higher creativity alternation between the higher differentiation tendencies of the Transcendental Psyche and the higher integration tendencies of the Embodied Soul.

Generally speaking, the more centered a self-actualizing person becomes, the more fluidly he can shift from one polarity to another, or from one side of a polarity to its opposite side, before he even receives any warning messages. Self-actualizing people know how to obtain the most richness, the greatest confrontation of novelty, and the highest sense of adventuresome excitement from each day without sacrificing the more conservative tendencies of the embodied soul which facilitate harmony and continuity of core Beingness. But such a delicate dialectical balancing between spiritually individuated and animal instinctual forces cannot become an intrinsic part of the core self until the higher creativity alternation has emerged. It is this alternation between the two poles of this supreme polarity of internal unification which permits a middle-in-mode interior life style most of the time.

Printed by VIGANÒ & EARZAGHI - Monza